LIFE
BEFORE
BIRTH

LIFE
BEFORE
BIRTH

*The Moral and Legal
Status of Embryos
and Fetuses*

BONNIE STEINBOCK, PH.D.
*University at Albany,
State University of New York*

New York   Oxford
OXFORD UNIVERSITY PRESS

Oxford University Press

Oxford New York
Athens Auckland Bangkok Bombay
Calcutta Cape Town Dar es Salaam
Delhi Florence Hong Kong Istanbul
Karachi Kuala Lumpur Madras Madrid
Melbourne Mexico City Nairobi Paris
Singapore Taipei Tokyo Toronto

and associated companies in
Berlin Ibadan

Published by Oxford University Press Inc.,
198 Madison Avenue, New York, New York 10016

Oxford is a registered trademark of Oxford University Press.

Library of Congress Cataloging-in-Publication Data
Steinbock, Bonnie.
Life before birth: the moral and legal status of embryos and
fetuses / Bonnie Steinbock
p. cm. Includes bibliographical references and index.

ISBN 0-19-505494-6 (cl) ISBN 0-19-510872-8 (pbk)
1. Unborn children (Law). 2. Abortion—Law and legislation.
3. Abortion—Moral and ethical aspects. 4. Fetus—Research—Moral
and ethical aspects. 5. Prenatal care—Moral and ethical aspects.
I. Title.
K642.S74 1992
363.4'6—dc20 91-46293

9 8 7 6 5 4 3 2 1

Printed in the United States of America
on acid-free paper

For David,
whose love makes all things possible

Acknowledgments

In writing this book, I have benefited from the help of many people. I thank the people who were kind enough to send me opinions, briefs, and other background material. They include K.J.S. Anand, Sharon Beckman, Nance Cunningham Butler, Charles Clifford, Ronald Cranford, Leonard Finz, Lynn Paltrow, and Fenella Rouse. A number of people made time in their busy schedules to give me interviews, either in person or on the telephone. I am especially grateful to Dr. Anand, Frances Berko, and Herman Risemberg.

I have been influenced by more people than I can name here. Many of them are given credit in the endnotes. I extend a general thank-you to all those with whom I have had conversations at professional meetings, conferences, and at the Hastings Center. I have profited a great deal from these informal contacts. I am particularly grateful to Daniel Callahan, Kathleen Nolan, and all the members of the Hastings Center Maternal-Fetal Relations Project. The lively discussions at our meetings helped shape Chapter 4.

I am especially indebted to two people. John Arras has been very generous with his time and knowledge, and is my sounding board and source of many ideas.

His perceptiveness and wit are a constant delight. I never met the late Nancy Rhoden, but I telephoned her regularly, for information, legal expertise, and philosophical wisdom. Her untimely death has deprived bioethics of a brilliant scholar, and me of a good friend.

Special thanks are due those who were willing to read the manuscript. My colleague Robert Meyers read Chapter 1 several times. Each time the chapter improved as a result of his written and oral comments. John Arras read Chapters 1, 2, 4, and 6. As usual, his comments were invaluable. John Robertson read the entire manuscript at a stage when it was so unwieldy that I considered naming it *Jaws*. His perceptive and trenchant comments helped to shorten and improve the book considerably.

Without the help of my former student, Lowell Fass, the book would never have seen the light of day. Lowell gave countless hours of his time, helping me master WordPerfect and printing the manuscript. His patience, skill, and generosity are greatly appreciated. I also benefited greatly from the term paper that Lowell wrote on *Johnson Controls, Inc.* Thanks also to Sharon Crawmer for taking time away from her own work to print and copy for me. I owe the book's title to Sidney Callahan, whose intelligence, warmth, and charm make her a delightful opponent on the topic of abortion. Jeffrey House of Oxford University Press was the ideal editor: he encouraged, but never *nudzhed*.

I am very grateful to Dorilee Stilsing (''Nanny''), whose superb care of my infant son, Sam, gave me the time and peace of mind to write the book. Thanks are also due to my older children, Nicholas and Sarah, for their patience with what often seemed to them a ridiculously long project. (''I can write a book in a day,'' Sarah scoffed, while Nick asked incredulously, ''Haven't you finished that book yet?'') I owe a special thank-you to my parents, Elmer and Natalie Steinbock, who came to Albany every summer from California, and ran errands, baby-sat, and did whatever they could to allow me to write. The book is dedicated to my husband, David Pratt, without whose help, support, and encouragement I could not have written it.

I have saved till last Joel Feinberg, who has been the greatest inspiration and whose influence is apparent on every page. His work provided the impetus and theoretical framework for this book. I have learned more from him than from anyone. For that, and his friendship, I am very grateful.

Contents

Introduction, 3

1. *The Interest View, 9*

    I. Consciousness as Necessary and Sufficient for
the Possession of Interests, 14
*Is Consciousness Necessary for Having Interests? /
Is Consciousness Sufficient for Having Interests?*

    II. The Interests of Nonconscious Individuals, 24
*Dead People / Permanently Unconscious People /
Anencephalic Infants*

    III. Future People, 37

    IV. Potential People: Embryos and Fetuses, 40

2. *Abortion, 43*

    I. Criteria for Moral Status, 46
The Conservative Position / The Person View

    II. The Argument from Potential, 59
*The Logical Problem / A Future Like Ours /
Contraception and the Moral Status of Gametes /
The Moral Significance of Potential Personhood*

    III. Possible People, 71
The Parfit Problem

    IV. The Argument from Bodily Self-Determination, 76
Thomson's Defense of Abortion / Roe v. Wade

V. The Moral and Legal Significance of Viability, 82
Practical Problems with a Sentience Criterion / Late Abortions

3. *Beyond Abortion: The Legal Status of the Fetus,* 89
    I. Recovery for Prenatal Injury in Torts, 91
    *Against Third Parties /The Irrelevance of Viability / Preconception Torts /
    Against the Mother / The Woman's Right of Privacy / Automobile Liability*
    II. Prenatal Wrongful Death, 100
    Wrongful-Death Actions / The Implications for Abortion
    III. The Criminal Law, 104
    Prenatal Neglect / Homicide
    IV. Wrongful Life, 114

4. *Maternal-Fetal Conflict,* 127
    I. Moral Obligations to the Not-Yet-Born, 128
    Risks to the Fetus
    II. Legal Obligations to the Not-Yet-Born, 133
    *Extending Child-Abuse Laws / Criminal Penalties for Fetal Abuse /
    Jailing the Pregnant Addict / Fetal-Protection Policies in the Workplace /
    Compulsory Medical Treatment of Pregnant Women*

5. *Fetal Research,* 165
    I. Fetal Research in America: History and Politics, 167
    II. Fetal-Tissue Transplants, 171
    *The Scientific Evidence / The Right-to-Life Objections /
    A Feminist Objection / Abortion for the Purpose of
    Procuring Fetal Tissue*
    III. Research on the Living Fetus, 186
    *Benefits from Fetal Research / Moral Objections / Research on Living Fetuses
    Ex Utero*

6. *Embryo Research and the New Reproductive Technologies,* 195
    I. *In Vitro* Fertilization and Embryo Transfer, 197
    *The Biological Status of the Extracorporeal Embryo / Discarding Surplus
    Embryos / The Risks of Abnormality / Politics and IVF Research*
    II. Embryos in Laboratory Research, 203
    *Detecting Genetic Disease in Embryos / Respect for Embryos as a
    Form of Human Life / Creating Embryos for Research*
    III. Dispositional Problems, 211
    The Rios Case / Davis v. Davis

Notes, 221
Index, 251

LIFE
BEFORE
BIRTH

Introduction

Our thinking about embryos and fetuses has changed dramatically in recent years. Hardly a day passes without newspaper coverage of some new development regarding prenatal life. Most obvious, perhaps, is the debate over abortion, but we have also been confronted with a host of other issues. Consider just a few. An estranged couple in Tennessee had a legal battle over control of the frozen embryos they had created while married in hopes of having a child. A Florida appeals court upheld the first conviction in the nation of a woman charged with delivering cocaine to her newborn baby through the umbilical cord. In Washington, D.C., a young woman dying of cancer was compelled by a court to undergo a cesarean section in an attempt to save her 26–week old fetus. Both the woman and her fetus died. A federal court of appeals upheld the "fetal protection policy" of Johnson Controls, Inc., prohibiting women with childbearing capacity from working in high-lead-exposure positions in its battery division. The Supreme Court reversed, declaring that fetal protection policies discriminate against women and are prohibited by the Civil Rights Act. Doctors in Colorado implanted a small amount of fetal brain tissue obtained from an abortion into the brain of a man suffering from Parkinson's disease. His condition is reported to be significantly improved. A pregnant woman in Massachusetts was charged with vehicular homicide after she drove while intoxicated and crashed her car, killing her eight-and-a-half-month-old fetus. All of these issues raise the question of the moral status of the unborn: are embryos and fetuses part of the pregnant woman or are they persons? Are they sources of tissue, research tools, or "preborn children"?

The legal status of the unborn seems equally unclear. For example, the legalization of abortion in 1973 was based in part on the unborn's never having been recognized in law as a full legal person. At the same time, fetuses have been considered as persons for the purposes of insurance coverage, wrongful-death suits, and vehicular homicide statutes. The legal status of the unborn thus appears to vary from jurisdiction to jurisdiction, from context to context, according to our purposes.

Medical and technological advances have compounded confusion over the status of the unborn. The threshold of viability—the point at which the fetus can survive outside the womb—has been pushed back into the second trimester of pregnancy. The same fetus might be a candidate for legal abortion and aggressive life-saving intervention. The emergence of perinatology and fetal surgery have made the fetus a patient in its own right. Recently, a surgical team at the University of California at San Francisco performed an unprecedented operation and successfully corrected a diaphragmatic hernia in a fetus. While such surgery is regarded as miraculous by couples whose unborn babies would otherwise certainly die, it is also troubling, as it creates the potential for conflict with the pregnant woman. A few courts have authorized compulsory cesarean sections, where this was deemed necessary to preserve the life or health of the fetus. Some commentators have suggested that, as *in utero* surgery becomes standard treatment, it could be legally imposed on pregnant women for the sake of the unborn. In a few states, women who used illegal drugs during pregnancy have been charged with delivering drugs to minors, or with prenatal child abuse. At the same time, abortion—which pro-lifers dub "the ultimate child abuse"—is not only legal, but a constitutionally protected right.

In short, there seem to be inconsistencies, both in morality and the law, in our treatment of the unborn. Some consider this evidence of confusion, or even hypocrisy. I once heard a politician dismiss an anti-smoking campaign that emphasized the effects of cigarette smoking on fetuses. With heavy sarcasm, he said, "Yet the anti-smoking lobby doesn't oppose abortion, which I suppose is also detrimental to fetal health."

This book is an attempt to show that at least some of these alleged inconsistencies and contradictions can be dispelled. The key is a theory of

moral status—that is, a theory about which kinds of beings c
object of moral concern. The question of moral status is fundame
the above-mentioned issues. None of them can be resolved, or
quately understood, without a plausible account of moral status. Consider,
for example, an issue that often comes up during the abortion debate—
namely, religion. Those who defend the right to abortion often argue that
the state has no right to impose the religious views of one group on all
citizens. This presupposes the fetus's lack of moral standing, and so will
be regarded as question-begging by those who believe that abortion violates
the unborn's right to life.

In Chapter 1, I present a theory of moral status, "the interest view."
In subsequent chapters, I apply this theory to problems involving embryos
and fetuses. However, I do not restrict myself to the status of the unborn
in the first chapter, because I want to present a general theory of moral
status. The reason for giving a general theory is to avoid "cooking the
evidence." That is, the theory should not be driven by the purposes to
which it is put. It should be independently plausible. For this reason, I
consider the implications of the interest view for animals, dead people,
permanently unconscious people, and future generations, as well as for the
unborn.

The basic idea of the interest view is that all and only beings who have
interests have moral status. Chapter 1 explains and defends this thesis, and
gives an account of interests as conceptually connected with sentience (the
ability to experience pain and pleasure) or conscious awareness. Mere things—
rocks, planets, automobiles—are not conscious or sentient and so do not
have interests. Nor do plants, although, unlike mere things, they are alive.
Plants have their own natural growth and development, independent of human designs and purposes. However, plants lack interests because it does
not matter to plants what is done to them. It is this notion of *mattering* that
is key to moral status. Beings that have moral status must be capable of
caring about what is done to them. They must be capable of being made,
if only in a rudimentary sense, happy or miserable, comfortable or distressed. Whatever reasons we may have for preserving or protecting nonsentient beings, these reasons do not refer to their own interests. For without conscious awareness, beings cannot have interests. Without interests,
they cannot have a welfare of their own. Without a welfare of their own,
nothing can be done for their sake. Hence, they lack moral standing or
status.

The exposition of the interest view in Chapter 1 is aimed primarily at
philosophers. It not only presents the interest view, but defends it against
possible objections. This takes us into such rarified areas as the theory of

belief and problems of identity. These issues are important to a thorough defense of the interest view, but they are unlikely to be of great interest to nonphilosophers, who can get a good enough idea of the interest view by reading the beginning of Chapter 1, stopping at the section titled "Is Consciousness Necessary for Interests?" and then skipping to the last section, "Possible People: Embryos and Fetuses." Some readers may be more interested in the specific practical problems I discuss than in the underlying theory. This book should be of value to these readers as well. They are advised to skip Chapter 1 and go directly to the chapters where these problems are discussed. They will find enough of the interest view incorporated in the subsequent chapters to make the general approach clear.

My primary concern, however, is to develop a view that can help dispel some of the apparent inconsistencies in our attitudes toward the unborn. I think that the interest view is useful in this respect. For example, it explains why the right of recovery for prenatally inflicted injuries does not conflict with a right to abortion. If an abortion is performed before the fetus becomes sentient (probably toward the end of the second trimester), the fetus is killed, but not harmed, paradoxical as this may sound. For to be harmed is to have one's interests set back or thwarted. Without thoughts or feelings or awareness of any kind, the embryo or fetus has no interests. Without interests, it cannot be harmed. It has the potential to develop into the kind of being that will have interests, but, as I argue in Chapter 2, this potential does not give it the actual interests necessary for moral standing. We may choose to respect embryos and preconscious fetuses as powerful symbols of human life, but we cannot protect them for their own sake. Without interests, beings do not have a welfare of their own.

The idea that the unborn do not have legally protectable interests has a long history in Anglo-American law. Chapter 3 reviews the legal status of the unborn in areas outside abortion, considering such issues as prenatal torts and wrongful-death actions, the fetus as homicide victim, and wrongful-life suits. An important distinction, only relatively recently acknowledged by the courts, is between the fetus per se and the not-yet-born child. That is, although fetuses do not have legally protected interests, born children do. One of their important interests is an interest in healthy, unimpaired existence. Children who are born maimed may be condemned to a lifetime of suffering and limitation. Prenatal injury clearly harms such children. If the injury is due to negligent or intentional wrongdoing, they deserve to be compensated. Recognizing this, and allowing surviving children to recover damages for prenatal torts, poses no conflict with permitting abortion.

Along the same lines, we can reconcile abortion and maternal obligations to the unborn. The interests of preconscious fetuses do not have to be considered in the decision to abort, since preconscious fetuses do not have interests. However, if a woman decides not to abort, but to carry the fetus to term, she is morally required to think about the effects of her actions on the baby who will be born. Drinking heavily, smoking cigarettes, using crack cocaine—all of these can harm the child she bears, and therefore I claim in Chapter 4 that there is a prima facie moral obligation not to engage in these dangerous behaviors. Whether a woman should be blamed for the harm she causes her unborn child depends on the choices she had, and the extent to which her behavior was free. Whether we should allow children to sue their mothers, whether we should jail pregnant drug users, or impose additional criminal penalties for drug use during pregnancy—these are far more complicated matters. They go beyond the interest principle, raising both philosophical and pragmatic questions. How much intervention into people's lives should be tolerated? How successful are coercive measures likely to be in the protection of the "not-yet-born"?

The symbolic value of the fetus becomes important in Chapter 5, where fetal research is discussed. On the interest view, preconscious fetuses are not human subjects whose consent must be secured in order to use them in experiments. Restrictions on such research cannot stem from concern for fetal welfare. However, nonsentient fetuses can be respected as a symbol of human life, and restrictions may legitimately be placed on fetal research and the use of fetal tissue, so long as this respect does not interfere with the real interests of actual people.

If preconscious fetuses lack moral status, then it goes without saying that so do fertilized human eggs. However, even very early embryos may be a potent symbol of human life, and thus deserving of respect. The frivolous use of human embryos in research or for commercial purposes is as unacceptable as the frivolous use of fetuses or fetal tissue. On the other hand, if important human interests can be satisfied through embryo research, then such research should be conducted and supported. One of the most difficult questions raised by embryo research and the new reproductive technologies concerns the disposition of extracorporeal embryos. The solution depends on whether such embryos are regarded as "preborn children," property, or something else. These issues are discussed in Chapter 6.

The interest view can help us develop a consistent, coherent legal conception of the unborn. This avoids a completely ad hoc approach that is intellectually unsatisfying, likely to generate cynicism, and incapable of offering guidance as new questions arise. It will by now be clear that while the interest view plays a fundamental role in finding answers to the dilemmas posed in this book, it is not the only factor. Matters like abortion, maternal–fetal conflict, fetal research, and the new reproductive technologies raise a host of issues, such as the function of the state and the proper province of law; the importance of privacy and the need for communal values; the role of women in society and the importance of the traditional family. I will discuss these issues as they arise, but I will not do so on the basis of an overarching moral or political theory. Some philosophers may find this unsatisfactory, but I am not convinced that a basic moral theory is necessary for doing applied ethics. In this I am relieved to find myself aligned with Joel Feinberg, who freely confesses to the absence of a "deep structure" theory in his important work *Harm to Others*. "Progress on the penultimate questions," Feinberg notes, "need not wait for solutions to the ultimate ones." [1]

This book is not intended to give a startlingly original conception of the status of the unborn. Instead, it attempts to elicit a view that is implicit in our legal traditions and ordinary moral thinking. Some philosophers may find this disappointing. They would prefer a novel theory, however counterintuitive. I believe, however, that a view that is espoused by many different people who have all thought long and hard about a topic is more likely to be true, or at least plausible. I have found variations on the interest view in philosophical works, law review articles, and judicial opinions, and I have cited these where appropriate. I hope in this book to give the view a firmer grounding and to make it more plausible to those who remain unconvinced. My aim is to provide a theoretical basis for some of our intuitive judgments and convictions, which can also help us to reach answers to new problems in bioethics in a coherent and consistent way.

1 | The Interest View

Moral problems typically involve conflicts between parties. These conflicts often arise because the interests of the individuals clash or cannot be mutually satisfied. For example, smokers' interest in smoking where they please conflicts with nonsmokers' interest in not being subjected to smoke. One factor relevant to a moral resolution of such conflicts is the relative importance of interests. Which is a more pressing claim, health or liberty? Equally important is the *moral status* of the claimants. That is, we need to know which beings count morally. Whose interests are we required to take into consideration from "the moral point of view"?[1]

I believe that the correct account of moral status is provided by "the interest view." The interest view maintains that the possession of interests is both necessary and sufficient for *moral status*. In a sense, this is trivially true. To have moral status is to be the sort of being whose interests must be considered from the moral point of view. Obviously, only beings with interests can have their interests considered. But the point is not trivial. The focus on interests requires us to consider the being itself—what is important to it—rather than what makes it valuable or significant to others. Gold, for example, is valuable, but that fact does not endow gold with moral status.

As many readers no doubt realize, the interest view is based on Joel Feinberg's "interest principle,"[2] which Feinberg proposed as an answer to the question "What kinds of beings can have rights?" However, my concern is not with the logic of rights-ascription, but with the more basic question of moral status. The question of who counts morally is more basic in that it is an issue for all moral views, even those that reject rights. Feinberg's central insight—that interests are essential to rights—can be applied to moral status as well. Interests are the content of rights; without interests, there would be nothing for rights to protect. Equally, if a being has no interests, it can have no claim against others, nothing that they are required to consider from a moral perspective. The possession of interests is therefore a minimal condition for both rights and moral status. All beings who can have rights have moral status. For to say that someone has a moral right to something is to say that he or she has a moral claim against others that they act (or refrain from acting) in certain ways. And to say that someone has a moral claim to the attention or concern of others is just another way of asserting moral status or standing.

All moral theories agree that people have moral status, that their claims must be considered from the moral point of view. Indeed, the willingness to consider, impartially and dispassionately, the claims of other people is definitive of taking the moral point of view. However, moral views differ both in their extension of moral status to entities other than people, and in the justification for assigning moral status to entities. For example, the Judeo-Christian tradition and Anglo-American law hold that moral status is primarily, if not exclusively, held by *human beings*. It is humans who count and whose interests must be considered. While there has been considerable debate about when a human life begins and when it ends, the significance of humanity to moral status is not disputed in commonsense morality. The importance of being human is simply taken for granted by most people.

The special moral status of human beings has been challenged in recent years by a number of philosophers.[3] They maintain that it is unjustified to base moral status on anything as arbitrary as membership in a particular species. They view the widespread acceptance of superior human moral status as due partly to the religious belief that God created man in his own image, and partly to human arrogance and complacence. Whatever its cause, "speciesism" is alleged to be as unjustified as racism or sexism.

In the next chapter, I will argue that the special moral status of human beings can be justified. For now, I want to point out that, even within commonsense morality, human beings are not the only ones who count or matter morally. It is not permissible morally to do anything one likes to animals, for example. Cruelty to animals is both morally wrong and legally prohibited. While it has been suggested that the basis for this moral and legal prohibition is the avoidance of cruelty to human beings,[4] or the offense to human sensibilities,[5] a more plausible explanation concerns the direct effect of such cruelty on the animals themselves. Certain treatment *hurts* animals: that is what makes it wrong. So animals do count. Whether they count as much as human beings—whether, that is, they have *equal* moral status—is a topic to which I will return in the next chapter. But animals do count, and any plausible account of moral status must reflect this.

A far more inclusive principle for determining moral status is suggested by Albert Schweitzer's ethics of reverence for life.[6] Schweitzer holds that life is sacred. It is good to cherish and maintain life; it is evil to destroy and check life. Admittedly, expressed this way, no claim about moral status necessarily follows. Life might be seen simply as a value to be promoted, like beauty or truth, without any suggestion that living things are entitled to our moral concern. However, Schweitzer's characterization of life as a "will-to-live" and his claim that ethics consists in "the necessity of practicing the same reverence for life toward a will-to-live, as toward my own," suggests a kind of golden-rule approach toward all living beings. Because we want to live, we should respect the claim of others to live. Animals and plants may not "want" to live, in the sense of having conscious desires, but they still strive to exist and that is why we ought to respect their lives. All living beings count, in Schweitzer's view. He says:

> A man is really ethical only when he obeys the constraint laid on him to help all life which he is able to succour, and when he goes out of his way to avoid injuring anything living. He does not ask how far this or that life deserves sympathy as valuable in itself, nor how far it is capable of feeling. To him life as such is sacred. He shatters no ice crystal that sparkles in the sun, tears no leaf from its tree, breaks off no flower, and is careful not to crush any insect as he walks. If he works by lamplight on a summer evening, he prefers to keep the window shut and to breathe stifling air, rather than to see insect after insect fall on his table with singed and sinking wings.[7]

Every living being, no matter how seemingly insignificant, thus has a claim to our moral attention and concern. Of course, we cannot completely avoid killing, if we are to survive. But we can avoid killing and inflicting suffering unnecessarily. Interestingly, Schweitzer does not oppose the use of animals in laboratory experiments, as do many of today's animal liberationists. He simply requires scientists "to ponder in every separate case whether it is really and truly necessary thus to sacrifice an animal for humanity."[8] The willingness to sacrifice animals for humanity, when truly necessary, but not, presumably, human beings for animals, even if equally necessary, indicates acceptance of a moral-status scale that ranks human life as more valuable than other forms of life. Thus, Schweitzer's ethic is closer to commonsense morality than it may appear at first sight. Its main departure from ordinary morality lies in its insistence that people should be willing to make significant sacrifices of comfort and convenience to avoid killing living things.

How plausible is the ethic of the reverence for life? It seems to me a well-intentioned confusion of distinct moral principles. For example, reluctance to break off an ice crystal might express appreciation for natural beauty, or a feeling that human beings should leave the natural environment undisturbed, as far as possible, in recognition of the delicate balance of ecosystems. It cannot exemplify reverence for life, since ice crystals are not alive. Similarly, Schweitzer's condemnation of the unnecessary use of animals in scientific experimentation is better explained by a principle that it is wrong to cause needless suffering than by reverence for life. The use of live cells that are discarded after the experiment is over does not provoke moral outrage, nor does Schweitzer suggest that it should.

If the ethic of reverence for life implies that it is seriously wrong to destroy any living thing, it is implausible. After all, all sorts of things are alive, including bacteria and viruses. I doubt that anyone seriously believes that we should have moral qualms about using antibiotics. Bacteria are not the kind of beings that can have moral claims against us. But why is this? The interest view provides an answer. Only beings with interests can have claims against moral agents. Interests are compounded out of beliefs, aims, goals, concerns. Biological life alone does not endow a being with interests. Permanently nonsentient, nonconscious beings cannot have interests. Without interests, they cannot have moral status.

Admittedly, most of us feel that there is something wrong with the wanton destruction of some nonsentient life-forms, such as trees and flowers. We might stop a child from peeling the bark off a birch tree, saying, "Don't do that; it will kill the tree." When vandals lopped the heads off hundreds of tulips, days before the annual Tulip Festival in Albany, New York, many people were morally outraged. Perhaps this can be explained by a moral principle that condemns vandalism in general, and particularly the wanton destruction of beautiful things that give many people pleasure. However, it might be argued that the killing of living flowers is worse than vandalism directed at nonliving things. Perhaps the fact that a thing is alive gives it a value that no nonliving thing has. (I am not sure that this is true. After all, one can always plant more tulips. If a work of art is destroyed, it is usually nonreplaceable.) But even if living things do have a special value, the mere fact that something is alive does not endow it with moral status. If that were so, then weeds as well as tulips would have a claim to our moral attention and concern. The ethic of reverence for life is simply too broad. It does not provide a reasonable account of moral status. The interest view, which is broader than the Judeo-Christian tradition but narrower than the ethic of reverence for life, is a much more plausible candidate.

In Section I, I argue first that the capacity for conscious awareness is a necessary condition for the possession of interests. This rules out both functional objects and organic beings, such as plants, bodily organs, and presentient fetuses. Next, I argue that conscious awareness is also a sufficient condition for having interests, opposing those philosophers who maintain that possession of language is essential to the having of interests. I believe that nonlinguistic beings, like animals and babies, can have interests, and so, moral status. In Section II, I apply the interest view to the postconscious and the never-conscious. Postconscious beings include the dead and those in persistent vegetative states. I argue that the interests they once had can exert a claim on us even after they are no longer alive or conscious. The never-conscious include anencephalic infants. Their moral and legal status has practical significance because of the possibility that they could be used as organ donors. The interest view seems to imply that this is morally permissible; however, the matter is complicated both by factual disagreements and the symbolic status of even the most radically impaired infants as family members.

Section III considers future people. At first glance, their situation seems to be exactly the reverse of that of dead people: the interests they will have can have a claim on us even before they come to exist. More precisely, this is so only in what have been termed "Same People Choices"—that is, choices that do not affect the identity of the people who will come into existence. The possibility of "Different People Choices"—that is, choices that do affect the identity of the people who come into existence—creates a problem with maintaining that future people can be harmed. However, so long as we restrict ourselves to Same People Choices, there is no problem in maintaining that people can be harmed by actions that occur before they were born or even conceived. This has implications for the moral and legal responsibilities of pregnant women to their future children (see Chapter 4). Section IV considers the moral status of potential people: embryos and fetuses.

I. CONSCIOUSNESS AS NECESSARY AND SUFFICIENT
FOR THE POSSESSION OF INTERESTS

The restriction of interests to beings capable of conscious awareness stems from a certain conception of what it is to have interests. Feinberg usefully analogizes having an interest in something to having a "stake" in it: "In general, a person has a stake in X . . . when he stands to gain or lose depending on the nature or condition of X."[9] I am better off if the things in which I have a stake, such as my health, my career, my assets, my family, flourish or prosper. Their flourishing is in my interest.

> One's interests, then, taken as a miscellaneous collection, consist of all those things in which one has a stake, whereas one's interest in the singular, one's personal interest or self-interest, consists in the harmonious advancement of all one's interests in the plural. These interests . . . are distinguishable components of a person's well-being: he flourishes or languishes as they flourish or languish. What promotes them is to his advantage or *in his interest;* what thwarts them is to his detriment or *against his interest.*[10]

This way of thinking about interests connects them to what we care about or want, to our concerns and goals, to what is important or matters to us. How large a stake people have in the advancement of their careers, financial success, physical health, or spiritual development depends on how important these things are to them.

If we think of interests as stakes in things, and understand what we have a stake in as defined by our concerns, by what matters to us, then the connection between interests and the capacity for conscious awareness becomes clear. Without conscious awareness, beings cannot care about anything. Conscious awareness is a prerequisite to desires, preferences, hopes, aims, and goals. Nothing matters to nonsentient, nonconscious beings. Whether they are preserved or destroyed, cherished or neglected, is of no concern to them. Therefore, when we care for things, or do what is necessary to keep them in mint condition, we are not acting out of concern for *them.*

This point is underscored when we think of devices that are used to get us to think of inanimate objects as having a welfare of their own. For example, children's books and cartoons often portray inanimate objects such as locomotives, automobiles, toasters, radios, and vacuum cleaners as feeling pride, envy, loneliness, or despair. In such stories, the little train does mind when it rusts or is not used; the radio is terrified of having its tubes removed. We are meant to feel sorry for the neglected train and relief when the radio is saved. But such feelings are appropriate—or possible—on the assumption that the object has feelings and concerns of its own. If the object lacks feelings and concerns, we cannot be upset or aggrieved on its behalf. We cannot hope that it is restored and used, for its own sake. Mere things do not have a sake of their own, because what happens to them is of no concern to them at all.

Of course, the fact that it does not matter to "mere things" what is done to them does not mean that it does not matter at all. There are good reasons to preserve, protect, and maintain all sorts of things, from beautiful paintings to natural wildernesses. An obvious reason for preserving a beautiful painting is the interest of people in looking at it. However, the reasons for taking care of things need not stem only from the actual interests of people (and other interested beings). Perhaps there are things people ought to be interested in, although they are too ignorant or insensitive to realize this. Environmentalists attempt to awaken our interests in remote wildernesses, and get us to appreciate the natural world, even though we may never observe parts of it, or have any direct interest in its preservation. They may even maintain that preservation of the natural environment has *intrinsic value*. If this means that the natural environment is something that sensitive, intelligent people *ought* to appreciate, a proponent of the interest view can agree. All the interest view denies is that the environment has a stake in its own preservation. The obligation to preserve wilderness areas is not one that we can owe *to* the wilderness. We can have obligations *regarding* mere things, but these obligations are not *to them*.[11] We have no obligations to them because it does not matter to them how we treat them. It is not *for their sake* that we take steps to preserve them, but for the sake of beings who have interests, such as existing people or animals, or future generations.

On the view I have been presenting, a being can have interests only if it can matter to the being what is done to it. Interested beings can be made happy or miserable; they can feel pleasure or pain. Of course, they do not always know what will make them happy or sad. They can often be wrong about what is in their interest. I am not claiming that if someone asserts that he does not care about X, then X is not in his interest. For X may be necessary for him to achieve Y, about which he does care, and he may be ignorant or willfully blind about the connection between X and Y. All I am claiming is that if nothing at all can possibly matter to a being, then that being has no interests. Its interests therefore cannot be considered, and so the being lacks moral status.

Although the connection between consciousness and interests seems to be a natural and intuitive one, it is not universally accepted. The idea that all and only beings capable of conscious awareness have interests has been criticized as being too restrictive, and not restrictive enough. Those who regard it as too restrictive maintain that consciousness is not necessary for the possession of interests. Those who regard it as not restrictive enough believe that conscious awareness is not sufficient for the possession of interests. I discuss these objections in turn.

Is Consciousness Necessary for Having Interests?

Regan's Argument

Tom Regan denies that consciousness is necessary for the possession of interests.[12] He thinks that even mere things, like a violin or an automobile, can have interests. The failure to realize this, he alleges, stems from a failure to recognize an ambiguity in the word "interest." One sense of interest (interest$_1$) refers to those things that are *in the interest* of a being—that is, those things that promote its welfare or good. Another sense of interest (interest$_2$) refers to the things individuals *take an interest in*—that is, the objects of their desires, preferences, aims, and goals. Regan agrees that only conscious beings, who have desires, preferences, and the rest, can have interests$_2$. But it does not follow, and, in Regan's view, is not true, that only conscious beings can have interests$_1$. All that is necessary for having interests$_1$ is a good or sake of one's own. Whatever promotes or produces that good will be *in* the thing's interest. Feinberg's mistake, according to Regan, is thinking that there can be only one kind of good of one's own, "namely the kind of good that we tend to equate with the integrated satisfaction of our desires—i.e., happiness."[13] Mere things cannot be happy or unhappy, but they can nevertheless have a good of their own. Their good or welfare is promoted by those things that enable them to be good instances of their kind. This is reflected when we say, for example, that having the oil changed every three thousand miles is good for a car. It's good for the car because it enables the car to run well. Similarly, excessive humidity is bad for oil paintings because it can damage them.

Feinberg acknowledges that we do often speak this way of what is good or bad for a thing, but he denies that this implies that the thing in question has interests *of its own*. Instead, the reference is to the interests of, for example, the car's owner, who wants a car that runs well, which in this context means something like "uses oil efficiently and doesn't need to be serviced too often." If running well were not something car owners had an interest in, this would not be a criterion of goodness in cars. In other words, to say that periodic oil changes are good for a car is an elliptical way of saying that periodic oil changes enable the car to perform in ways that advance the interests of people.

Regan thinks that this analysis confuses goodness and value. "That a car fulfills our purposes is not what makes it a good car; it is not even one of the good-making characteristics of a car."[14] Rather, a car fulfills our purposes because it is good; and it is good because it has good-making characteristics. To say that a car fulfills our purposes explains why we *value* or choose it; it does not explain what makes the car *good*.

Since human purposes do not explain what makes a car good, Regan thinks that the good-making characteristics of a thing must be independent of human interests and purposes. A good car would not cease to be good, he points out, just because people lost interest in driving cars. Regan concludes that talk of what is good for the car does not refer obliquely to what people want, but rather to the car's *own* good. Thus, he identifies what makes a car good (its good-making characteristics) with the car's good or welfare.

There are two errors in Regan's argument for ascribing to mere things a good of their own (and thus interests that advance that good). First, he confuses the application of good-making characteristics with their genesis. It is true that a good car would not cease to be good simply because people lost interest in driving cars. It would still be a good car insofar as it met the standard of goodness for cars. The reason for this is that standards, *once created,* can be applied independently of the actual interests and purposes of people. It does not follow that the standards themselves have an origin independent of human purposes. *People* determine the standards or criteria of goodness in functional objects, according to human interests and purposes.

Regan's second error is in confusing a thing's *being good* with its *having a good*. Functional objects can, of course, *be* good (or bad), depending on whether they meet (or fail to meet) the criteria for goodness. To say that they *have* a good, by contrast, is to suggest that they have a stake in fulfilling the good-making criteria. But mere things have no such stake. A car doesn't care whether it runs well or breaks down. If it cannot possibly matter to a being how it is treated, it is absurd to claim that we should give it such treatment *for its own sake*. And if we cannot treat it in certain ways for its own sake, then it makes no sense to ascribe to it a good or sake of its own.

The case is very different for interested beings, beings to whom it can matter how they are treated. They can not only *be good* in the sense of meeting standards set by human beings, but they have a good or welfare of their own that is independent of human purposes. In fact, what is good for such beings, what is in their own true interests, may even conflict with the standards of goodness created by human beings. Consider the clipping of the ears of certain breeds of dogs. This is done because clipped ears are thought to have aesthetic value. An unclipped boxer won't win any prizes; such a dog will be considered "no good." But clipped ears have nothing directly to do with the *dog's* own welfare or well-being. Of course, a prize-winning dog may be treated better, and so indirectly benefit from having its ears clipped. However, not all dogs whose ears are clipped enter competitions, and not all who enter win. So most dogs are unlikely to benefit even indirectly by having their ears clipped. Clipping their ears does not promote their health or comfort; on the contrary.

Now compare clipping the dog's ears with having it vaccinated against distemper. It is in the owner's interest to have his animal vaccinated, since owners usually want healthy animals. But it is also in the dog's own interest, since a dog that gets distemper will experience considerable discomfort, and probably die. We might reasonably reproach an owner who neglected to have his dog vaccinated by saying, "It isn't fair to the dog. Even if you don't care if the dog dies, you should vaccinate him for his *own* sake."

This example shows us how standards of goodness can diverge from what is "good for" an animal. Such a divergence is impossible in the case of functional objects, because they have no good apart from the standards created by human interests and purposes. It is only when a being can have this kind of good that it makes sense to attribute to it a good or welfare or sake *of its own*. Feinberg does not, as Regan thinks, *confuse* interests$_1$ and interests$_2$. Rather, he correctly maintains that the ability to have interests$_2$ is necessary for the ability to have interests$_1$. It is only if treatment can matter to a being that it can be said to have a sake or welfare *of its own*.

The Natural-Function View

It is possible to accept the above criticism of Regan and still argue that conscious awareness is not necessary for the possession of interests. That is, one might agree that mere things cannot have interests that advance their own good because things do not have a good or welfare of their own, independent of human interests and purposes. However, one might argue that organic beings, unlike mere things, have natural functions that are not determined by human interests. Their good is achieved when they fulfill their natural function. Whatever enables them to achieve this function is in their interest. So organic beings have interests$_1$, even though they may not have interests$_2$.

The natural-function view has a certain plausibility. We do not need to attribute imaginary mental states to hearts or livers, as we do to toasters and vacuum cleaners, to talk about doing things for *their* sake. For example, smoking is bad for the heart. Giving up cigarettes promotes cardiac health. Thus, we might tell someone to "Stop smoking—for your heart's sake." Why should we not say that certain things (such as not smoking, moderate exercise, and a low-cholesterol diet) are in one's heart's interest? This is true even if the individual in question has no interest$_2$ in giving up smoking, exercising, or eating properly. The possibility of divergence in the case of conscious beings between interests$_1$ and interests$_2$ is one reason for developing an analysis of interests$_1$ based not on interests$_2$, but rather on natural functions.

Plants are another example of nonconscious beings that may be thought to have interests$_1$ and a welfare of their own. Unlike mere things, they are living beings with natural tendencies of growth and development. Plants can live or die, be healthy or sick. And what counts as healthy or thriving or flourishing is not determined solely by human interests and purposes, but stems from the plant's own biological nature. Human interests may even diverge from what is "good for" the plant with respect to its natural development and growth, as when a bonsai is created.

Unlike mere things, then, both plants and bodily organs have what may be called "autonomous goodness"—that is, a good that stems from their own nature, as opposed to the purposes imposed by people. However, having autonomous goodness is not the same as having "a welfare of one's own." The difference can be illustrated by thinking about when it does, and does not, make sense to act "for the sake of" a being. I suggested earlier that it is perfectly intelligible to admonish someone to stop smoking "for your heart's sake." By saying this, we are reminding the smoker that his habit damages his heart, and suggesting implicitly that it is in his interest to maintain cardiac health. But what if the smoker is ninety-two? He may maintain that it is *not* in his interest, all things considered, to stop, since at his age the advantages to be gained by quitting are not worth the deprivation of pleasure. Such a position need not be the result of ignorance, self-deception, or a weak will. It may be a perfectly rational attitude. If so, can we nevertheless recommend to him that he ought to stop anyway, "for his heart's sake"? Surely this would be absurd. The reason, I suggest, is that one's heart does not have a sake of its own. The expression "Do it for your heart's sake" makes sense only in a context where proper cardiac functioning contributes to the well-being of its owner.

By contrast, a dog, for example, has a sake of its own. Because of this, we can tell its owner that he ought to have his dog vaccinated, for the dog's own sake. What explains this difference between dogs and hearts? Both are organic beings, and both have "autonomous goodness" in the sense that what is good for them does not depend on human interests and purposes. But dogs, unlike hearts, have a stake in their own well-being. When they are sick, they don't feel well, and they cannot do the things they enjoy doing. For this reason, it matters to the dog whether it is sick or healthy, and therefore it makes sense to suggest that steps be taken to preserve its health for its *own* sake.

What about plants? Plants are organic wholes, and not parts of organisms, like hearts and livers. Is this difference important for the possession of interests or moral status? I cannot see why it should be. Plants, like bodily parts and mere things, lack conscious awareness. Without conscious awareness, they cannot have interests$_2$—desires, plans, hopes, goals. They cannot take an interest in anything, including their own health, lives, or well-being. Of course, plants have a well-being: they can be healthy or sick, alive or dead. The question is whether this well-being amounts to "a welfare of their own." It might be objected that plants do have a welfare of their own in a way that mere things and bodily organs do not. Functional objects are good insofar as they meet the criteria of goodness, and these are determined by us, according to our purposes. Admittedly, we do not determine standards of goodness for bodily organs, but nevertheless the proper functioning of an organ is determined by the role it plays in the health of the entire organism. Thus, the welfare of a heart, for example, is not completely independent of the welfare of the whole human body. The situation seems to be different for plants, which are autonomous beings, substances with lives of their own. What constitutes a plant's well-being, what makes it a good specimen of its kind, is entirely independent of human wants and purposes. Because their well-being does not depend on external purposes, some may feel inclined to say that plants have a welfare *of their own.*

However, the expression "a welfare of one's own" is intended to emphasize the stake that conscious, sentient beings have in their own well-being. It matters to sentient beings how you treat them. This simply does not apply to plants. Plants are totally indifferent to treatment that furthers or hinders their well-being. Morally, this is a crucial difference. Feinberg makes the point this way: "Having no conscious wants or goals of their own, trees cannot know satisfaction or frustration, pleasure or pain. Hence, there is no possibility of kind or cruel treatment of trees. In these morally crucial respects, trees differ from the higher species of animals." [15]

Defoliating a forest with Agent Orange may be *morally* wrong—that is, there may be moral reasons why people should not do this—but it is not a wrong *to* the trees. In order to preserve this difference between people and animals on the one hand, and plants on the other, I suggested earlier that we label the kind of well-being of which plants are capable "autonomous goodness." This captures the idea that the well-being of plants is independent of human purposes, while reserving the idea of "a welfare of one's own" for beings who have a stake in their own well-being. Whatever reasons we have to promote a plant's good, enabling it to flourish or thrive, these reasons do not derive from the plant's own concerns, aims, or goals. This does not, as I have tried to indicate, rule out an "environmental ethic," but it does mean that such an ethic cannot be based on "golden-rule" or "fair-play" reasons. Such reasons require us to put ourselves in the other's place, to take the other's point of view. This is literally impossible in the case of plants, because plants do not have a point of view. To acknowledge moral reasons to preserve or protect plants is not to say that the plants have claims against us, or that we are morally obligated *to them* to protect them. But moral status involves these kinds of assertions, and that is why plants, like bodily parts and mere things, do not have moral status.

Animals, on the other hand, can have interests. As Feinberg notes, "Many of the higher animals at least have appetites, conative urges, and rudimentary purposes, the integrated satisfaction of which constitutes their welfare or good." [16] Because they have a welfare of their own, we can not only preserve animals, as we can forests, but treat them humanely. Sentient beings can be given treatment which is good for them, for their own sake.

Is Consciousness Sufficient for Having Interests?

Some philosophers deny that animals have interests. R.G. Frey, for example, argues that animals lack the cognitive equipment necessary for interests—namely, wants and beliefs. [17] He acknowledges that animals can have *needs*—that is, whatever is necessary for them to survive or function well—but then, so can plants and even mere things. Needs are not the same as interests, and are not sufficient for moral status or rights.

Frey's argument is this: To want something is to have certain beliefs— in particular, the belief that one does not now have what one wants. Animals cannot have beliefs, according to Frey, because to have a belief is to believe that a certain sentence is true. Only creatures with linguistic ability can regard sentences as true. Since animals lack linguistic proficiency, they cannot have beliefs. Without beliefs, they cannot have wants; without wants, they cannot have interests. Without interests, they cannot have rights. Equally, they lack moral status.

I think we must agree that the ability to have wants implies the ability to have beliefs. The question is whether only language-users can have beliefs. An alternative model attributes beliefs to animals on the grounds that this is the best way to explain their behavior. This intuitive or common-sense belief-desire model arises out of our attempt to explain human behavior. In countless examples, the only remotely plausible explanation we can offer is in terms of the subject's beliefs and desires. The situation is quite parallel for at least higher animals. As Stephen Stich says:

> . . . it would be remarkable indeed if a theory could be produced which explains the behavior of higher animals without appeal to beliefs and desires, and if this theory could not be adapted to explain human behavior as well. In light of the evolutionary links and behavioral similarities between humans and higher animals, it is hard to believe that belief-desire psychology could explain human behavior, but not animal behavior. If humans have beliefs, so do animals.[18]

However, a problem arises when we attempt to specify just *what* a non-language-user believes. If we cannot say what the animal believes, how can we use the belief to explain its behavior? Donald Davidson makes the point this way:

> We identify thoughts, distinguish between them, describe them for what they are, only as they can be located within a dense network of related beliefs. If we really can intelligibly ascribe single beliefs to a dog, we must be able to imagine how we would decide whether the dog has many other beliefs of the kind necessary for making sense of the first. It seems to me that no matter where we start, we very soon come to beliefs such that we have no idea at all how to tell whether a dog has them, and yet such that, without them, our confident first attribution looks shaky.[19]

We are presented, then, with a dilemma. On the one hand, it seems as reasonable to think that a belief-desire psychology can explain the behavior of higher animals as it is to think that such a theory can explain the behavior of people. On the other hand, we seem quite unable to say what it is that an animal believes, and thus unable to explain its behavior in terms of its beliefs and desires. Stich suggests that the dilemma of animal belief arises because we have two very different conceptions of belief. On the one hand, we take beliefs to be functional states that interact with desires to produce action. Viewed this way, we attribute beliefs to creatures whose behavior is amenable to explanation on the belief-desire model. On the other hand, beliefs are states with content; they are propositional attitudes. If a state is a belief, it must be a belief *that* something or other; we expect there to be some way of expressing its content.

The problem, according to Stich, is not that we lack information about animal behavior and reactions, and thus animal concepts. Even with complete information, we still would not be able to specify precisely what the animal *believes*. The reason is that we are not clear about the nature of belief. How central to our concept of belief is the having of specifiable content? "Is a belief-like state which lacks a specifiable content simply a somewhat peculiar belief, or is it, in virtue of lacking content, no belief at all?"[20] Stich writes, "But what are we to say of a belief whose content we cannot specify? Under what condition is it true or false? There is, it seems, no obvious account of truth for such beliefs. In depriving beliefs of expressible content we have also deprived them of truth values."[21] To paraphrase a song from *Showboat,* beliefs without truth values ain't no beliefs at all.

The problem of truth is a difficult one. But I do not think that the solution is this extremely restrictive theory of belief. It rules out not only animals, but also prelinguistic children, to whom we unhesitatingly ascribe all sorts of wants and preferences.[22] Admittedly, we are often uncertain *why* a child wants something—that is, what it is about the object that makes it appealing. However, it seems perverse to maintain that a child who is crying and reaching for an object doesn't want anything because we are not capable of specifying precisely what he wants.

Even if one accepts the restrictive Davidsonian account of belief, I do not think that Frey's conclusion that animals do not have interests (or rights or moral status) follows. Whether propositional content is necessary for full-fledged beliefs, it is not necessary for interests$_2$. "Belief-like states" will do. So long as animals experience their treatment as painful or pleasant, it matters to them how they are treated. Sentient beings thus have at least one interest$_2$: an interest in not experiencing pain. This is sufficient to make them candidates for moral concern.

Once we demonstrate that animals can have interests, and so can meaningfully be ascribed moral status, the next question is whether they *do* have moral status, whether they are *entitled to* moral concern. To put the point another way, given that we *can* treat sentient creatures kindly and humanely, why are we *required* to do so? The only answer, it seems to me, is that pain is objectively bad. This answer is given by both utilitarians, such as Jeremy Bentham and Peter Singer, and Kantians, like Thomas Nagel. In *The Possibility of Altruism,*[23] Nagel points out that we tend to regard our own pain as objectively bad—that is, as giving others and not just ourselves reasons for action. If we then shift our perspective and see things from another's point of view, we will regard ourselves as having reasons provided by his pain. It is our ability to do this that makes us susceptible to arguments of the form "You wouldn't like it if someone did that to you." The success of such arguments does not depend on our thinking that the other *will* do whatever it is to us. The argument is not a prudential one.

Rather, its success depends on our acknowledgment of objective reasons for action.

If the pain of other people provides us with at least some reason for doing certain things, it would seem that the pain experienced by nonhumans would also yield objective reasons for action. Pain is pain, no matter who feels it. So long as a being is sentient—that is, capable of experiencing pleasure and pain—it has an interest in not feeling pain, and its interest provides moral agents with prima facie reasons for acting. Sentience, then, is sufficient to give a being moral status.[24]

I should stress that the interest view gives only a minimal condition for having moral status—namely, the possession of interests. It does not locate beings on a scale of moral importance. In particular, it is silent as to whether all beings who have moral status have it equally. Perhaps such features as species membership, rationality, and potentiality are relevant to moral status, providing principled reasons for counting the interests of some beings more heavily than others. I will return to this issue in the next chapter.

So far I have argued that mere things and nonconscious living things fall below the moral-status line; animals and people lie above it. It is now time to turn to more problematic cases: individuals who used to be, but will never again be, conscious, those who will never attain consciousness, and those who have the potential for conscious awareness.

II. THE INTERESTS OF NONCONSCIOUS INDIVIDUALS

Can the dead have interests? Or people in persistent vegetative states? These questions may seem remote from the topic of this book: the moral and legal status of embryos and fetuses. However, the topics are importantly connected. By understanding how the dead can have interests, we also come to understand how not-yet-born and even not-yet-conceived individuals can have interests, and thus a claim to our moral concern.

Dead People

Dead bodies—corpses—do not have interests. A corpse is a piece of decaying organic matter, without feelings, thoughts, or experiences of any kind. Without feelings and thoughts, it is impossible to have a stake or interest in anything. At the same time, most people have desires about what is to happen to their bodies, their property, their family and friends, or their own reputations after they are dead. They take an interest in what happens in the world even after they are no longer around to know about it. Thus it seems that dead people both do and do not have interests. How are we to resolve this apparent inconsistency? Feinberg says, "I would like to suggest that we can think of some of a person's interests as surviving his death, just as some of the debts and claims of his estate do, and that in virtue of the defeat of these interests, either by death itself or by subsequent events, we can think of the person who was, as harmed."[25] The interests that survive are not the interests of the decaying corpse (that, as Feinberg says, would be absurd), but rather of the once-living person who is no longer with us. Feinberg refers to the once-living person as the "antemortem person" and the dead body as the "postmortem person." It is antemortem persons who have surviving interests, and who can be harmed and wronged.[26]

But how, it may be asked, can interests, which are derived from and linked to wants, continue to exist after the person who has those wants is dead? To explain this, Feinberg uses W. D. Ross's distinction between want-fulfillment and want-satisfaction.[27] The fulfillment of a want is the coming into existence of that which is desired. The satisfaction of a want is the pleasant feeling of gratification that normally occurs in the mind of the desirer when he believes that his desire has been fulfilled. Want-fulfillment and want-satisfaction are logically distinct. The fulfillment of wants does not always bring satisfaction. As George Bernard Shaw put it in *Man and Superman,* "There are two tragedies in life. One is to lose your heart's desire. The other is to gain it." Nor does a feeling of satisfaction imply that one's wants have actually been fulfilled, since the feeling may result from being deceived.

Dead people, as the Rolling Stones might say, can't get no want-satisfaction. But that does not mean that they cannot have their wants fulfilled after they have died. Their wants are fulfilled just in case events happen after their death as they wanted or planned while they were alive. The fulfillment of these wants is as much a part of their good as the fulfillment of wants while they are alive.

Admittedly, dead people cannot know that their wishes were carried out, their families provided for, their reputations intact. Nor can they know if their wills are violated, their families impoverished, their reputations destroyed. But why should their mere lack of knowledge of these events imply that they have not been harmed? This does not seem to be true of living people who are unknowingly victimized. If ignorance does not prevent the living from being harmed, neither can it prevent the dead from being harmed.

A more troubling aspect of Feinberg's account has to do with the appearance of retroactivity. The antemortem person is harmed and wronged after his death by betrayals, broken promises, defamatory lies, and the like.

But how, it may be asked, can an event that occurs after a person's death harm the living person he was before he died? How can an event that occurs at one time cause harm to someone living at an earlier time? Feinberg's answer is that posthumous harms do not entail backward causation because they do not entail physical causation at all.[28] The occurrence of the harmful posthumous event *makes it true* that the antemortem person is harmed; it does not retroactively cause him to be harmed. Feinberg maintains that the subject of posthumous harm has been harmed all along, or at least at the point when he acquired the interest that would be defeated. It is just that until the harmful event actually occurs, no one could know of his harmed condition.[29]

The claim that the antemortem person is harmed all along, by virtue of the future defeating of his interests, seems very counterintuitive. It does not appear to square with our judgments about living people. We do not ordinarily think that someone who will fall off her bicycle or break her ankle in six weeks is *now* in a harmed condition in virtue of that future harm. Why, then, should we maintain that antemortem persons are now in a harmed condition, due to events after their death?

Feinberg's account can be made more plausible if we distinguish between propositions that ascribe properties timelessly and propositions that ascribe properties in the present. Whatever harms will befall me are timelessly true of me. That is, supposing that I will break my ankle in six weeks' time, then it is true of me now that I break my ankle on such and such a date (six weeks from today). This does not imply that I am harmed *now*, six weeks before the accident. I am not harmed "all along." Rather, I have "all along" the property of being harmed at a particular time. This does not involve a belief in predestination, since the claim is not that breaking my ankle is something that will or must occur, but only that if it does occur, then the statement of its occurrence is timelessly true.[30]

Though the puzzles raised by posthumous harming are admittedly difficult, I do not think they are insurmountable. The common saying that the dead are beyond harming refers, I think, to the fact that the dead cannot be hurt, angered, or distressed. But their surviving interests can be defeated, and when this happens, the subject of posthumous harm is the antemortem person, for it is the antemortem person who cared about what would happen after he died. If, after my death, the cause to which I have devoted my life fails, if the security I have worked to provide for my children is destroyed, if my own reputation is blackened, the interests I have now in these things are defeated, and I am harmed.[31]

Permanently Unconscious People

There are currently estimated to be between 5,000 and 10,000 patients in the United States in persistent vegetative states (PVS).[32] Some maintain that withholding or withdrawing any treatment necessary to sustain life is murder. Others would allow some forms of treatment to be stopped (e.g., respirators), but oppose the removal of nasogastric feeding tubes. Still others argue that we should regard PVS patients as already dead. I will argue that this involves too great a conceptual shift. Nevertheless, the interest view supports the conviction that we are not required to sustain the lives of those who will never again be conscious.

First, some relevant facts. PVS patients have suffered severe neurological destruction of the cerebral hemispheres, which contain the function of consciousness or awareness, as well as voluntary action. Because of the damage to their brains, they are permanently unconscious. However, they are not, as is often mistakenly maintained, "brain dead." Brain death involves the death of the whole brain. When the whole brain is dead, the functions of both the cerebral hemispheres and the brain stem, which controls vegetative functions, cease permanently. When brain death occurs, there is no eye movement, no pupillary response to light, no cough, gag, or swallowing reflex, no spontaneous respiration. The heart can continue to beat, since this is not completely dependent on the integrity of the brain stem.[33]

By contrast, the brain stem of patients in a persistent vegetative state remains relatively intact. They can breathe, often unassisted by a respirator. Their eyes are open at times, and periods of wakefulness and sleep are present. This differentiates them from comatose patients, whose eyes are shut, and who remain in a sleeplike state. The pupils of PVS patients respond normally to light. They often have an intact involuntary swallowing reflex, which theoretically allows them to be fed by mouth. However, this is extremely burdensome on those caring for them, and so most PVS patients are tube-fed. They often have intact gag and cough reflexes as well, which helps account for their ability to survive for many years.[34]

Is it possible for PVS patients to experience anything, even if they cannot communicate their experiences to us? Most neurologists (but not all) think that this is not possible. As the American Academy of Neurology expressed it in an amicus curiae brief in the Paul Brophy[35] case:

> No conscious experience of pain and suffering is possible without the integrated functioning of the brainstem and cerebral cortex. Pain and suffering are attributes of consciousness, and PVS patients like Brophy do not

experience them. Noxious stimuli may activate peripherally located nerves, but only a brain with the capacity for consciousness can translate that neural activity into an experience. That part of Brophy's brain is forever lost.[36]

PVS patients sometimes grimace and cry out, and so appear to be in pain. However, most neurologists maintain that these "stereotyped" reactions are merely reflexes, and not evidence of discomfort.

It may be objected that we cannot be certain what PVS patients experience. How can doctors be so sure that these patients do not feel pain? For years the conventional medical wisdom was that newborn infants cannot experience pain. It is only very recently that evidence of pain in newborns has been recognized as "overwhelming."[37] If doctors could confidently claim that pain behavior in newborns was not evidence of pain, maybe they are making the same mistake about PVS patients. How do they know that responses to noxious stimuli are just reflex responses?

In part, the answer given by neurologists is conceptual: "Pain and suffering are attributes of consciousness . . . ." The notion of "unconscious pain" is difficult, if not impossible, to understand. If pain requires consciousness, and if consciousness is not possible without a functioning cerebral cortex, then PVS patients cannot feel pain.

Further evidence that PVS patients do not experience pain is provided by a new diagnostic test, the PET (positron emission tomography) scan. "This test measures in a quantitative fashion the metabolic rates of glucose and oxygen in various parts of the brain, including the cerebral cortex, an important index since consciousness cannot be sustained below certain quantifiable levels of metabolism."[38] In addition, the PET scans of PVS patients are similar to the PET scans of patients who have been anesthetized for surgery. We know that anesthetized patients do not feel pain, because they can tell us so after the operation. Their subjective experience confirms what we expect to be the case based on objective data. It is reasonable to conclude that PVS patients also do not experience pain.

It must be acknowledged that current tests for persistent vegetative state are not completely reliable, even when carefully performed and interpreted.[39] There have been a few cases of patients who have recovered consciousness after a year of being in a vegetative state from hypoxia (lack of oxygen to the brain). Tests done on these patients indicated such severe brain damage as to make recovery impossible.[40] Despite such cases, most neurologists are quite confident about their ability to diagnose PVS. They argue that a few diagnoses that proved to be wrong do not show either the criteria or methods of application to be unreliable, only fallible.

It seems, then, that we can assume that there is such a thing as persistent vegetative state, a condition of permanent and irreversible nonconsciousness. What are we to say about the interests of those who are still alive, yet conscious no longer? Permanently unconscious bodies, like corpses, do not have interests, a sake, or welfare of their own. Routine nursing care, such as turning over and oral hygiene, is not done for the sake of the PVS patient. Someone who is permanently unconscious does not suffer from bedsores, a dried-out mouth, parched lips, or a swollen tongue. However, these conditions make the patient look awful. It may be assumed that the once-conscious person would not want to look grotesque, and so would prefer to have routine nursing care as long as life is sustained. Moreover, a neglected and uncared-for appearance of the patient is extremely distressing to family members. Similarly, the administration of analgesics doesn't reduce discomfort in the patient, since she can no longer feel pain. However, analgesics may inhibit reflex responses that resemble pain behavior and that are upsetting to family members. For this reason, pain medication may be indicated, again not for the patient's sake, but for that of the family. As one neurologist puts it: "My patient is really the family."[41]

The only interests PVS patients have are those that have survived their permanent loss of consciousness. Antevegetative persons can have surviving interests just as antemortem persons do. However, no one has an interest in continued existence in a permanently unconscious state. It is the experience of life that makes life valuable to its possessor. Without the possibility of experiences, now or in the future, life has no value to the one who lives. The biographical life of the PVS patient is over, even though he is not biologically dead.[42] Sustaining his biological life is not something we can do for his sake or to benefit him. Whatever reasons there may be for continuing treatment, or refusing to turn off the machine (such as concern for the family's feelings or fear of setting a bad precedent), they do not refer to the interests of the patient.[43]

Admittedly, there are a few people who would want to be kept alive if there was *any* chance, no matter how remote, of regaining consciousness. They reason that they are no worse off alive and in a persistent vegetative state, since there is no pain or discomfort, and—who knows?—they just might beat the odds and regain consciousness. Such people might plausibly maintain that keeping them alive is in their interest, and that this could be done for their sake. So long as keeping such people alive does not impose unreasonable burdens or costs on others, their wishes should be respected.[44] However, it should not be assumed that keeping someone alive in a persistent vegetative state does not harm his (antevegetative) interests. Most people do not regard the prospect of living in a vegetative state with equanimity. The idea of existing as a permanently nonconscious body fills many people with distress and horror. They would want more than a logical possibility of regaining consciousness. They would not regard themselves as "no worse off" for being maintained in a persistent vegetative state simply because they are not in pain. The interest in *not* being artificially maintained belongs to the conscious individual who existed before the injury to his brain (the antevegetative person), and it survives his or her permanent loss of consciousness. We have as much reason to respect this sort of surviving interest as any other.

Anencephalic Infants

Anencephaly is a devastating and observable neurologic malformation. The cerebral hemispheres are usually completely absent, as is most of the cranial vault. A variable amount of brain stem and cerebellum is present. The eyes are usually present, but the face is severely malformed. The prevalence rate of anencephaly has been steadily declining over the past several decades, as maternal screening for neural-tube defects has become more common. Its occurrence rate is around 0.3 per 1,000 births, with some two-thirds being stillborn.[45] What should be the moral and legal status of anencephalic infants? Should they have the same moral status as other human beings? Or is it morally permissible to consider them, as we do the dead, as potential sources of organs?

This is not an idle question. "In the United States, approximately 300 to 500 children die annually of end stage renal disease, about 400 to 800 children succumb to liver failure, and 400 to 800 die at birth or shortly thereafter of certain forms of congenital heart disease."[46] Many of these children are candidates for transplantation surgery. Some 40 to 70 percent of children under two years of age who are on transplant waiting lists die before donors can be found.[47] The need for small organs is considerable, and the supply scant. The sorts of injuries, such as highway accidents, that can destroy the brain while leaving other organs intact are much rarer in infants than in adults and children. This has led some to look to anencephalic infants as possible donors.

Anencephalic infants are possible donors because they are both permanently unconscious and terminally ill. Regardless of the degree of therapeutic efforts, most die within days of birth. However, it is not possible to wait until the infants die to remove their organs, because their solid organs usually undergo irreversible hypoxic injury during the process of dying and become unsuitable for donation by the time of death.

Because brain-stem function is initially demonstrable in live-born anencephalic infants, they do not meet the legal requirements for total brain death called for by the Uniform Determination of Death Act (UDDA). It has been suggested that the law be changed to allow the organs of live-born anencephalics to be used without a requirement of total brain death. Others have suggested that anencephalics, though live-born humans, are not persons, and therefore not subject to the same protections as other human persons. In the absence of any change in the law, some investigators have attempted to modify the medical care of live-born anencephalic infants, to determine whether organ viability can be maintained until total brain death. However, this has not proved to be feasible.[48]

If anencephalics are to be a source of organs, current law will have to be changed. Legislative proposals to facilitate this have taken two forms. The first is to modify the standards set forth in the UDDA and similar state laws so that they encompass anencephalic infants. This approach was taken by California senator Milton Marks in February 1986. Apparently moved by a story of a couple frustrated by their inability to donate the organs of their anencephalic baby to an infant at the University of California Medical Center, Senator Marks introduced—but later withdrew—a bill that would have amended the UDDA by classifying an infant with anencephaly as dead. Alexander Capron succinctly states the problem with this approach:

> Adding anencephalics to the category of dead persons would be a radical change, both in the social and medical understanding of what it means to be dead and in the social practices surrounding death. Anencephalic infants may be dying, but they are still alive and breathing. Calling them "dead" will not change the physiologic reality or otherwise cause them to resemble those (cold and nonrespirating) bodies that are considered appropriate for post-mortem examinations and burial.[49]

A slightly different approach is to retain the whole-brain standard of death in general, but to make an exception of anencephalics only. This approach has been taken by Michael Harrison, a pediatric surgeon at the University of California San Francisco Medical Center. Harrison argues that the whole-brain definition of death was drafted to protect the comatose patient whose injured brain might recover function. This simply does not apply to anencephaly, in which the physical structure necessary for recovery is absent. This leads Harrison to suggest that we might treat "brain absence" as equivalent to brain death for legal purposes.

The "brain-absence" approach has been criticized on both scientific and policy grounds. Ronald Cranford and John Roberts maintain that it is medically inaccurate to call anencephalics "brain absent," as a variable amount of brain stem and cerebellum is present.[50] Other commentators argue that while anencephaly may be *clinically* distinct, it is not *conceptually* different from other devastating neurological impairments. There is no reason to limit the functional equivalence of brain death for the purpose of harvesting organs for transplantation to anencephaly. Why not take organs from infants with holoprosencephaly, hydranencephaly, and certain trisomies, as well as PVS patients?[51] Indeed, as Capron points out, hydranencephalics (whose cerebral hemispheres have been largely or entirely destroyed *in utero* by infection) would be more attractive sources of organs than anencephalics, as they tend to survive for longer periods of time, and so have more-developed and larger organs. Shewmon et al. argue that making an exception for anencephalics could be used to justify taking organs from "incompetent patients in the final stages of a terminal illness or even prisoners on death row, whose organs would be much more suitable for transplantation than those of anencephalics and whose execution could be timed according to the availability of an optimally matched recipient." They go on to say:

> Specifically, using this kind of logic, half of all the infants who die of congenital kidney, heart, and liver disease would be better used as organ sources to preserve the lives of the other half, rather than letting them all die along with their transplantable organs. Even though this sounds preposterous, the experience at transplantation referral centers indicates that the enthusiasm for using anencephalics does indeed quickly extend to other categories of dying infants.[52]

The point here is a psychological one. The suggestion is that making an exception of anencephaly is likely to put us on a slippery slope that would endanger the lives of other handicapped or terminally ill people. Perhaps the best answer to slippery-slope arguments has been given by philosopher Samuel Gorovitz. Speaking as an experienced skier, Gorovitz points out that it is often possible to start down a slippery slope and then stop.[53] Instead of automatically avoiding slippery slopes, educational and legal measures can be taken to ensure that the feared results do not occur. For example, it could be specified that only anencephalic infants are to be used as transplant donors.

This raises a conceptual question, distinct from the psychological issue of whether using anencephalic infants as organ donors is likely to lead to thinking of all terminally ill infants as potential donors. The conceptual question is whether anencephaly is sufficiently different from other neurological disorders to justify making it a unique exception to the whole-brain concept of death. Those who regard anencephaly as unique maintain that there are several features that differentiate the anencephalic infant from infants with less severe neurological disorders. Anencephalic infants, it is argued, have an "utterly hopeless prognosis"; they are "permanently unconscious and terminally ill"; and "the diagnosis can be easily established both *in utero* and at birth with an extraordinarily high degree of certainty."[54] However, there is no consensus among the experts about any of these characteristics.

Some commentators are positive that anencephalics lack the capacity for experience of any kind. Arthur Caplan writes, "There is no question that such children are incapable of any cognitive activity or any form of sentience."[55] Cranford and Roberts agree. "Because these infants are permanently unconscious and can experience no pain or suffering, and, therefore, can never be aware of what happens to them, a strong argument can be made that, like other permanently unconscious patients, they have no interest in treatment, i.e., treatment can no longer benefit or harm them."[56]

However, some commentators are skeptical of the claim that anencephalics can experience nothing. Shewmon et al. concede that while the capacity for experience is undoubtedly missing in those with craniorachischisis (a congenital fissure of the skull and spine), such infants are invariably stillborn, and their organs unsuitable for donation. "Whether those with relatively intact brain stems have any subjective awareness associated with their responsiveness to the environment is inherently unverifiable, but what is known about the functional capabilities of the brain stem, particularly in newborns, suggests at least keeping an open mind."[57] They argue that decerebrate newborns are neurologically much more similar to normal infants than to decerebrate adults. Therefore, it is not possible to apply adult-derived neurophysiological principles in support of the claim that a functioning cortex is necessary for consciousness or pain perception in newborns. In addition, according to Shewmon et al., ". . . decerebrate (anencephalic or hydranencephalic) human newborns with relatively intact brain stems can manifest a surprising repertory of complex behaviors, including distinguishing their mothers from others, consolability, conditioning, and associative learning, although irritability and decreased ability to habituate are also common."[58]

The ability to distinguish one's mother from others is good evidence of conscious awareness. How else can this ability be explained? In addition, in light of the fact that it is only recently that physicians have acknowledged the capacity of perfectly normal newborns to feel pain, we should be cautious of claims that there is "no question" that anencephalics are nonconscious and nonsentient. More research might clarify the issue. Until then, it would seem only prudent not to make radical changes in organ-donation policy.

Other areas of factual disagreement concern the reliability of diagnosis, the imminence of death, the medical suitability of anencephalic infants to be organ donors, and the number of potential recipients. While Cranford and Roberts suggest that "hundreds or thousands" of newborns or infants can benefit from receiving organs from anencephalic infants,[59] D. A. Shewmon[60] places the number much lower. Nearly two-thirds of all anencephalics are stillborn, and their organs cannot be used. Moreover, as the use of AFP screening and amniocentesis becomes more common, more fetuses with neural-tube defects will be aborted. Taking these facts into consideration, Shewmon estimates the annual number of live anencephalic births in the United States to be just over 300.[61] Of these 300, most are be born prematurely, and have intrauterine growth retardation, making them unsuitable as organ donors. In addition, a number of anencephalic infants have associated gross malformations of their organs. Finally, there is the difficulty of finding an appropriate recipient. Looking ten years into the future, even anticipating improvements in matching donors and recipients, transportation, and transplantation techniques, Shewmon projects the annual number of infants in the country who would benefit from anencephalic organs to be less than fifty. He concludes:

> Such present and future projections ought to be borne in mind in discussions of the impact of anencephalic organ harvesting upon the many hundreds of children who die each year from congenital kidney, heart, and liver disease, before we expend great effort in modifying diagnostic criteria for brain death, changing statutory definitions of death, or relaxing fundamental principles of transplantation ethics in order to obtain anencephalic organs.[62]

Clearly, there will need to be greater consensus on the factual issues before the wisdom of allowing donation from live-born anencephalic infants can be determined. If anencephalic infants are conscious and sentient, they should be treated like any other sick and dying newborns. Certainly they should not be seen as living organ donors merely because they lack cognitive potential and are certain to die soon. At the same time, if anencephalics are totally lacking in conscious awareness, they have no interests that can be considered. Nothing, not prolongation of life or so-called "comfort care," can be done for their sake. To insist that they nevertheless be treated like other sick and dying infants who *can* be benefited and harmed is to ignore a crucial, morally relevant difference.

Alexander Capron ignores this difference when he says:

> . . . if society wants to adopt a policy of sacrificing living patients for their organs, it seems very strange—and a very bad precedent—to start with the most vulnerable patients. Unconsenting, incompetent patients who

have never had a chance to express their views about whether, if near death but not yet dead, they would want their bodies cut up for purposes of organ donation, are the *least* suitable source.[63]

If anencephalic infants are nonconscious and nonsentient, they are *not* "the most vulnerable patients"; they are not vulnerable at all. To be vulnerable, one must be capable of being harmed. To be capable of being harmed, one must have interests that can be thwarted, set back, or defeated. Without some form of conscious awareness, a being can have no interests and is immune from being harmed.

It might be objected that the same can be said of permanently unconscious adult patients. Capron fears that the retrieval of organs from living anencephalics would lead to the "nightmarish scenario" that took place in Robin Cook's novel *Coma,* in which vital organs were removed from comatose patients. Of course, in the novel, patients were deliberately *made* comatose in order to serve as organ sources. The nightmare is not that their vital organs were removed after they became comatose; the nightmare is that they were made irreversibly comatose. They would be no better off had they been put into persistent vegetative states but allowed to keep their vital organs.

Nevertheless, I think we can agree with Capron that organs should not be harvested from PVS patients. To begin with, organs should not be retrieved even from *dead* bodies without consent. People often have strong feelings about what should be done with their corpses, and these surviving interests should be respected. If consent, based on the preferences of the deceased, is necessary for organ donation *after* death, how much more stringent should consent requirements be for organ donation *before* death, when there is always the possibility of misdiagnosis, and the chance of killing a patient who might have regained consciousness. This explains why even people who are happy to donate their organs after they die may not want their organs taken should they enter a persistent vegetative state. Their wishes should, of course, be respected. However, the wishes of anencephalic infants cannot be respected. This is not because, as Capron suggests, they have never had a chance to *express* their views, but because they lack the capacity to *have* views on this, or any other, matter. Thus, there can be no obligation to determine what they would have wanted. Indeed, doing so does not even make sense.[64]

A complete and irreversible lack of consciousness would differentiate anencephalics from most other severely impaired newborns. It might not distinguish anencephalics from hydranencephalics or iniencephalics, if they too completely lack sentience and awareness. If they do, then hydranencephalics and iniencephalics also lack the capacity for interests and moral status. The mere fact that they tend to survive for longer periods is not morally significant if they are completely unconscious. However, it does not follow that if we make an exception of anencephalic infants, we are logically committed to making an exception of hydranencephalics and iniencephalics as well. The more exceptions allowed to the UDDA, the greater the danger of misdiagnosis and of confusing permanent unconsciousness with a less severe neurological condition. This is one reason for making anencephaly the only exception to the UDDA. In addition, if some physicians have doubts about the capacity for sentience in anencephalics, many more have doubts about sentience in less devastating disorders.

Sometimes it is said that infants who lack the capacity for conscious awareness are not "persons" and that this is the reason why they may be killed. In my view, the introduction of the question of personhood needlessly confuses the issue, for two reasons. First, there is no philosophical or moral consensus on the requirements of personhood. There isn't even agreement on the relevant characteristics—for example, whether being human is necessary or sufficient for being a person. Some philosophers place the standard so high that even normal newborns do not qualify, while others consider fertilized human eggs to be people. It is unlikely that any argument for using anencephalic infants as organ donors based on their lack of personhood will be successful.

Second, the term "person" is not purely descriptive, but normative, and more, honorific. When we call a newborn baby a "person," we are not so much describing its capacities as expressing the idea that it is a family member. The same is true of anencephalic infants. Like all other babies, they have parents and a place in a network of human relationships. On this basis alone, such babies can be considered to be "persons." To deny that anencephalic infants are people suggests that such babies are not important, not our children, not worthy of being treated with dignity and respect. A more accurate characterization acknowledges that they are people who, due to their devastating neurological deficit, cannot be benefited or harmed. Nothing can be done for *their* sake, although their parents can love them and mourn their deaths. The parents who have attempted to donate the organs of their anencephalic infants have not done so because they regard their infants as worthless or undeserving of respect. Rather, they feel that respect is best shown by donating tissues and organs so that others may live. If so, then, as Caplan says, "it seems hollow sentimentality to prohibit such gifts on the grounds that it is repugnant to certain sensibilities to do so."[65]

III. FUTURE PEOPLE

The situation of future generations appears to be just the reverse of that of dead and permanently unconscious people. The interests they will have in the future can exert a claim on us now, even before they come into existence. If people today pollute the atmosphere and drinking water, despoil the environment, and deplete natural resources, that is likely to have disastrous effects on the lives of those who come later. Their actual future interests will be harmed; they will suffer because of our decisions today. The same reasons we have not to inflict harm on present existing people apply to future existing people. We can have moral obligations to them, and they can have rights against us. Because they have interests, future people qualify for moral status.

Objections to the claim that future people have moral status are of three kinds. The first two, often not carefully distinguished,[66] are fairly easily rebutted. The third objection poses much greater problems.

The first objection is a logical argument. It maintains that future generations do not have moral status because they do not exist. If they do not exist, nothing is true of them. They have no properties at all, and so do not have interests, moral status, or rights. However, the fact that future people do not now exist does not deprive them of the ability to have properties. Tomorrow does not now exist, and yet all sorts of things can be said about tomorrow: it will be cloudy, it is graduation day, it is the day we're going on a picnic, etc. Furthermore, these features possessed by future dates can provide us with reasons for acting. ("Better buy some bread for sandwiches.") Expected events in the future can have an impact on what we ought to do now. In the same way, the needs and interests of future people can provide us with reasons for acting.

The second argument is an empirical one. It is that we cannot have obligations to future generations because we do not have sufficient information about their lives and needs. For example, we might make enormous sacrifices to conserve fossil fuels for the sake of future generations, only to learn (or perhaps we never would learn) that solar power will be the sole energy source at some point in the future. It is absurd, according to this view, to posit obligations if we cannot specify the content of those obligations. This cannot be done without detailed knowledge of the kinds of lives that will be led.

In contrast to the logical argument, this objection allows that we can make sense of obligations to future generations, or of doing things for their sake. It says only that we do not have enough information to know what to do. This point has some force. The further away future people are in time, the less we can know about their lives and needs. It would be silly to try to guide environmental policies based on the needs of people a thousand years from now. However, it is possible to predict some of the needs of the next few generations. We can reasonably expect that they will continue to drink water and breathe air. It is facetious to maintain that we have no idea what the effects of today's policies will be on future people. Admittedly, we may get it wrong. We may make unnecessary sacrifices or, worse, pursue policies that are detrimental to the interests of future people. There is always the possibility of well-meaning mistakes. But this is true of our relations with existing people as well, and so is not a reason for denying the moral status of future people.

So far, the claim is only that present nonexistence does not disqualify a future actual person from a place on the moral-status scale. I have not addressed the knotty problem of how much future people ought to count, or how strong their claims are, as opposed to the claims of presently existing people. My point is simply that the interests of people who will exist can have a claim on us now, so that it is possible now to do things that will harm and wrong people who do not yet exist.

It is precisely this claim that forms the basis of the third objection. This objection says that we cannot be morally required to consider the interests of people living hundreds of years from now, because it is impossible for us *to affect their interests.* This is not simply because future people do not yet exist, nor is it because we lack knowledge about the conditions of their lives. Rather, the claim is that people in the distant future are often radically inaccessible. They cannot be harmed or benefited by what we do today because their very existence may be determined by the actions we take, or fail to take, now.

This problem with future people has been explained by Derek Parfit, and thus is often termed "the Parfit problem." (Parfit himself calls it "the Non-Identity Problem"; others refer to it as "the identity problem.") To understand the problem, a distinction must be drawn between two kinds of choices. Most of our moral thinking involves what Parfit calls "Same People Choices." In Same People Choices, whatever we choose, all and only the same people will ever live. "Some of these people will be future people. Since these people will exist whatever we choose, we can either harm or benefit these people in a quite straightforward way."[67] Thus, there is no conceptual problem with having obligations to future people in Same People Choices. As Parfit notes:

> Remoteness in time has, in itself, no more significance than remoteness in space. Suppose that I shoot some arrow into a distant wood, where it

wounds some person. If I should have known that there might be someone in the wood, I am guilty of gross negligence. Because this person is far away, I cannot identify the person whom I harm. But this is no excuse. Nor is it any excuse that this person is far away. We should make the same claims about effects on people who are temporally remote.[68]

However, future people differ in one crucial respect from spatially distant people. We can affect their identity. This fact produces a problem.

Suppose we are trying to decide on an energy policy. Most people agree that we should consider the long-range impact of our choices. That is, we should not think simply about the effect on ourselves and our children. We should also consider the impact of our current choices on people living hundreds of years from now, so far as we can predict this. Many people would urge that we should conserve resources now, even if this means a slight lowering in our standard of living, in order to prevent serious shortages for people in the further future. To deplete resources now will have harmful effects on generations yet to come.

However, Parfit points out, the choice we make, whether to conserve or deplete, is itself likely to affect which people get born. It is not true that, whichever policy we choose, the same particular people will exist in the further future. Over time, the choice of one policy, rather than another, is likely to affect who marries whom, and when they have children. Thus, different people will be born, depending on which policy we choose. Parfit says, "We can plausibly assume that, after three centuries, there would be no one living in our community who would have been born whichever policy we chose. (It may help to think about this question: how many of us could truly claim, 'Even if railways and motorcars had never been invented, I would still have been born'?)"[69]

We have, then, two possible sets of future people: the people who will be born in 300 years if Conservation is chosen, and the people who will be born in 300 years if Depletion is chosen. If we choose Depletion, the standard of living in 300 years will be very low, much lower than if we'd chosen Conservation. However, it is not true that our choice of Depletion causes anyone to be worse off than he would have been if we had chosen differently. And, on a plausible conception of harming, to harm someone is to make him worse off than he would otherwise have been. Since choosing Depletion makes no one worse off than he would otherwise have been, the choice of Depletion, paradoxically enough, *harms no one*. If we choose Conservation, the future will contain the Conservation-people, living decently in a Conservation-environment. If we choose Depletion, the future will contain the Depletion-people, living in a not-so-nice Depletion-world.

The point is that they are two distinct populations. There is no way that we can choose Conservation and arrange for the same people to be born as would have been born had we chosen Depletion. The opportunity to have a decent standard of living simply is not open to the Depletion people. It's a not-so-nice life or no life at all.[70]

The Parfit problem most obviously has implications for policy planning in the areas of conservation and energy. But it also has implications for issues in this book, including abortion, "wrongful-life" cases, and the new reproductive technologies. Recognition of the Parfit problem forces us to reexamine the concept of harming (see Chapter 3), and to search for other principles to explain why certain choices would be morally wrong, even if, strictly speaking, they harm no one (see Chapter 2).

Same People Choices do not pose the perplexing problem raised by Different People Choices. So long as individuals will exist at a future time, regardless of what we choose, those individuals can be harmed or benefited by what we do. They have a claim to our moral concern. Futurity alone does not deprive someone of moral status. However, all claims and rights of future people are premised on their actual future existence. It is only on the assumption that they will exist that they can have interests that exert claims on us. Merely possible future people do not have interests. Unlike future actual people, merely possible people cannot be harmed or benefited, made miserable or happy. Thus, we cannot owe it to them to bring them into existence. There is no right to be brought into existence, only a right to have one's interests considered if one comes into existence.[71]

IV. POTENTIAL PEOPLE: EMBRYOS AND FETUSES

The ability of embryos and fetuses to have interests raises both factual and conceptual questions. The factual issue concerns the emergence of conscious mental states. Mindless, nonsentient creatures cannot have interests. Precisely when fetuses attain conscious awareness is controversial and perhaps indeterminable, but it seems unlikely that fetuses have experiences of any kind before the second trimester, and quite likely that they begin to have sensations of some kind at some point during the third trimester. Embryos (the unborn during the first eight weeks of gestation) at least do not have interests. At the same time, they are living things. They can survive or die; develop normally or become deformed; be healthy or sick. Like plants, embryos have autonomous goodness, but they do not have a welfare of their own.

It might be thought that if embryos and fetuses do not have welfares of their own, then it does not matter what is done to them. In Chapters 5 and 6, I argue that this does not follow. As potential persons, embryos and fetuses have a symbolic value that precludes using them in unnecessary experiments or for purely commercial gain. However, this symbolic value is less important than the actual interests of born human beings in life and health.

Although embryos and early fetuses do not have interests, they will acquire interests once they are born, or even late in pregnancy, once they become sentient. Their future interests can be damaged by events that occur while they are still in the womb, or even before conception. Smoking, drinking alcohol, or using drugs such as heroin or cocaine during pregnancy can cause a child to be born with serious impairments. The decision to engage in these risky activities during pregnancy is a Same People Choice. Doing these things can injure a child who otherwise would have been born healthy. Thus, to smoke or drink or take drugs is to run the risk of harming one's baby. That future baby has moral claims against its mother that she not engage in risky activities likely to cause it harm. In Chapter 4, I discuss the nature and extent of women's obligations to the children they decide to bear, as well as the question of whether any of these obligations should be legally enforced.

In the next chapter, I use the interest view to defend a pro-choice position on abortion. I argue that abortion does not harm or wrong embryos or preconscious fetuses. Lacking the capacity for awareness of any kind, early-gestation fetuses do not have interests of their own. The pro-life attempt to present embryos and early-gestation fetuses as if they were just like babies, who clearly do have interests, is therefore seriously misleading, I contend. Fetuses have only "contingent" rights and claims—contingent, that is, on future existence as interested beings.

To defend this pro-choice position, I will have to respond to those who maintain that there is a *noncontingent* right to be born, based on the humanity of the unborn and/or its potential personhood. I argue that while these features may be relevant in determining the relative moral standing of beings on the moral status scale, neither potential personhood nor biological humanity by itself in the absence of conscious awareness confers moral status. At the same time, it does not follow that abortion is necessarily morally neutral. There may be moral objections to abortion, stemming from values and ideals concerning sexuality, marriage, and parenthood. However, such personal values and ideals should not be the basis of legal restrictions or public policy.

2 | Abortion

Nearly two decades after the Supreme Court ruled in *Roe* v. *Wade*[1] that a woman has a constitutional right to terminate her pregnancy, abortion remains one of the most divisive and emotionally charged issues in America. Pro-lifers march with posters of macerated fetuses; pro-choicers use a bloody coat hanger as their symbol of the days of illegal abortions. But behind the drama and the emotion are claims that can be subjected to philosophical scrutiny. Is the unborn a human being, with a right to life like any other human being, as pro-lifers maintain? If it is, then very few abortions, if any, could be justified. For we do not generally think that it is morally permissible to kill children because they are unwanted or illegitimate or severely handicapped. On the other hand, if the fetus[2] is not a child, but only part of the pregnant woman's body, then restrictive abortion laws would be as difficult to justify in a pluralistic society as laws against contraception. For restrictive abortion laws impose enormous physical, emotional, and financial burdens on women. Even legal moralists, who hold that society has the right to enforce its moral beliefs through law, could not justify the imposition of such heavy burdens. Only the assumption that the unborn is a human being like any other, entitled to the law's protection, could justify the prohibition of abortion. Thus, the moral status of the unborn is central to the abortion debate.

Some writers on abortion are skeptical of any attempts to resolve the abortion question by investigations into the moral status of the unborn, because people's views on the status of the unborn are rarely independent of their opinions about abortion. Sociologist Kristin Luker argues persuasively that what really divides pro-choice and pro-life activists are their differing views on the meaning and value of sexuality, motherhood, and the proper role of women.[3] Their attitudes on these issues determine their views on abortion, which in turn determine how they think about the fetus. For this reason, according to philosopher Ruth Macklin, any attempt to derive the morality of abortion from a conception of the unborn is bound to be question-begging.[4]

It must be acknowledged that our conceptual views are not immune from social, political, and psychological influences. The radically different world-views of pro-choicers and pro-lifers undoubtedly affect their thinking about embryos, and whether they see them as clumps of cells or very small babies. But recognition of such influences does not preclude rational assessment of the arguments.

Few writers on abortion come to the topic with a fully open mind, and I am no exception. I believe that the decision to have an abortion is one that belongs to the pregnant woman—not the state, not her doctor, not her husband. My pro-choice position is based on two independent considerations: the moral status of the fetus and the pregnant woman's moral right to bodily self-determination. I believe that both are necessary to an adequate treatment of abortion, yet many writers on abortion focus on only one aspect, while ignoring or downplaying the other. Thus, some opponents of abortion talk about the fetal right to live, or the wrongness of depriving a potential human being of its future life, without even mentioning the fact that a particular woman must carry and bear the fetus for it to have a future life.[5] On the other side, some feminists regard the inquiry into the status of the fetus as irrelevant to the problem of abortion.[6] The central questions, from a feminist perspective, are not about the abstract individual rights of fetuses but how to create the social conditions that make possible the fulfillment of reproductive responsibilities. Sandra Harding says that we must go "beneath the surface of the abortion dispute" and ask such questions as:

> Why are adult women not treated by law or custom as full social persons
> with equal rights . . . ? How can a woman or a child exercise her "right

to life'' or "freedom of choice" in the face of poverty, unemployment, racism, legal and individual sexism, and the whole gamut of material conditions attributable to these material restrictions on social personhood?[7]

But these questions, important as they are, do not go "beneath the surface of the abortion dispute." *They change the subject.* The issue is whether abortion is a morally permissible choice. This question would remain, even if poverty, racism, or sexism were eliminated. In such a world, there would presumably still be contraceptive failures and unwanted pregnancies. It goes without saying that women ought to be recognized as fully autonomous choosers; the question is whether abortion is a choice that autonomous choosers are morally permitted to make. It is hard to see how one can answer this question without responding to the claim that abortion is the killing of a human being, with a right to life.

The interest view responds to this claim by arguing that embryos and early fetuses lack moral status. We are not morally required to consider their interests because, prior to becoming conscious and sentient, fetuses do not *have* interests. The defense of this claim requires some factual investigation as to when sentience occurs. More important, I will need to explain why sentience is essential to moral status. After all, if allowed to grow and develop, the nonconscious, nonsentient fetus will become conscious and sentient. It has been argued that its potential to acquire these characteristics gives the fetus a present interest in continued existence, and makes abortion seriously wrong.

In Section I, I defend the sentience criterion for moral status against its main contenders: genetic humanity and personhood. In Section II, I discuss the claim that the fetus has moral standing in virtue of its potential to develop into a person, and argue that potential personhood by itself does not endow a being with interests or moral status.

Section III takes up the moral standing of merely possible persons. I defend a "person-affecting restriction" (PAR), which maintains that only existing beings, whether past, present, or future, can be harmed. Merely possible people cannot be benefited or harmed, nor do they have moral claims against us. I then discuss several purported counterexamples to the PAR, and try to show why they do not require its abandonment.

In Section IV, I offer a pro-choice argument based on the pregnant woman's right of bodily self-determination or privacy, as it has been deemed in the law. I conceive of the right of bodily self-determination as a fundamental moral right. It includes the right to decide what happens in and to one's body, as well as the right to bodily integrity. The moral right of bodily self-determination is the basis for several common law rights, including the right to refuse medical treatment and the right to informed consent. In addition, the discovery of a constitutional right of privacy is most plausibly explained by the assumption of a fundamental moral right of bodily self-determination. The pro-choice argument I offer here has both moral and legal significance. It is based on Judith Thomson's famous and influential article, "A Defense of Abortion."[8] Thomson argues that no one is morally obligated to make large sacrifices to allow another person to use his body, not even if this is needed for life itself. I point out some problems with basing a general defense of abortion on this claim, but suggest that these problems disappear if the fetus is not assumed to be a person, with a right to life. In other words, I combine Thomson's argument on the right of individuals to bodily self-determination and autonomy with the interest view's conception of the fetus. This results in a view very similar to that taken by the Supreme Court in *Roe* v. *Wade*. Section V discusses the significance of viability, and argues that it is late gestation rather than survivability per se that has moral significance.

I. CRITERIA FOR MORAL STATUS

The Conservative Position

The most extreme antiabortion position holds that a fertilized human ovum is a human being, with a right to life, like any other human being. This is often called the "extreme conservative" position. The argument for this view has two parts. First, the conservative points to the fact that the fetus is indisputably genetically human. Moreover, it is not merely a human cell, like any cell in a human body. At fertilization, the egg and sperm combine to form a new genotype. The fertilized egg, or single-celled zygote, has the full complement of twenty-three pairs of chromosomes, one in each pair from each parent. From this single cell develop all the different types of tissue and organs that make up the human body. Fertilization thus marks the spatiotemporal beginning of a new human being. As John Noonan expresses it, "The positive argument for conception as the decisive moment of humanization is that at conception the new being receives the genetic code. It is this genetic information which determines his characteristics, which is the biological carrier of the possibility of human wisdom, which makes him a self-evolving being. A being with a human genetic code is man."[9]

The second part of the conservative argument maintains that, after fertilization, there is no event or change in the unborn that has such moral significance that it would enable us to say, "*Now* we have a human being, but before this event it was not human.'' Traditionally, birth has been held to mark the beginning of human life. At birth, the fetus is separated from its mother and is no longer physiologically dependent on her. Birth as a dividing line has the advantage of being objective and definite. Your birth certificate marks the day, hour, and even minute you were born. However, the conservative denies that birth has such enormous moral significance. There is not much difference between a newborn moments after birth, and a fetus moments before it is born. How can a change in location have such a drastic effect on moral status?

The conservative then moves backward through pregnancy, dismissing other suggested landmarks. Consider, for example, viability, defined by the Supreme Court in *Roe* v. *Wade* as the time when a fetus is "potentially able to live outside the mother's womb, albeit with artificial aid." [10] Why should the fetus's ontological, moral, or legal status depend on its capacity for independent life? The argument might be that before the fetus can survive independently of the mother, it is really only a part of her body, like an organ or a limb. By contrast, a viable fetus, though *within* the body of the mother, is not merely a part of her body. A mere bodily part is not capable of living on its own. A viable fetus can be separated from its mother and remain alive. The conservative responds that it is a mistake to identify *independent* existence with *separate* existence. The nonviable fetus admittedly cannot exist independently of its mother, but it is nevertheless a separate individual, with its own genetic code. It is not merely a part of the pregnant woman's body. Moreover, the conservative denies that independent existence has the moral significance ascribed to it by the viability criterion. Babies and young children are also dependent on the care of others for their survival. As Noonan puts it, "The unsubstantial lessening in dependence at viability does not seem to signify any special acquisition of humanity." [11] Moreover, people dependent on iron lungs or respirators are not less human, less worthy of protection, than the rest of us.[12]

Nor does the conservative find moral relevance in any earlier stages, such as quickening. Quickening refers to the mother's ability to perceive fetal movement. Probably the view that human life begins at quickening stems from the biologically inaccurate view that the fetus is not alive before it moves. Since we now know that even the single-celled zygote (indeed, even the sperm or ovum) is alive, there is no reason to base moral status on the fetus's ability to move (motility), and even less reason to make its moral status depend on its mother's alertness in detecting movement.

The fetus begins to look recognizably human between 12 and 16 weeks gestation age (g.a.).[13] Its eyes are obvious, though it does not yet have eyelids. It still has ear slits rather than ears. Its hands, still encased in an enveloping membrane, have well-demarcated fingers and thumbs. It may not look much like a baby, but it is clearly a *human* fetus. By contrast, it is difficult to distinguish a human fetus at 8 weeks g.a. from a cat or pig fetus of the comparable gestational age. There is clearly a difference in appearance between an early fetus and a more developed one, but does this difference have moral significance? The conservative denies that it does, on the ground that this suggests that deformed human beings (such as the Elephant Man) who do not look like other people lack human moral status.

Finally, it has been suggested that human life begins when brain waves first appear, at about 8 weeks g.a. The rationale for this view is that it provides a symmetry between the criterion for the end and the beginning of life. Both are marked by the absence of brain function. The most extreme conservative gives no more significance to the emergence of brain waves than to any other developmental stage in the life of the unborn. If the embryo is not killed, it has a good chance of acquiring brain waves, human form, the capacity for movement, viability, and every other human feature. Therefore, the extreme conservative concludes, *no* stage or feature can have decisive moral significance, such that abortion is permissible before the fetus attains it, but not after. Every successive stage is just development from the beginning.

As I said earlier, there are two parts to the extreme conservative position. First, it attaches moral significance to the genetic humanity of the fetus; second, it argues that this humanity is present from conception onward. Either part can be challenged independently. For example, Baruch Brody takes what might be called a modified conservative position. Like Noonan, Brody bases the moral status of the unborn on its being human. However, he does not agree that humanity begins at conception. Brody argues that a functioning brain is essential for being human. When the brain stops functioning, the person dies and goes out of existence. On the same reasoning, the fetus "comes into humanity" when its brain begins to function.[14] In other words, the beginning of brain function marks a radical discontinuity in the life of the unborn. The human being who begins when brain function starts is not identical with the embryo whose brain has not yet begun to function.

Even if one accepts the thesis of radical discontinuity (a thesis that most conservatives would reject as inconsistent with the reality of continuous physical development), it is not clear why this should be marked by the emergence of brain waves. The beginning of brain function, taken as a physiological occurrence, is not different from any other change in the fetus. The significance of brain function lies rather in its connection with mental states, such as conscious awareness. Brody suggests this when he says, "One of the characteristics essential to a human being is the capacity for conscious experience, at least at a primitive level. Before the sixth week, as far as we know, the fetus does not have this capacity. Thereafter, as the electroencephalographic evidence indicates, it does. Consequently, that is the time at which the fetus becomes a human being." [15]

The phrase "capacity for conscious experience" is ambiguous. It might refer to the physiological ability of a being to have conscious experiences *at some point* in its development. The fetus at six weeks after conception (eight weeks g.a.) certainly has the capacity for conscious experience in this sense, but so does the single-celled zygote. Obviously, this is not what Brody intends. In another sense of "capacity," a being has the capacity for an experience x if x occurs, given the appropriate stimulus. A frog has the capacity to feel pain if, on being subjected to certain kinds of stimuli, the frog feels pain. However, in this sense of "capacity," neither a zygote nor a 6-week-old fetus has the capacity for conscious experience. The emergence of brain waves is only a necessary, not a sufficient, condition of conscious experience.

What further development is necessary for the fetus to feel pain, arguably the most primitive form of conscious experience? Painful sensations are transmitted on nerve fibers and interpreted in the cerebral cortex. Development of the fetal neocortex begins at 8 weeks of gestation, and by 20 weeks each cortex has a normal complement of 109 neurons. The cortical neurons undergo profuse arborization and develop synaptic targets for the incoming thalamocortical fibers and intracortical connections. K.J.S. Anand and P.R. Hickey, researchers at Children's Hospital in Boston, explain the significance of this development for pain perception:

> The timing of the thalamocortical connection is of crucial importance for cortical perception, since most sensory pathways to the neocortex have synapses in the thalamus. Studies of primate and human fetuses have shown that afferent neurons in the thalamus produce axons that arrive in the cerebrum before mid-gestation. These fibers then "wait" just below the neocortex until migration and dendritic arborization of cortical neurons are complete and finally establish synaptic connections between 20 and 24 weeks of gestation. [16]

Anand and Hickey's research was aimed at proving that neonates and preterm babies can feel pain. However, it also seems to indicate that pain perception much earlier than the end of the second trimester is highly unlikely. Admittedly, the evaluation of pain in the fetus is difficult, both because pain is a subjective phenomenon and because we do not have access to the fetus *in utero* to perform behavioral tests. Nevertheless, from what we do know about the physiology of pain perception, it seems reasonable to conclude that the fetus during the first trimester, and probably well into the second trimester, is not sentient. The neural pathways are not sufficiently developed to transmit pain messages to the fetal cortex until 22 to 24 weeks of gestation. If the early fetus is not sentient, it is unlikely to have conscious awareness of any kind. Certainly the ability to feel pain would precede more highly developed cognitive states, such as thoughts, emotions, and moods.

To summarize, brain function has no significance if taken as a purely physiological development in the fetus. Brain function is significant only because it is a necessary condition for mental states, such as sentience, conscious awareness, beliefs, and memories. However, brain function is not a sufficient condition for even the most rudimentary mental states. Thus, Brody's claim that the emergence of brain waves marks the beginning of human life is not tenable. If the capacity for conscious experience is a necessary condition of humanity, the fetus does not become human until sometime toward the end of the second trimester. This criterion for moral status supports a liberal, rather than a conservative, stance on abortion.

Recent advances in our knowledge of embryology have led to another modified conservative position, one that is consistent with the rejection of abortion. This position also maintains that there is a radical discontinuity in the life of the unborn, occurring at *implantation,* or the embedding of the embryo in the lining of the uterus. Implantation begins approximately on the sixth day following fertilization, and takes about a week. Mary Warnock notes, "Both the internal and external processes of development are crucial to the future of the embryo. If the inner cell mass does not form within the blastocyst, there is no further embryonic development; while if implantation does not occur the blastocyst is lost at or before the next menstrual period." [17]

The chances of an embryo's developing into a fetus improve significantly after implantation occurs. This is one reason for choosing implantation as "the decisive moment of humanization." Another reason is that implantation coincides with the formation of the "primitive streak," which is the precursor of the spinal cord. After the primitive streak forms, embryonic fission, which produces identical twins, cannot occur. As Mary Warnock put it in a television interview, "Before fourteen days the embryo hasn't yet decided how many people it is going to be." [18] The chance of twinning, admittedly very small, makes it impossible to say that at fertilization there exists a unique human being. There could be two or three or more. However, once the primitive streak has formed, and implantation has taken place, there is only one, unique individual, and he or she has a pretty good chance of developing into a viable baby.

Adoption of the implantation criterion for humanity would rule out all surgically induced abortions, as well as abortions induced by the RU 486 pill, since these all occur after implantation. However, the implantation criterion could permit such abortifacient techniques as a "morning-after" pill or menstrual extraction. Indeed, some devices ordinarily thought of as "birth control," such as the IUD, may prevent conception by preventing implantation. They are actually, therefore, very early abortifacients.

So far, we have looked at two challenges to the conservative claim that there is no nonarbitrary, morally relevant postfertilization event that marks the beginning of a human life. One challenge argues that the beginning of brain function marks a morally significant event, on the ground that the fetus after brain function begins is not identical to the fetus prior to brain function. The other challenge maintains that implantation has moral significance, because the numerical identity of the unborn is decided then.

A quite different objection to the conservative position maintains that the assumption that genetic humanity is relevant to moral status is radically confused. I will refer to this objection, and the stance on the status of the fetus that comes out of it, as "the person view."[19]

The Person View

Warren: The Irrelevance of Genetic Humanity

Proponents of the person view maintain that the conservative position is based on a conceptual error, a confusion between two senses of the word "human." A human fetus is undeniably genetically human. However, this sense of "human" lacks moral relevance, according to person-view proponents, such as Mary Anne Warren.[20] It is not genetic human beings who have a special moral status and a right to life, but *persons*. Now, as a matter of fact, all the people we know are genetic human beings. This leads us to confuse the moral and genetic senses of the word "human." The confusion is cleared up when we realize that there could be nonhuman persons, such as the cinematic character E.T. E.T. is a person because he resembles us in morally important ways. He is conscious, self-conscious, rational (indeed, far more rational than humans), a moral agent, and a language-user. It is in virtue of his possession of these characteristics that he deserves the respect due to persons, and cannot be treated as a mere thing. The person view goes on to maintain that personhood, and the special moral status it involves, cannot be based on anything so arbitrary as species membership, but must instead be defined in terms of the possession of certain psychological and cognitive capacities, including consciousness, self-consciousness, reasoning, self-motivated activity, and language. Warren concedes that possession of all these capacities may not be necessary for personhood, but a being who possessed none of these characteristics is clearly not a person. So a fetus, at least in early or midgestation, is clearly not a person. Even a late-gestation fetus, who has some degree of conscious awareness, has fewer of the person-making characteristics than does a mammal or even an adult fish. Warren concludes that it is not seriously wrong to kill fetuses. In fact, abortion is "morally neutral," comparable to having one's hair cut.[21]

This comparison outrages many people, even those who support a woman's right to choose abortion. Warren seems to be saying that the decision to have an abortion is "no big deal," and this trivializes the complex feelings many woman have had in connection with abortion. To compare abortion to having one's hair cut is to ignore the physical, emotional, and cultural significance of pregnancy. Nevertheless, one could argue that, whatever the *psychological* significance of the decision to terminate a pregnancy, the decision is still not a matter of *moral* concern. This suggests that actions have moral significance only if they harm or wrong persons. If the fetus is not a person, then the decision to abort it is not a moral one. This seems to me to be an excessively narrow conception of morality. A wider conception views morality as being about the right way to live, or about being the right sort of person. In making certain choices or acting on certain reasons, one might be acting as a shallow, thoughtless, uncaring kind of person would act. To act in such ways is not morally neutral, even if one's choice does not harm or wrong any person.[22]

A more worrisome objection to the person view is that it apparently justifies not only abortion but also infanticide. A newly born infant is not significantly different from a late fetus in terms of person-making characteristics. A newborn is conscious and sentient, but then, so is a late-gestation fetus. More important, so are many nonhuman animals. Advocates of the person view are thus faced with the following choice. If they set the requirements for personhood low enough to include newborns, they will have to acknowledge the personhood of late-gestation fetuses and most animals. Infanticide will be wrong, but so will killing animals for food. On the other hand, if they require more than mere sentience for personhood, neither animals nor human babies will be persons. This accords with the commonsense view about animals, but conflicts strongly with most people's views about the wrongness of killing babies.

Warren suggests that the opposition to infanticide can be justified on consequentialist grounds. Parents ought not to be allowed to opt for the death of a newborn, even if they do not want to raise it, because there are other people ready and willing to adopt the child, and who would be "deprived of a great deal of pleasure" if the child were destroyed. Even if a child is considered to be unadoptable because she is severely physically or mentally handicapped, it is still wrong in most cases to kill her, because most people would prefer to pay taxes to support orphanages and state institutions for the handicapped rather than to allow unwanted infants to be killed.

This concession to ordinary moral thought is unsatisfying. If killing babies is seriously morally wrong, the reason cannot be merely that most people in fact prefer that babies live. What if the market for adoptable babies vanished because new reproductive technologies enabled anyone who wanted a child to have one of her own? What if people stopped being willing to spend money on orphanages and state institutions for handicapped infants? It seems that Warren would have to agree that under such conditions it would be perfectly all right to destroy unwanted infants, a conclusion that is enormously counterintuitive. Warren's attempt to explain what's wrong with killing babies leaves out entirely the idea that infanticide, like other homicides, is a wrong to the child who is killed, because it deprives the child of his life. It treats the destruction of an infant as if it were merely the destruction of a valuable commodity. As Jean Elshtain suggests, this puts infanticide "about on the level of having one's stereo and Beatles' albums stolen."[23]

Of course, the mere fact that a conclusion is counterintuitive does not prove an argument wrong. Perhaps there really is nothing wrong with killing babies, aside from the distressing effect on sensibilities. This is the approach favored by Michael Tooley, another proponent of the person view. He maintains that the opposition to infanticide is not based on rational principle. It is a mere taboo, like the taboo against masturbation or oral sex. These practices are not morally wrong simply because some people—or even the majority of people—are revulsed by them. However, while I acknowledge that feelings are no substitute for reasons, the existence of strong and widely held feelings against the implications of a view provide us with a motivation for finding an argument against it.

One objection to Warren's analysis is that it suffers from the same defect she discovered in the conservative position. Just as there is ambiguity in the word "human" between its genetic and moral senses, so there is ambiguity in the word "person" between its descriptive and normative senses. In its descriptive sense, the word "person" refers to a being with certain psychological traits, such as consciousness, self-consciousness, and rationality. In its normative sense, a person is someone with full moral standing, and, in particular, a right to life. Warren simply assumes that all and only descriptive persons are normative persons; indeed, she takes it as "self-evident." Missing from her account is an explanation of the moral significance of the capacities that make someone a descriptive person. Without this explanation, the person view is as arbitrary as the genetic-humanity criterion.[24]

We need an argument that justifies the special moral standing of descriptive persons. Such an argument might go like this. The moral significance of rationality and self-consciousness lies in their connection with moral agency. A moral agent is someone who is responsible for his or her own actions, who can be held accountable, praised, and blamed. This requires the ability to consider the merits of possible courses of action, decide which is the best thing to do, and to act on that judgment. Such activity is possible only for intelligent, reflective, and self-aware beings. In addition, moral agents are capable of moral reasoning, which involves detachment from one's own personal perspective and interests. Because of their ability to engage in moral discourse, to modify their behavior in response to rational considerations, to refrain from injurious behavior if others are likewise willing to refrain, moral agents occupy a unique moral status. H. Tristram Engelhardt, Jr., defends the superior moral standing of descriptive persons, or "persons in the strict sense," as he calls them, this way:

> This central place of persons in the strict sense in moral reflection flows from the very notion of a moral community. If one views ethics as a means of resolving moral disputes in a fashion not based upon force, but rather upon peaceable negotiation, in a context where the participants are held accountable for their actions, the only original members of that community, of the moral world, will be persons in the strict sense: entities who are self-conscious, rational, and self-determining and therefore accountable for their choices, and who have interests.[25]

This argument links descriptive and normative personhood. It provides a rationale for treating all descriptive persons, whatever their species, as normative persons, entitled to respect and moral concern. But it does not follow that *only* descriptive persons have this moral status. There may be good reasons for extending the moral status of descriptive persons to all human beings. Conservatives who insist that a human embryo is a person need not be *confused* about the distinction between genetic humanity and moral humanity. Instead, they could be maintaining that genetic humanity is sufficient for normative personhood. Ruth Macklin comments, "If there

is any confusion here, it is to be laid at the door of those like Warr
apparently forgetting her avowal that the concept of a person is i
moral concept, treats it as a purely descriptive notion. . . . What a
tionists are doing . . . is *proposing* that the fetus be considered a person,
and therefore, a creature to be treated as a member of the moral community.''[26]

The most likely basis for the conservative proposal that fetuses be treated
as members of the moral community is some version of the argument from
potential. The argument from potential says that fetuses deserve to be treated
now as if they were persons because if they are allowed to grow and develop—in other words, are not aborted—they eventually will acquire all the
properties of descriptive persons. This differentiates human fetuses and
newborns from, say, guppies. Potentiality arguments pose the greatest difficulty for pro-choicers; I will return to this subject shortly. But first I want
to consider another attempt to show that abortion is not seriously morally
wrong, based on an argument that fetuses cannot have a right to life.

Tooley: Persons and the Right to Life

Like Mary Anne Warren, Michael Tooley maintains that all and only descriptive persons have a right to life. But whereas Warren takes this to be
self-evident, Tooley has an argument. Tooley begins by espousing Feinberg's interest principle (see Chapter i). According to the interest principle,
all and only beings that can have interests can have rights. Tooley takes the
interest principle one step further, arguing that particular rights are connected with specific sorts of interests. That is, an individual cannot have a
particular right *R* unless that individual is capable of having some interest *I*
that is furthered by its having right *R*. Tooley calls this the "particular-
interests principle."

The particular-interests principle is supposed to explain and defend certain widely held moral views. For example, most people would maintain
that it is worse painlessly to kill a normal adult human being than to torture
one for five minutes. Though both acts are seriously wrong, they are not
equally wrong. But most people would regard it as much worse to torture
a newborn kitten for five minutes than to kill it painlessly. How is this
difference to be explained? The particular-interests principle suggests an
explanation: "Though kittens have some interests, including, in particular,
an interest in not being tortured, which derives from their capacity to feel
pain, they do not have an interest in continued existence, and hence do not
have a right not to be destroyed."[27]

To have an interest in not feeling pain, a kitten need only have the desire that a particular sensation cease. "The state desired—the absence of a particular sensation—can be described in a purely phenomenalistic language, and hence without the concept of a continuing self."[28] By contrast, the desire protected by a right to life is a desire for one's own continued existence. To have this desire, one must possess a bundle of fairly complex concepts, including the concept of something's continuing to exist and the concept of a continuing subject of experiences. In addition, the desire for one's own continued experience is a desire that *this* subject of experiences should continue to exist. Thus, to have the desire for continued existence, one has to be able to think of oneself as a subject of continuing experiences. Tooley concludes that only beings who have this concept can have a right to life.

Two responses might be made to this argument. It might be argued that a desire to live does not require the concept of oneself as a continuing subject of experiences. All that is necessary is the capacity to have desires in general, and a preference for survival, which can be expressed behaviorally. Plants cannot have a desire to live, because they do not have desires at all. But conscious, sentient beings who struggle to avoid death may be said to want to live, and so to have an interest in continued existence.

A different response makes use of the distinction noted in Chapter I between two senses of "interest." Whatever promotes a being's good or welfare is *in* its interest; I called these interests$_1$. By contrast, the things one wants or pursues, the things in which one *takes* an interest, are interests$_2$. Keeping this distinction in mind, one might respond to Tooley's argument by agreeing that only a being with a concept of itself as a continuing subject of experiences can want to go on existing as the being it is. Only beings with self-concepts can have an interest$_2$ in continued existence. But it doesn't follow that only beings with a self-concept can have an interest$_1$ in continued existence. Rights can surely protect interests$_1$ as well as interests$_2$. So, if continued existence is *in* a being's interest, it can have a right to life, even if it cannot *take* an interest in its own continued existence. Is there any reason to deny that life can be in the interest of animals, babies, and other individuals without self-concepts?

Tooley responds with a version of the radical-discontinuity argument. Imagine, Tooley says, a preconscious embryo that develops into a person, Mary. Mary has a happy life, and is glad her mother did not abort her. So it may be said that it was in Mary's interest that the embryo from which she developed was not destroyed. However, Tooley argues, it is a mistake to think that therefore nondestruction is in the *embryo's* interest. The embryo is not a subject of consciousness. It does not have any interests at all, and so cannot have an interest in its own continued existence.

Now consider a human baby that is sentient and has simple desires, but is not yet capable of having a desire for its own continued existence. If it will develop into an individual with a happy life, can't we say that it is in the baby's interest not to be killed? Tooley denies this. He says that we mistakenly attribute to the baby an interest in continued existence because we wrongly identify the baby with the adult person she becomes. We then think that because it is in the adult Mary's interest that she was not destroyed when she was a baby, that it must also be in the baby Mary's interest not to be destroyed. After all, baby Mary just *is* adult Mary, when she was younger. However, Tooley maintains that such an identification is justified only if there are causal and psychological connections between adult Mary and baby Mary. In the absence of any such connections, it is "clearly incorrect to say that Mary and the baby are one and the same subject of consciousness, and therefore it cannot be correct to transfer, from Mary to the baby, Mary's interest in the baby's not having been destroyed." [29]

Tooley's argument is open to several objections. First, it assumes, implausibly, that there are no causal and psychological connections between a baby and the adult person she becomes. Most psychologists believe that the treatment one receives as an infant affects the development of one's personality. Parents who were once warned against "spoiling" babies are today encouraged to meet their infants' needs not only for food, but for comforting and loving.[30] It is believed that this creates not only happier *babies,* but happier, more secure, more well-adjusted *adults*. This would be impossible if there were not causal and psychological connections between the infant and the adult she becomes.

Second, even if there is a radical discontinuity between a baby and the adult it becomes, it does not follow that the baby cannot have an interest in its own continued existence. Granted, the baby cannot *take* an interest in its continued existence. It lacks the concepts necessary for that desire. Still, life can be *in* the baby's interest. Life is in a being's interest if the experiences that comprise its life are, on the whole, enjoyable ones. Such a life is a good to the being in question. Infants, even very young ones, can enjoy their lives. They can take pleasure in a variety of activities and experiences. This being the case, we can certainly preserve their lives for their own sake. The same is true for animals and severely mentally retarded humans. It is only when life is miserable that we begin to doubt whether continued existence is a benefit. If this is right, then a self-concept is not necessary to have an interest (an interest$_1$) in continuing to exist. All that is necessary is the ability to enjoy one's life.

A conscious, sentient newborn ordinarily has a life worth living, a life he enjoys, a life that is a good to him. Continuing to live is certainly *in* the baby's interest, because of the value to him of his life *right now*. A right to life protects his interest₁ in his life. I conclude that there is no conceptual bar to ascribing to newborns a right to life.[31] Nor is there any conceptual bar to ascribing a right to life to the nearly born fetus. A late-gestation fetus is conscious and sentient. It is possible that it has pleasurable experiences. If so, it has an interest in continuing to live, an interest that can be protected by a right to life. By contrast, embryos and preconscious fetuses do not have lives that they value, lives that are a good to them. Life is no more a good to an embryo than it is to a plant or a sperm. Thus, the importance of sentience is not primarily that abortion causes pain to the sentient fetus. That problem might be taken care of with an anesthetic. The relevance of sentience is that a sentient being can have a life it values, and that we can protect for its own sake.

Some antiabortionists consider it callous and unfeeling to deny moral status to the preconscious fetus. But the charge of callousness makes sense only if we persist in thinking of embryos and fetuses as being just like babies, only smaller. In fact, I think that this is how many opponents of abortion do regard the fetus. For example, the film *The Silent Scream* purported to show a 12–week fetus struggling to get away from the abortionist's scalpel, and opening its mouth in "a silent scream." Critics of the film charged that normal fetal movements were speeded up to make it look as if the fetus were recoiling in pain. But even if the film was not doctored, such movements are not by themselves evidence of pain. A mimosa plant shrinks from touch, but no one claims that the mimosa feels pain. The reason is that a plant lacks the nervous system necessary for the experience of pain. Similarly, the fetal nervous system at 12 weeks is not sufficiently developed to carry and transmit pain messages. Insofar as opposition to abortion is based on factual error, or worse, deliberate misrepresentation of the facts, it must be rejected out of hand.

A more sophisticated conservative position acknowledges that zygotes, embryos, and early fetuses do not suffer from being aborted, nor does death deprive them of happy lives. Nevertheless, it maintains that even a zygote has an interest in not being killed. This interest in continued existence does not derive from the kind of life it has *now,* but rather on the kind of life it *will* have, if it is allowed to develop and grow. Such arguments are known as arguments from potential. If successful, they can support the conservative proposal that genetic humans ought to be treated as normative persons.

II. THE ARGUMENT FROM POTENTIAL

There are different versions of the argument from potential, but the basic idea is that it is wrong to kill, or otherwise prevent the development of, a human fertilized egg because it possesses the potential to be a descriptive person. As Stephen Buckle expresses it, "It is, potentially, just like us, so we cannot deny it any rights or other forms of protection that we accord ourselves." [32] A fertilized egg does not now have any of the properties of a person. It isn't even sentient. But this does not matter because, left alone and allowed to develop, the zygote will become a person. Buckle says, "The fertilized egg is not 'just like us' only in the sense that it is not *yet* just like us. Therefore, the argument concludes, we should not interfere with its natural development towards being a rational, self-conscious being. On its strongest interpretation, the argument is thought to establish that we should treat a potential human subject as if it were already an actual human subject." [33]

The Logical Problem

A standard objection to the argument from potential is that it involves a logical mistake. The mistake consists in thinking of a "potential person" as a kind of person, and, on this basis, ascribing to "potential persons" the rights of other persons. But potential persons are not persons; they do not now have the characteristics of persons. As Stanley Benn makes the point, "For if A has rights only because he satisfies some condition P, it does not follow that B has the same rights now because he *could* have property P at some time in the future. It only follows that he *will* have rights *when* he has P. He is a potential bearer of rights, as he is a potential bearer of P. A potential president of the United States is not on that account Commander-in-Chief." [34]

It is a logical error to think that potential personhood implies possession of the rights of actual persons. However, the argument from potential need not be based on this logical mistake. Like the defender of the genetic humanity criterion, the defender of the argument from potential can be understood as making a normative proposal: that potential persons *ought* to have the same rights as actual persons. Understood this way, the argument is not based on a logical confusion, but is rather in need of defense. Why should beings who are potentially "just like us" be entitled to the same protection as we are?

A Future Like Ours

Don Marquis argues that abortion is seriously immoral, for the same reason that killing an innocent adult human being is immoral.[35] What makes killing wrong is not primarily the effects on other people, or the threat to the fabric of society. What makes killing wrong is the effect on the victim. The loss of one's life is one of the greatest losses one can suffer. The loss of one's life deprives one of all the experiences, activities, projects, and enjoyments that would otherwise have constituted one's future. When I am killed, I am deprived of all of the value of my future. Abortion deprives the fetus of its future, a future just like ours. Hence, abortion is prima facie seriously morally wrong.

Marquis maintains that this is not an argument based on the wrongness of killing potential persons, since the central category is not *personhood* at all, but the category of having a valuable future like ours. However, if we ask what it is that makes "a future like ours" valuable, the answer is likely to be in terms of our capacity to enjoy our lives and derive meaning from them, to envisage a future and to make plans about it, to have relationships with others. In other words, the very capacities that make us people are what enable us to have a valuable future. So the notion of personhood, and the special wrongness of killing persons, is implicit in Marquis's account.

On the interest view, only beings that have already begun to experience their lives have an interest in the continuation of their lives. Only sentient beings can be harmed or wronged by being killed. Marquis calls this the *discontinuation account*. He concedes that it is intelligible, but holds that it is inferior to his "future-like-ours" account of the wrongness of killing. The value of one's present life is irrelevant, Marquis argues. What matters is the future of which one is deprived by death. Whether one has immediate past experiences or not does not work in the explanation of what makes killing wrong.

How are we to decide between the interest view, which incorporates a discontinuation account, and Marquis's "future-like-ours" view? It must be admitted that certain examples pose serious difficulties for the interest view. Consider the following example. Imagine that an infant is born in an unconscious condition. Her brain stem is intact, and so she breathes on her own. However, the part of the brain controlling consciousness is damaged. The baby cannot suck and needs to be tube-fed. The rest of her brain is structurally normal. Imagine further that there is a treatment that can cause the damaged part of the brain to regenerate, allowing the baby to become conscious. If she is treated, she will go on to a normal babyhood. If she is left untreated, she will die within a few weeks. Would we not regard such treatment as *in the best interest* of the child? Doesn't she have a right to the treatment? If she is allowed to die, isn't she harmed, and indeed wronged?

The answer seems to be "yes," and yet an affirmative answer conflicts with the sentience criterion of the interest view. For the brain-damaged baby is not, and never has been, sentient. She does not have a life that is a good to her; she does not have any enjoyable experiences. Yet the ability to have pleasurable experiences was the basis for ascribing to a normal newborn an interest in its own continued existence. If we think that treatment that enables the brain-damaged baby to become conscious is in her interest, this seems to imply that she has an interest$_1$ in becoming a being with interests$_2$. Why is this not also true of the fertilized egg? Neither the baby nor the zygote has a biographical life yet, but both have the potential for one. If we think that the unconscious baby can be a victim, how can we deny "victimizability" to the zygote?[36]

One possibility is to accept the conclusion that the baby has no interests, and hence no sake or welfare of her own. Life is not in *her* interest, though there are plenty of other reasons to sustain her life and give her the treatment that will enable her to become conscious. For example, this would be in her parents' interest. They have an interest in having a normal, healthy child, but the child herself has no interest in her own coming to exist as a conscious, sentient being.

This seems very counterintuitive. It is hard to think of a fully developed, otherwise healthy baby as not having a welfare of her own, simply because she is temporarily unconscious. Moreover, treating the baby might conceivably not be in the interest of her parents. They might have their own reasons for refusing treatment—if they were Christian Scientists, for example. If they refused treatment, allowing the baby to die, wouldn't they be guilty of child neglect, just as they would be for refusing lifesaving medical treatment for a conscious child?

Another possibility is to look for differences between the unconscious baby and zygotes that justify different moral status and treatment, differences that allow us to regard the baby, but not the zygote, as victimizable. The most obvious differences between the baby and the embryo are physiological. A fetus is still in the process of becoming a human being, and a zygote is in the very first stage. By contrast, the unconscious neonate in our example is a fully developed baby, physically similar to any other baby. Moreover, the baby in our example could easily be a normal baby. Everything is already in place. She is not merely a potential person, as is an embryo or a fetus. She's a *baby*, albeit one who needs treatment. Because she is so close to being a normal baby, it is virtually impossible to treat her as anything else. In other words, although, strictly speaking, she does not have interests of her own, we treat her as if she did, because she is so close to having them. We extend human moral status to the temporarily unconscious neonate because she is like a normal infant in all respects save one, and that deficiency can be easily remedied. A zygote, on the other hand, is nothing like a baby. As the biologist Clifford Grobstein says, "Biologically, the preembryo [the fertilized egg prior to implantation] and the newborn are so different—separated by nine months of development but a billion years of evolution—that it seems almost bizarre to think of them having the same status."[37]

There is another difference between the brain-damaged infant and the fetus that is relevant to moral status. In order for the fetus to achieve consciousness, it needs the woman to act as its life-support system. The brain-damaged baby is already born. It needs medical attention to become conscious, but this can be provided without making demands on the body of another person. Society can therefore recognize the baby as a human person and member of the moral community without infringing on anyone's privacy or bodily self-determination.

Thus, the extension of human moral status to the unconscious neonate does not commit us to granting similar status to zygotes, embryos, or preconscious fetuses. At the same time, as the fetus develops, it gets closer to becoming an individual that will have moral claims on us. It seems reasonable that the considerations offered to justify terminating a pregnancy should be stronger at the end of pregnancy than at the beginning. This moderate or gradualist approach to abortion is compatible with the interest view.

Contraception and the Moral Status of Gametes

The strongest objection to the argument from potential is that it seems to make contraception, and even abstinence, prima facie morally wrong. If the objection to abortion is that it deprives the zygote of "a future like ours," why, it may be asked, cannot the same complaint be made of contraceptive techniques that kill sperm, or prevent fertilization? Why don't gametes have "a future like ours"? Why aren't unfertilized eggs and sperm also potential people? John Harris makes the point this way:

> To say that a fertilized egg is potentially a human being is just to say that if certain things happen to it (like implantation), and certain other things do not (like spontaneous abortion), it will eventually become a human being. But the same is also true of the unfertilized egg and the sperm. If certain things happen to the egg (like meeting a sperm) and certain things happen to the sperm (like meeting an egg) and thereafter certain other

things do not (like meeting a contraceptive), then they will eventually become a new human being.[38]

So, if abortion is seriously wrong because it kills a potential person, then the use of a contraceptive is equally seriously wrong. In using a spermicide, one commits mass murder! Indeed, even abstinence is wrong, insofar as it prevents the development of a new human being. Very few defenders of the potentiality principle are willing to accept this conclusion.[39] They must then give reasons why a zygote, but not a sperm or ovum, is a potential person.

Defenders of the potentiality criterion sometimes appeal to an enormous difference in probabilities. John Noonan points out that the chances of any particular sperm becoming a person are remarkably low. There are about two hundred million spermatozoa in a normal ejaculate, of which only one has a chance of developing into a zygote. By contrast, he estimates the chances of a zygote developing into a person to be about 80 percent. The difference is still impressive, even if we adjust Noonan's estimate to reflect more recent information on the miscarriage rate. A 1988 study found that 31 percent of all conceptions end in miscarriage, usually in the early months of pregnancy and often before women even know they are pregnant. Even this study probably underestimated the miscarriage rate by an unknown amount, since some fertilized eggs are so defective that they never make chorionic gonadotropin, the hormone that pregnancy tests measure, and are miscarried within days of fertilization.[40] This suggests that a given zygote's chance of becoming a person is about 50 percent, rather than the 80 percent chance Noonan gives it. Still, the zygote's one-in-two chance is a lot better than a sperm's one-in-two-hundred-million chance. The odds of an ovum's developing into a person are better than those of a sperm, but still much worse than those of a fertilized egg. If we think of potential in terms of statistical likelihood, a zygote has greater potential than a gamete. But it is not clear that the odds matter. Although the chances of any particular sperm becoming a person are infinitesimal, why should that prevent its being a potential person? Is not every entrant in a lottery a potential winner, even if the odds of winning are extremely low? Every gamete, it may be said, has the potential to develop into a person, even though very few do.

Rosalind Hursthouse maintains that thinking about potentiality in terms of the chance or opportunity to become a human being embodies "a confusion about the concept of potentiality."[41] It is not the odds of a fetus's becoming a human being that make it a potential human being, but rather the fact that this is the result of "natural development" or what the fetus will become if nothing external intervenes. Richard Warner makes a similar point: "All things being equal, the zygote will grow into a person. On the other hand, the ovum or sperm qua itself is neither growing nor developing no matter in what sort of environment one should find it or put it into. A gamete will not, by itself, grow into anything other than what it already is—a gamete."[42]

The notion that an X is a potential Y only if an X will grow into a Y "all by itself" does not seem generally applicable. The orange powder known as "Tang" is a potential orange-flavored drink, but the powder doesn't turn into a drink all by itself. Someone has to intervene and add the cold water. So why should the fact that a gamete cannot become a person without external intervention deprive it of potential personhood? This seems especially so in light of the new reproductive technologies, such as *in vitro* fertilization, or IVF (see Chapter 6), in which fertilization takes place outside the body, in a petri dish. The resulting embryo is then transferred to the uterus of a female. The IVF embryo cannot become a person without considerable human intervention. Yet surely the embryo created in a laboratory is as much a potential person as the embryo produced by the normal human reproductive process.

Defenders of a potentiality principle sometimes try to differentiate between a gamete and a zygote by saying that, prior to fertilization, no particular individual exists. It is at conception, not before, that the particular human being *who I am* comes into existence. The child's question "Where was I before I was born?" has an answer: you were in your mother's womb. But the question "And where was I before that?" has no answer. Before I was conceived, I did not exist. Had the sperm and egg that combined to make me fused with any other egg or sperm, I would never have existed at all. So the zygote is identified with me, in a way that neither the egg nor the sperm is.

To this it might be retorted that while neither the egg nor the sperm is a particular potential person, each is potentially *some* person—namely, the person it will develop into if it fuses with another gamete. Why should its potential personhood be diminished by the fact that it is impossible to say, in advance, *which* person it will be? As Peter Singer and Karen Dawson say, "Potentiality is one thing: uniqueness is something quite different."[43]

Stephen Buckle argues that, on one conception of morality, potentiality and uniqueness are connected. He suggests that those who debate the moral relevance of potentiality often seem to be at cross purposes because they are appealing to different interpretations of the concept of potentiality. The consequentialist conception of potentiality focuses on future outcomes: the production of future persons. Consequentialists who accept the argument from potential maintain that abortion is prima facie wrong, though justifiable if the alternative (not having an abortion) produces a worse state of affairs, all things considered. For example, terminating *this* pregnancy may enable a woman to have a child at a time when she could care for it better. The argument also applies to contraception and even abstinence, as ways of preventing future people from coming into existence. From a consequentialist standpoint, there is no crucial difference between the fertilized egg, on the one hand, and the sperm and unfertilized egg, on the other. "This is so because the sperm and unfertilized egg, when considered jointly, also have the potential *to produce* a future human subject, even though that potential is not *activated* until fertilization occurs."[44]

A different conception of potentiality, and a different reason for regarding it as morally significant, is associated with a deontological approach to ethics. Buckle refers to this version of the argument from potential as the "respect for capacities of individuals" argument. According to this version, ". . . respect is due to an existing being because it possesses the capacity or power to develop into a being which is worthy of respect in its own right; and respect is due to such a being because it is *the very same being* as the later being into which it develops. The already-existing being is a being which has the potential *to become* a being worthy of respect in its own right."[45] It is the identification of the zygote with the later person that both makes the zygote a potential person and entitles it to respect and concern. Neither the sperm nor the egg has the same genetic code as the being who develops from their union, so neither is the same being as the fertilized egg.

It might be objected that, although the sperm and egg do not individually have the potential to become a person, when considered together, they do. Why must a potential entity be composed of a single object? We can speak of the potential of a team or an army; why not the potential of the sperm and the egg? Buckle argues that this response is misplaced. It works if we take potential to refer to the potential *to produce,* but will not do as an argument about the potential *to become.*

This is because the potential *to become* attaches only to distinct individuals that preserve their identity over time. It therefore attaches only to entities that, if they are composed of distinct parts, nevertheless can be classed as a distinct single individual. To satisfy this condition, the several and distinct parts must in some way constitute a complex *whole.* Where a collection of discrete entities is not organized into a whole, there is no individual to possess the potential *to become,* no individual that develops through the actualization of the potential.[46]

"In the case of the sperm and egg," Buckle says, "there is no complex unity, no overarching organization. Such unity or organization arises only with fertilization (in fact, only with the completion of the fertilization process at syngamy)."[47] Although the sperm and egg, considered jointly, have the potential *to produce* a human subject, they do not have the potential *to become* a human subject.

Is there any reason to prefer one conception of potentiality over another? An argument against the consequentialist conception is that it is objectionably broad; it does not distinguish potentiality from mere possibility. Feinberg suggests that the reason for holding the line at conception is that if we acknowledge the sperm to be a potential person, this may lead to the view that the entities that combined still earlier to form that spermatozoon are also potential people. "At the end of that road is the proposition that everything is potentially everything else, and thus the destruction of all utility in the concept of potentiality. It is better to hold this particular line at the zygote."[48] There are, it seems, conceptual reasons for adopting the "becoming," rather than the "producing," notion of potentiality. But does this conception have the moral significance the conservative thinks it does? What makes it seriously morally wrong to kill entities that can *become* persons, but not at all morally wrong to destroy entities that can *produce* persons?

At this point, the debate seems to be at a standstill. Antiabortionists are convinced that there is an enormous moral difference between the product of conception and the ingredients of conception. Their opponents are convinced that the difference is one of degree, and lacking in moral importance. Neither side is obviously right or wrong. Yet the success of the argument from potential hinges on differentiating the zygote from its component gametes.

The interest view rejects the argument from potential as providing a basis for moral status. Potential people have no more moral status than merely possible people. Just as there is no obligation to bring possible people into existence, there is no obligation to enable potential people to develop into actual people. Does this mean that embryos and presentient fetuses are valueless, that they have no more moral significance than gametes? Michael Tooley takes this position:

> . . . the destruction of a human organism that is a potential person, but not a person, is prima facie no more seriously wrong than intentionally refraining from fertilizing a human egg cell, and destroying it instead. Since intentionally refraining from procreation is surely not seriously wrong, neither is the destruction of potential persons.[49]

For Tooley, abortion and contraception are morally equivalent.

Many people will reject this equivalence as obviously wrong. There is no question that abortion is for most women psychologically and emotionally different from contraception. Few women experience abortion as just another way to avoid motherhood. Abortion is the end of a specific pregnancy, and this termination can be psychologically distressing, even when it is felt to be necessary. Pregnancy affects a woman's body in concrete, noticeable ways, preparing her to carry and bear a child. The child she would have, if she did not abort, is thus likely to have for her a reality that no merely possible person can have. Some women are pleased at finding that they *can* bear a child, even if they realize that having a child at this point in their lives is unwise. In ending the pregnancy, they are likely to have mixed feelings. In addition, pregnancy is imbued with certain cultural meanings. It is ordinarily a joyous experience, and one that is associated with congratulations, gift-giving, and special treatment. As one woman expresses it, "Sadness at not being able to celebrate pregnancy, to enjoy the sense of specialness it brings, is an understandable response." [50] Once we understand this, we can see why so many women (and men) do not have the same attitude toward abortion as they do toward contraception. Unless one's religion forbids it, contraception is likely to be regarded as morally neutral, a sensible preventive health habit, like flossing your teeth. It has none of the sadness or sense of loss that often accompanies abortions. A view that equates abortion and contraception is remote from the experiences of most people.

Does this matter? Some philosophers deny that it does. They argue that people's intuitions or felt convictions have no moral significance. They remind us that some people "experience" blacks and women to be inferior to whites and men. They maintain that we should not try to account for such feelings in our moral theories. The appropriate response to feelings that do not accord with moral theory is, "So what?"

I do not agree with this total rejection of moral feelings. It *may* be that a feeling is mere prejudice, incapable of being supported by good reasons. I think that this can fairly easily be shown of racist and sexist views. But from the fact that some strong convictions are indefensible, it does not follow that all are. A morality that is radically divorced from our deepest feelings, and disconnected from our experiences and emotions, cannot be practical or action-guiding. For all the reasons I have given above, I think we are justified in regarding abortion as morally more serious than contraception, and for thinking that abortion is a moral issue in a way that contraception is not. Still, I would not go so far as Rosalind Hursthouse, who argues that abortion is a choice that a completely wise and virtuous person would rarely make, because it usually displays a callous and light-minded attitude toward life. [51] This is unfair. A great many abortions occur because of contraceptive failure. A woman who is responsibly using a reliable contraceptive, and nevertheless gets pregnant, should not be labeled callous or light-minded. At the same time, this characterization might fit a woman who does not use contraceptives, repeatedly becomes pregnant, and has several abortions. I knew a sixteen-year-old girl who was about to have her third abortion. I asked her what seemed to be the problem. "Oh," she responded, "I can never remember to put in a diaphragm, and the pill makes me fat." We can acknowledge that her attitude toward sexuality, pregnancy, and potential human life is immature and superficial, without implying that the unborn has moral status. Abortion may be morally undesirable, in a way that contraception is not, without its being a *wrong to* the unborn.

The Moral Significance of Potential Personhood

On the interest view, embryos and preconscious fetuses lack moral status, despite the fact that they are potentially people. Does potentiality have *zero* moral relevance? I do not think we have to say this. Potential personhood cannot, by itself, give a being moral status. The fact that a being has the capacity to develop into a person does not mean that it has any interest in doing so, or any interests at all, for that matter. And without interests, a being can have no claim to our moral attention and concern. But what about beings that have moral status, in virtue of their being interested beings, and *also* are potential persons?

Babies

Human babies are not just sentient beings. They are also potential persons. Their potential descriptive personhood is a good reason for regarding their lives as more important, morally more valuable than the lives of sentient beings who are not potential persons, such as animals. Just as it is reasonable to value the life of a person over a nonperson, it is equally justifiable to value the life of a sentient potential person over the life of a sentient being who lacks this potential. So potential personhood, while it cannot get someone onto the moral-status scale, so to speak, can determine one's relative place on that scale. Extending normative personhood, and a serious right to life, to human infants does not commit us to extending the same moral status and right to life to nonhuman animals.

However, it must be acknowledged that some infants do not have the potential to become descriptive persons. They lack the capacity to have complex lives. Where should we place such infants on a moral-status scale?

Is the fact that they are *human* of any moral significance, when humanity is severed from the potential to become a descriptive person? Are there good reasons, in other words, to extend normative personhood to humans who will never have the complex capacities of descriptive persons? I think there are. These reasons stem from the parent–child relationship. Parents are supposed to care for their children, sick or healthy, handicapped or normal. A handicap, even a very severe one, does not take away an infant's status as *someone's child*. The fact that an infant is unlikely to develop into a complex, reasoning being should not, and usually does not, lessen his parents' love and concern for him. Nor does the infant's lack of potential remove parental obligations. So while the greater potential of human beings differentiates us from other species, and justifies our special human moral status, the absence of this potential in an individual infant does not radically change its status. He or she is still part of a network of relationships, which creates duties of care. The basic obligation owed to children is that adults, whether their parents or state-appointed guardians, will look out for them and act in their best interest. This does not necessarily mean that all severely handicapped infants must receive life-prolonging treatment. A few, such as anencephalics, may be so impaired that they do not have interests at all. If so, then nothing can be done in their interest or for their sake (see Chapter 1). Most severely handicapped children do have interests, but a few have lives that are so filled with pain, or so devoid of the things that make life worth living, that acting in their best interest may mean allowing them to die. In rare cases, it may even mean killing them. This is not because severely handicapped newborns do not have the same right to life as other normative persons. Rather, their right to life is not violated if they are genuinely "better off dead." (See Chapter 3 for a discussion of "wrongful life.")

Sentient Fetuses

What is the moral status of sentient fetuses? They have begun to have experiences, and so it is at least possible that they enjoy their lives. Obviously, the range and nature of their enjoyment is not very great, but perhaps late fetuses, like babies, are capable of sensuous pleasure, from sucking their thumbs, from the warmth of the womb, from the sound of their mothers' heartbeats, from motion as the mother moves around. Certainly in newborn nurseries the temperature is kept quite high, on the ground that this is what the baby was used to before birth. The ability to calm infants by motion is often attributed to this being a replication of the uterine environment. Studies have been done correlating fetal activity with extrauterine sound, leading researchers to claim that fetuses can not only hear inside the womb, but that they enjoy some kinds of sounds more than others. If all of this is right, then it seems plausible to say that late fetuses have, or have begun to have, lives in the biographical sense. Death deprives them of their lives, and so is a harm to them. Thus, it seems that life is *in* the interest of the conscious fetus, and it, like a newborn, can have a right to life.

On the other hand, fetuses, unlike born babies, dwell inside pregnant women. This has been dismissed by conservatives as "mere geography," but the geography is not insignificant. Any attempt to protect the life of a fetus may conflict with, or even endanger, the interests of the pregnant woman, including her life or health. There is a possibility of conflict that simply does not exist in the case of the newborn. For this reason, we cannot simply extend the right to life possessed by all human newborns to sentient fetuses.

To summarize, sentience is sufficient for minimal moral status. The interests of all sentient beings—persons, animals, conscious fetuses, and babies—must be considered. However, some sentient beings may have lives that are more valuable than others. They occupy a higher place on the moral-status scale. For example, we have good reasons for extending normative personhood, and a right to life, to human infants, stemming both from their relation to other human persons and from their potential personhood. We do not have these reasons to extend normative personhood to nonhuman animals. Conscious fetuses, though substantially similar to newborns, and thus entitled to some legal protection, are located inside the pregnant woman's body. This makes it impossible to give them full protection without violating her right to privacy or bodily self-determination (see Section IV of this chapter).

Embryos and preconscious fetuses are admittedly potential persons, but they do not have interests. Therefore, their interests cannot be considered in making the decision to abort. A pregnant woman who wishes to be responsible and conscientious in making a decision about abortion is not required to consider the child who might have been born. In order to justify having an abortion, she does not have to claim that her child would be miserable. She can acknowledge that, if she does not abort, the resulting child might well have a very happy life. Pro-lifers are quite right to cast scorn on the notion that all unplanned pregnancies result in unwanted children, or that all unwanted children necessarily have unhappy lives.[52] Instead, pro-choicers should respond that the happiness of the potential child is not determinative—indeed, not even relevant to the decision to abort. There is no obligation to bring happy people into the world, only an obligation to try to give the children one decides to bring into the world a decent chance at happiness.

It may seem obvious that there is no obligation to bring happy people into the world. How can someone who does not exist have any claim to our attention and concern? However, future people do not exist either and, as I argued in Chapter I, this does not prevent them from having claims against us. For this reason, philosophers like R.M. Hare have argued that merely possible people do count. We can harm people in the future by using up all the world's resources or by destroying the ozone layer, Hare notes; why can't we harm them by preventing them from being conceived? In the next section, I will argue that it is only future actual people who can be harmed, not merely possible people.

III. POSSIBLE PEOPLE

Nonexistence admittedly does not cause anyone to *suffer*. Nor can a non-existent person be *deprived* of existence, in the sense of having it taken away. But it may be argued that someone who is prevented from being conceived or born is *denied* existence, denied the chance to enjoy life. R. M. Hare puts the point this way:

> . . . if it would have been a good for him to exist (because this made possible the goods that, once he existed, he was able to enjoy), surely it was a harm to him not to exist, and so not to be able to enjoy these goods. He did not suffer; but there were enjoyments he could have had and did not.[53]

The point may be put another way. If death—no longer existing—can be a harm to the one who dies, why isn't nonexistence a harm to someone who never exists? Why should we have an interest in continuing to exist, but no interest in coming to exist in the first place? There seems to be an asymmetry that needs explanation.

Such an explanation can be given if we think about why we consider death to be a harm. Death is not merely nonexistence, but the termination of someone's life. Death ends all of one's plans, projects, concerns, and desires. Feinberg explains why death is a harm this way: "To extinguish a person's life is, at one stroke, to defeat almost all of his self-regarding interests: to ensure that his ongoing projects and enterprises, his long-range goals, and his most earnest hopes for his own achievement and personal enjoyment, must all be dashed."[54] None of this is true of never-existing people. The failure to bring them into existence does not thwart their plans, end their relationships, or destroy their hopes of achievement and happiness. Admittedly, it forecloses the possibility of there ever being these plans, hopes, and relationships, but that is a tragedy for no one. There is literally no one to feel sorry for, or guilty about, when people who might have existed are not brought into existence.

However, there remains an issue that requires investigation. I have been arguing that we have obligations to actual sentient beings, existing now and in the future, but no obligations to merely possible people. Actual people count; merely possible people do not.[55] Derek Parfit characterizes this as a "person-affecting view." Person-affecting principles maintain that only actions that harm actual people are wrong. Such principles can explain many of our moral views, because ordinarily the choices we face are Same People Choices (see Chapter I). We run into difficulties, however, with Different People Choices, where our choice itself affects *who* will exist. The recognition of Different People Choices may force us to reconsider the adequacy of person-affecting principles, and this could have implications for abortion.

The Parfit Problem

A Different Person Choice we discussed in the last chapter concerned a fourteen-year-old girl who chooses to have a baby. There seem to be compelling reasons why this would be a bad idea; some have to do with the likely effects on the girl's life, but others refer to the effect on the child. Teenage mothers tend to have babies who are low birthweight, which is associated both with a significantly higher mortality rate than that for full-term babies, and with learning disabilities in the future. The child of a teenage mother is also unlikely to get adequate mothering, as her mother is still a child herself. These considerations incline us to urge the fourteen-year-old to wait, and have a baby when she can give it a good start in life. Suppose she pays no attention, and goes ahead and has a child. Parfit points out that it is simply not true that it would have been better *for that child* if she had waited. If she waits, and has a child later on, it will be a different child.

The same problem arises with another kind of example, which Don Locke calls "the Fated Child."[56] In this example, a woman learns that if she conceives at a certain time, the resulting child will inevitably die of a heart attack around the age of twenty-five. If she waits a month, she will have a child with a normal life expectancy. Most of us would agree that it would be wrong to conceive the Fated Child. But why, exactly, would it be wrong? The answer cannot be that the child is disadvantaged by being conceived at that time. If the woman waits, she will have a different child. (It will be a child from a different ovum and sperm.) Assume that the Fated

Child has a worthwhile life, despite his premature death, that he does not object to his mother's decision. He is glad to be alive. So, how is her decision wrong?

To explain why it is wrong to have a Fated Child when she could have had a healthy child, we seem to have to appeal to what Locke terms "the Possible Persons Principle": "the principle that in judging the rightness or wrongness of an action or decision we need to take account not merely of those who actually do, or will, exist, but also of those who would have existed if there had been a different action or decision."[57] It is wrong to have a child with a limited life expectancy when, with a little restraint or foresight, one could have had a healthy child. But if we adopt the Possible Persons Principle (PPP) in order to explain what is wrong with conceiving a fated child, we will have to give up the Person-affecting Restriction (PAR). The PPP is, in effect, the rejection of the PAR, which requires that actions and decisions be judged only by their effect on those people who actually do exist. And if we give up the PAR, then we cannot say that abortion is morally permissible because it affects no actual person, and only actual people count.

Perhaps we do not have to reject the PAR. Perhaps having the Fated Child is wrong in itself, and not because the woman could have had a different, healthy child. Perhaps it is wrong to bring a child into the world under sufficiently adverse conditions, whether or not one could have a healthy child. In Chapter 3, I argue that it is wrong to cause children to be born when there is a substantial chance that they will have lives that fall below a decent minimum. This principle does not invoke the PPP, and so does not require us to give up the PAR.

However, is it clear that the Fated Child necessarily has a life so bad that it falls below a decent minimum? Dying at the age of twenty-five is tragic, but might not twenty-five years of healthy life compensate for the prospect of an early death? It's far from clear that the child would be better off never having been born. The case of the child born to a teenage mother is even clearer: such a life isn't ideal, but it is not so bad as to make life not worth living, or nonexistence preferable. Should we conclude, then, that there's nothing wrong with conceiving a Fated Child or having a baby at the age of fourteen? Or, if there is something wrong, is the wrongness to be explained entirely in terms of the effects on the parents and society generally? This seems to leave out the idea that having children under very adverse conditions is *unfair to them*, even when their lives are not necessarily going to be so bad as to make nonexistence preferable.

I believe that we can make sense of the idea that it is wrong to have children under very adverse conditions through appeal to a *principle of pa-*

rental responsibility. This principle maintains that in deciding whether to have children, people should not be concerned only with their own interests in reproducing. The fact that a fourteen-year-old girl may want very much to have a baby is no reason at all for her deliberately to conceive. If she is to act responsibly, she must think about the welfare of the child she will bear. She should ask herself, "What kind of life is my child likely to have?" Individuals who will make good parents—that is, loving, concerned parents—will want more than a decent minimum for their children. They will want them to have lives *well worth living.* They will refrain from bringing children into the world unless and until they can give them a decent chance at having a good life. On the principle of parental responsibility, it is wrong to bring children into the world with "the deck stacked against them."

The principle of parental responsibility involves an important asymmetry. It maintains that the fact that a child will be born under very adverse conditions is a strong, indeed perhaps decisive, moral reason against procreation. However, the fact that a child, if brought into existence, would have a happy life does not obligate its putative parents to have a child. It is never wrong, on this view, to refrain from becoming a parent, but it may be wrong to embark on parenthood. Parfit says that the Asymmetry, if it exists, must be explained. If the fact that a child would have a miserable life is a good or definitive reason not to have a child, why is the fact that a child would have a happy life *no reason at all* to have a child?

The interest view provides an answer to this question. It tells us that we should be concerned with the happiness or unhappiness of beings who have interests. It maintains that the point of morality is to make people (and other interested beings) happy, not to make more happy people. So, it is *prima facie* wrong to make people miserable, and equally wrong to cause them to exist, if they cannot be given a decent chance at having a happy life. By contrast, not causing a child to exist makes no one worse off. As Richard Brandt has said, "We must remember that *no person is frustrated or made unhappy or miserable by not coming to exist.* No one is *deprived* by non-birth as a sentient being."[58]

Mary Anne Warren expresses the point this way:

> . . . failing to have a child, even when you could have had a happy one, is neither right nor wrong . . . But the same cannot be said of *having* a child, since in this case the action results in the existence of a new person whose interests must be taken into account. Having a child under conditions which should enable one to predict that it will be very unhappy is morally objectionable, not because it violates the rights of a presently existing potential person, but because it results in the frustration of the interests of an actual person in the future.[59]

If one adopts the interest view, one will also accept the Asymmetry. But while the interest view can provide a rationale for the Asymmetry, it obviously cannot provide a rationale for itself. There may be a better theory of moral status, as Parfit suggests in his search for Theory X.[60] I do not claim that this is impossible. Rather, I have tried to show that the interest view, with its limitation of moral concern to beings who do exist, have existed, or actually will exist, is a plausible view, and that it does not necessarily lead to paradoxes or contradictions, as Parfit suggests.

I have suggested that a principle of parental responsibility can explain why it is wrong to have children under very adverse conditions, even when their lives are not necessarily "wrongful." What are the practical implications of such a principle? I am *not* arguing that only well-educated, materially well-off people should have children. Nor am I saying that it is wrong to have children who are less than "perfect." A principle of parental responsibility does not necessarily rule out having children who are in various ways at a serious disadvantage. The morality of having children under such conditions depends on whether the parents are able and willing to compensate for those disadvantages, to give the child a decent shot at a happy life. I doubt very much whether a fourteen-year-old girl will be able to do this. On the other hand, many parents are able to give seriously handicapped children the love and attention necessary to make their lives well worth living.

Sometimes this will not be possible. For example, I think a strong case can be made that HIV-infected women should not have children. Admittedly, the moral obligation of HIV-infected women to avoid conception is complicated by two factors. First, there is a pretty good chance that such women will *not* pass the virus on to their babies. Current studies indicate that the risk of actual perinatal HIV infection through any given pregnancy is somewhere between 20 and 30 percent.[61] Second, the severity of the disease varies widely. The most severely afflicted children present with adult-style opportunistic infections, such as *Pneumocystis carinii* pneumonia (PCP), during the first year of life. These children face painful death within a month or two after diagnosis. Such children have lives that clearly qualify as "wrongful." However, other children develop far milder manifestations, are diagnosed at a later date, and live much longer. John Arras says:

> Only a relatively small percentage (say, 10 to 20 percent) of those born HIV infected actually fit the worst-case scenario of early infection, chronic hospitalization, and death before the age of two.
>
> The rest will develop different and often less lethal manifestations of AIDS later on and will live longer, perhaps to the age of ten or beyond. The longer these children live with a tolerable quality of life, the more

their lives will be worth living. A child who lives at home, goes to school, and attends summer camp does not fall into the same category as a Tay-Sachs baby.[62]

Nevertheless, even the better-off AIDS babies have lives that are, in Arras's words, "decidedly grim." More than half will die before the age of seven, and the remainder must live under a cloud of impending death with progressively deteriorating immune systems. In addition, most HIV-infected babies are born to mothers (and fathers) who are themselves dying. Many of these parents are too sick to care for their own children, who are often abandoned in hospitals or put in foster care. When the medical and the social realities are considered, it is very unlikely that an HIV-infected woman will be able to provide her baby with a decent chance at a good life. In most cases, deliberately conceiving a child would be morally wrong.

Is it equally morally wrong for a pregnant woman to refuse an abortion if she is HIV-positive? Perhaps abortion might be morally obligatory if the resulting child were certainly doomed to an existence that was both extremely painful and so brief as to preclude the attainment of any compensating abilities or pleasures. However, such an existence is not necessarily or even likely to be the fate for a child born to an HIV-infected mother. In light of the moral and psychological differences between abortion and contraception that I discussed above, an attempt to derive from the moral obligation to avoid conception an obligation to abort seems unwarranted.

IV. THE ARGUMENT FROM BODILY SELF-DETERMINATION

Thomson's Defense of Abortion

In 1971, Judith Jarvis Thomson published a genuinely novel defense of abortion.[63] She noted that most debates about abortion center on the moral status of the fetus: whether it is a person with a right to life. This is because people have generally thought that if we accept the premise that the fetus is a person, it follows that abortion is always wrong. The argument goes like this: All persons have a right to life. The fetus is a person, and so it has a right to life. The mother has the right to decide what happens in and to her body, but the right to life is stronger and more stringent than the mother's right to decide, and so outweighs it. So the fetus may not be killed; an abortion may not be performed.

It is this argument that Thomson wants to challenge. She argues that even if we grant the personhood of the fetus, abortion is not necessarily wrong. For it is possible that in at least some cases abortion does not violate the fetus-person's right to life. This is initially puzzling. If the fetus has a right to life, and abortion kills it, then how can abortion fail to violate its right to life? Thomson suggests that our perplexity stems from a failure to understand the nature of rights in general and the right to life in particular. In a nutshell, her argument is that having a right to life does not entitle a person to whatever he or she needs to stay alive, and in particular does not entitle him to the use of another person's body.

To illustrate this point, Thomson creates the following example:

> You wake up in the morning and find yourself back to back in bed with an unconscious violinist. He has been found to have a fatal kidney ailment, and the Society of Music Lovers has canvassed all the available medical records and found that you alone have the right blood type to help. They have therefore kidnapped you, and last night the violinist's circulatory system was plugged into yours, so that your kidneys can be used to extract poisons from his blood as well as your own.[64]

The director of the hospital, while acknowledging that it was very wrong of the Society to kidnap you, nevertheless refuses to unplug you, since to unplug you would be to kill him. Anyway, it's only for nine months. After that, the violinist will have recovered and can be safely unplugged. Thomson questions whether it is morally incumbent on you to accede to this situation. It would be very nice of you, of course, but do you *have* to stay plugged in to the violinist? What if it were not nine months, but nine years? Or longer still? What if the director were to maintain that you must stay plugged in forever, on the ground that the violinist is a person, and all persons have a right to life? Thomson suggests that you would regard this argument as "outrageous," and says that this suggests that something really is wrong with the plausible-sounding right-to-life argument presented above.

The violinist example, fantastic though it is, preserves some of the features of the pregnancy situation without making at all doubtful the personhood of the "victim." Given that the violinist is a person, with a right to life, do you murder him, do you violate his right to life, if you unplug yourself? If not, then we have, it seems, a case of terminating the life of an innocent person that is not a case of violating his right to life.

The violinist example is intended to demonstrate Thomson's central theme, that the right to life does not necessarily include getting whatever you need to live. To take a less fanciful example, I may need your bone marrow in order to live, but that does not give me a right to it. Even if you *ought* to be willing to donate, even if your refusal is selfish and mean, it does not follow that I have a right to your bone marrow, or that you may legitimately be compelled to donate.[65] The right to life does not imply a right to use another person's body.

However, it may be objected that the fetus *does* have a right to use the pregnant woman's body because she is (partly) responsible for its existence. By engaging in intercourse, knowing that this may result in the creation of a person inside her body, she implicitly gives the resulting person a right to remain. This argument would not apply in the situation most closely aligned with the violinist example—pregnancy due to rape. A woman who is pregnant due to rape does not voluntarily engage in sexual intercourse, and so cannot be said to have implicitly given the fetus permission to use her body.

On this analysis, even if abortion is ordinarily a grave wrong, it is permissible in the case of rape. Many antiabortionists wish to make such an exception, but they have been hard-pressed, on their own argument, to account for it. For antiabortionists maintain that the fetus is an innocent person. How can it be right to kill the fetus because its father is a rapist? The Thomson argument gives an answer: the fetus whose existence is caused by rape has no right to use the pregnant woman's body. Killing it does not violate its right to life.

But what about most pregnancies, which do not result from rape but from voluntary intercourse? Given that the presence of the fetus is due in part to the woman's own voluntary action, can she now eject it at the cost of its life? Thomson responds by saying that even where the woman voluntarily engages in sex, she may not be responsible for the presence of the fetus. She argues that responsibility for an outcome depends on what one has done to prevent it. She suggests that if a person has taken all reasonable precautions to prevent something from happening, then she has not been negligent, and should not be held responsible for its having occurred. So whether the woman can be said to have given the fetus a right to use her body would depend on such variables as whether she was using a reliable contraceptive that happened to fail.

Some critics of Thomson have taken her to task for concentrating exclusively on rights. The real question, they say, is not what constitutes giving the unborn person a right to use one's body, but rather the conditions that make aborting the fetus morally permissible. Thomson responds by saying that since her intention was to examine the right-to-life argument, she can hardly be faulted for concentrating on rights. However, she acknowledges that we can have moral obligations to help people, even when they do not have rights against us. Suppose that the violinist needed your kidneys only for an hour, and that this would not affect your health at all. Even though you were kidnapped, even though you never gave anyone permission to plug him into you, still you ought to let him stay: "it would be indecent to refuse."[66] Similarly, if pregnancy lasted only an hour, and posed no threat to life or health, the pregnant woman ought to allow the fetus-person to remain for that hour. She ought to do this even if the pregnancy was due to rape, and the fetus has no right to use her body. This conclusion is based on the principle (which Thomson calls "minimally decent Samaritanism") that if you can save a person's life without much trouble or risk to yourself, you ought to do it. In the real world, however, pregnancies do not last for only an hour, and they do involve considerable sacrifices.[67] Thomson concludes, "Except in such cases as the unborn person has a right to demand it—and we were leaving open the possibility that there may be such cases—nobody is morally *required* to make large sacrifices, of health, of all other interests and concerns, of all other duties and commitments, for nine years, or even for nine months, in order to keep another person alive."[68]

Thomson's analysis apparently justifies abortion only in a relatively narrow range of cases. Many unwanted pregnancies occur because contraception was not used at all, or only occasionally. In such cases, the woman *is* (partly) to blame, and so the resulting fetus may be said to have been given the right to use her body. If so, then abortion violates its right to life, and is impermissible. Mary Anne Warren writes, "This is an extremely unsatisfactory outcome, from the viewpoint of the opponents of restrictive abortion laws, most of whom are convinced that a woman has a right to obtain an abortion regardless of how and why she got pregnant."[69]

It seems to me that Warren is right. A successful defense of abortion cannot be based solely on the woman's moral right to decide what happens in and to her body. This yields a defense of abortion in a relatively narrow range of cases—namely, those in which the woman is absolved of responsibility for the presence of the unborn. By the same token, a defense of abortion based solely on the claim that presentient fetuses lack moral status is vulnerable to potentiality arguments. The strongest argument in favor of a liberal abortion policy combines both these approaches. This was the approach taken by the United States Supreme Court in *Roe* v. *Wade*.

Roe *v.* Wade

The legalization of abortion in *Roe* v. *Wade* was based on two factors: the woman's right to privacy and the status of the unborn. First the Supreme Court held that the unborn have never been recognized in the law as persons in the whole sense: "In areas other than criminal abortion, the law has been reluctant to endorse any theory that life, as we recognize it, begins before live birth or to accord legal rights to the unborn except in narrowly defined situations and except when the rights are *contingent upon live birth.*"[70] Because the unborn is not a person within the language and meaning of the Fourteenth Amendment, it therefore does not have the right to life specifically guaranteed by that Amendment. So states are not permitted to prohibit abortion to protect the fetus's right to life. On the other side, the woman's constitutional right of privacy entitles her to make this most personal of decisions, without state intervention, at least throughout the first two trimesters. At the same time, the Court recognized legitimate state interests in protecting maternal health, in maintaining medical standards, and in protecting potential human life. "At some point in pregnancy, these respective interests become sufficiently compelling to sustain regulation of the factors that govern the abortion decision. The privacy right involved, therefore, cannot be said to be absolute."[71]

In the second trimester, states may regulate the abortion procedure in ways that are reasonably related to maternal health but may not forbid abortion. This changes after the fetus becomes viable, or capable of surviving outside the womb, albeit with artificial aid, sometime around the 28th week of gestation, possibly as early as the 24th week. "If the State is interested in protecting fetal life after viability, it may go so far as to proscribe abortion during that period, except when it is necessary to preserve the life or health of the mother."[72]

At this writing, *Roe* is still the law of the land, despite numerous attempts by state legislatures to restrict the right to abortion. In July 1989, in *Webster* v. *Reproductive Health Services*[73], the Supreme Court upheld various restrictions on abortion in a Missouri statute. Since *Webster,* every attempt to restrict abortion by states has been upheld by the courts. On July 18, 1991, the Louisiana legislature overrode a veto by Governor Buddy Roemer to pass the most restrictive abortion law in the nation. The law outlaws all abortions except to save the lives of pregnant women or when victims of rape and incest meet certain conditions. It makes no provisions for allowing abortions when a woman's health is threatened by her pregnancy.[74]

The Louisiana law was immediately challenged in court. On August 7, 1991, a federal district judge, Adrian G. Duplantier, ruled that the Louisiana statute was unconstitutional under *Roe* v. *Wade.* However, Duplantier also made it clear that he was personally opposed to *Roe* v. *Wade* and "wholeheartedly" agreed with Justice Byron R. White's dissenting opinion in that decision.[75] The Louisiana Attorney General, William V. Guste, Jr., said that he would try to appeal the ruling directly to the Supreme Court, bypassing the United States Court of Appeals for the Fifth Circuit. Mr. Guste hopes that the Supreme Court will overrule *Roe* v. *Wade* and hold the Louisiana law constitutional. The Louisiana law is one of four that opponents of abortion hope the Supreme Court will review and use as a basis for overturning *Roe* v. *Wade*. The three others are from Pennsylvania, Utah, and Guam.[76]

There are various possible bases for an overturning of the 1973 decision. Some critics of *Roe* v. *Wade* (such as Judge Robert Bork, the unsuccessful candidate for the Supreme Court in 1987) object to the "creation" of a right of privacy nowhere mentioned in the Constitution. Others, who accept a constitutional right of privacy, deny that the Constitution protects a woman's right to abort. They maintain that the right to abortion is "judge-made" and one upon which the Constitution is silent. An adequate discussion of these claims would take us far afield into the topic of constitutional interpretation and judicial decision-making.[77] I will simply say that I agree with those who maintain that the right of privacy is a fundamental right and a central American value that is implicit in the concept of ordered liberty.[78] Moreover, as Justice Brennan said in *Eisenstadt* v. *Baird*, "if the right to privacy means anything, it is the right of the individual, married or single, to be free from unwarranted governmental intrusion into matters so fundamentally affecting a person as the decision whether to bear or beget a child."[79]

Not all of *Roe*'s critics oppose the right to abortion. Rather, they think that the constitutional analysis in *Roe* is shaky. For example, Donald Regan claims that the right to abortion would have been given a sounder footing if it had been based on the right to "equal protection" instead of a right to privacy.[80] Regan uses Thomson's "Defense of Abortion" to present a convincing argument that it is unfair to require pregnant women to become "Good Samaritans" when similar burdens are not imposed on other members of society. This provides an argument against restrictive abortion laws that does not depend on a right to privacy nowhere mentioned in the Constitution.

The problem with basing the right to abortion solely on an "equal-protection" basis is that it implies that restrictive abortion laws are unconstitutional only if comparable burdens are not imposed on other members of society. Some have argued that restrictive abortion laws do not pose unique burdens on women; the law can impose comparable or greater burdens on men—for example, a military draft in time of war. Others think that all citizens *should* be legally required to undergo burdens or make sacrifices to save lives. They support Good Samaritan statutes that, if enacted, would undercut an equal-protection basis for the right to abortion. Moreover, basing the right to abortion solely on "equal protection" completely leaves out the element of governmental intrusion into one of the most private, most personal decisions a woman may ever face. In my view, such intrusion by the state is unjustified even if the pregnancy is relatively trouble-free and even if others in society are legally required to be Good Samaritans.

It is not necessary to choose between the argument from privacy and the equal protection argument. They can be used together to support a constitutional right to abortion. Indeed, it seems to me that this is implicit in the approach taken by Justice Blackmun in *Roe v. Wade*. For while Blackmun explicitly mentioned only the right to privacy, he elaborated the physical and psychological harms that the state would impose upon the pregnant woman by denying the choice of abortion as part of his defense of the claim that there exists a right of privacy "broad enough to encompass a woman's decision whether or not to terminate her pregnancy."[81]

Another objection to *Roe* v. *Wade* has to do with the significance of viability as the cutoff point after which states may, if they choose, prohibit abortion.

V. THE MORAL AND LEGAL SIGNIFICANCE OF VIABILITY

Why should viability mark the point at which states are entitled to override the pregnant woman's rights to self-determination and bodily autonomy? The *Roe* court offered the following as justification: "With respect to the State's important and legitimate interest in potential life, the 'compelling' point is at viability. This is so because the fetus then presumably has the capability of meaningful life outside the mother's womb. State regulation protective of fetal life after viability thus has both logical and biological justifications."[82]

A number of commentators have pointed out that this is no justification at all. The capacity for independent life does not *explain* the significance of viability; it merely gives the meaning of viability. As John Hart Ely has argued, ". . . the Court's defense seems to mistake a definition for a syllogism. . ."[83] In fact, it could be maintained that viability's logical significance is the opposite of what the Court implied: "Why should a fetus' capacity to live independently be a reason to forbid the mother from forcing it to live independently?"[84]

Law professor Patricia King defends viability as a reasonable criterion for certain kinds of legal protection.[85] She argues that birth was traditionally the point at which the fetus got protection because birth was once the point at which the unborn demonstrated its *capacity for continued existence.*

Today, the capacity for continued existence can be predicted before birth. There is no reason, therefore, to insist on live birth before offering at least some protection to the unborn. Moreover, the difference between a newborn and a viable fetus is negligible. So, if we are concerned to protect newly born human beings, we ought also to extend similar protection to viable fetuses.

At the time *Roe* was decided, viability was usually placed at about seven months (28 weeks g.a.), although the Court acknowledged that it might occur earlier, even at 24 weeks. Like all medical facts, this is subject to change, as technology progresses. In her dissent from *Akron,* Justice Sandra Day O'Connor argued that improvements in medical science are pushing the point of viability further back toward conception. The result, Justice O'Connor suggested, was that *Roe* was "on a collision course with itself."[86] As abortions become safer later in pregnancy, the time during which the State can regulate abortions out of concern for maternal health will increasingly be reduced. This would expand the right to choose abortion. At the same time, on grounds of protecting viable fetuses, states could regulate, and even proscribe, abortions earlier and earlier in pregnancy. This would greatly restrict the right to abortion. Thus, the trimester framework appears to expand and restrict the right to abort at the same time.

O'Connor's prediction that fetuses might become viable in the first trimester in the not-too-distant future is very unlikely. While the point of viability may be somewhat earlier than the one cited in *Roe* v. *Wade,* medical science appears to have reached a biological limit in its ability to save premature infants. If a baby is born before 23 or 24 weeks of pregnancy, it simply cannot survive, because its lungs are too immature to function, even with the help of respirators. Only about 10 percent of babies born at 23 weeks, even in the best newborn intensive-care units, can survive.[87] According to Nancy Rhoden, "Many experts believe that because of the extreme immaturity of a fetus of less than about 23 weeks, 22 or 23 weeks represents an absolute lower limit on fetal viability absent development of an artificial placenta."[88]

What if an artificial placenta were invented? Viability might then be possible immediately after conception. Even without an artificial placenta, it is now possible to recover an embryo by uterine lavage from one woman and then to transfer that embryo into the uterus of another (infertile) woman. This procedure, known as surrogate embryo transfer (SET), has already produced some live births. It might someday be possible routinely to salvage aborted embryos, freeze them, and then implant them into the uteruses of women capable of bearing children but not of becoming pregnant. These frozen embryos could be thought of as "viable," in the sense of being capable of existence independent of their genetic mother. Of course, an embryo cannot exist independent of *some* womb, but a womb, natural or artificial, might be thought of as "artificial aid," comparable to a respirator necessary to sustain the life of a very premature fetus.

If viability were pushed back into the first trimester, would it have the moral and legal significance assigned to it by the Court in *Roe* v. *Wade?* Nancy Rhoden presents a compelling argument that it would not. She suggests that the reason the Supreme Court focused on viability as the point at which states might prohibit abortion is that, in 1973, the capacity for independent existence *coincided with* late gestation. The Court did not realize the possibility of divergence between viability and late gestation because "in 1973 it was virtually inconceivable that a viable fetus would be anything other than one that was substantially developed and had survived to the last stage of pregnancy."[89] Rhoden argues that where *ex utero* survivability is divorced from late gestation, survivability no longer has moral significance.

Rhoden distinguishes between viability as simple technological survivability (which she calls "Viability$_1$") and viability as a normative concept ("Viability$_2$"). She says, "Viability as a normative concept thus has at least two major components. It is not merely technological, but rather encompasses the idea that the fetus is so substantially developed that it has a claim to societal protection."[90] Rhoden argues that Viability$_2$—"the complex, value-laden notion that once a fetus can survive *ex utero* and is substantially developed, its claim to societal protection increases"—is a necessary, although unarticulated, component of the *Roe* viability standard. She recommends that the *Roe* decision be revamped, and that legal protection be extended to the *late-gestation,* rather than technologically viable, fetus. She acknowledges that "late gestation" is a fuzzy concept, but believes it certainly does not occur before the midpoint of pregnancy (week 20). She believes that the point at which states can prohibit elective abortions "should remain approximately what it is today, and in no event should it creep earlier than the week 21–24 range."[91]

Rhoden's analysis is supported by the interest view, which explains more fully the significance of late gestation. It is only after the fetus has a fairly developed nervous system, probably around weeks 22 to 24, that it becomes conscious and sentient. The most important similarity between the newborn and the late-gestation fetus is sentience, because of the conceptual connection between sentience and interests. However, there are some practical problems with using sentience to limit legal abortions.

Practical Problems with a Sentience Criterion

Despite difficulties in determining whether a particular fetus is viable,[92] at least there is *some* consensus in the medical community about the probability that a given fetus will survive, assuming that we know its gestational age. By contrast, the onset of sentience is far more problematic and controversial. Scientists disagree about which neurological structures and events are essential for the capacity to feel pain. There is disagreement about the role of myelination and the development of the cerebral cortex in the perception of pain. So long as there are these debates, it is not possible to say with any degree of certainty precisely when sentience occurs.[93] We may, however, be able to set outer limits. Before 8 weeks g.a., sentience is not possible; after 28 weeks g.a., it is very likely. But that is a very large gray area. How, it may be asked, can we possibly base public policy on such an ephemeral notion?

Another possibility is to pick "brain birth," or when neocortical brain activity begins, as the moment when the fetus should be protected.[94] This proposal is based on the idea that it is intelligence that sets humans apart from all other creatures, and it is neocortical activity that endows human beings with higher intellectual functions. The neocortex first begins producing EEG waves between the 22nd and 24th weeks of pregnancy. On the "brain birth" view, when a fetus reaches the stage of development when recognizable neocortical activity begins, the state should be allowed to regulate and proscribe abortions to protect that human life, except where necessary to preserve the mother's life and health. Gary Gertler says:

> Human cognition is that characteristic which meets [the] necessary and sufficient conditions for being a person deserving of human rights. Since the inception of neocortical brain activity, or brain birth, is the beginning of cognitive capability, it is the point at which personhood protection should begin. Brain birth is not merely an index, sign, or litmus test of being human; it is a more basic trait that should be recognized as conferring personhood on whomever possesses it. All and only those beings that have neocortical brain activity have the right to basic human rights, in particular the right to full and equal protection against homicide.[95]

To account for the two-week margin of error in determining gestational age, and the "remote possibility" that an individual fetus might develop EEG brain activity before the 22nd week of pregnancy, Gertler suggests that we adopt the 20th week of gestation as the point at which the state would have the right to intervene and protect fetal life.

"Brain birth" as the beginning of human life is symmetrical with the proposal of some that we should consider human life to have ended when the neocortex ceases functioning. The brain-birth standard has the advantage of being objective (unlike sentience) and unaffected by developments in medical technology (unlike viability). However, it is subject to two criticisms. First, no state has so far defined death exclusively in terms of a lack of neocortical function. At present, we distinguish between people who are in persistent vegetative state and people who have died (see Chapter 1). So the argument from symmetry is not as strong as Gertler suggests.

Second, Gertler's view is vulnerable to the same criticism I made earlier against Brody. Since Gertler argues that cognition is what makes humans special, presumably he means by cognition something more than mere sentience or consciousness, since these are attributes we share with virtually all animals. What makes us special is our capacity for self-awareness and our ability to reason abstractly. (We may share this to some degree with chimpanzees, gorillas, and orangutans, but this is controversial.) However, no 22–week-old fetus is capable of reasoning or self-awareness. A fetus, even a very well-developed one, is less intelligent than an adult mammal, or even, as Warren has pointed out, an adult fish. In fact, even a newborn baby does not yet have "cognitive capability." Neither behavioral, nor neurophysiological, nor bioelectrical evidence provides any reason for attributing higher mental capacities to newborns. As Michael Tooley says, "The neuronal circuitry in the human brain undergoes, in general, tremendous development during the postnatal period. What is crucial, however, is that those networks, located in the upper layers of the cerebral cortex, that are thought to underlie higher mental functions, are not present at birth; their emergence takes place only over an extended period of postnatal development."[96]

If normative personhood depends on such characteristics as self-consciousness and the ability to reason, then newborn humans are not persons. *A fortiori*, neither are 22–week-old fetuses. If the *potential* for cognition suffices, then there seems to be no reason why younger fetuses or embryos, who are also potential persons, aren't also entitled to legal protection.

By contrast, the sentience criterion advocated by the interest view bases moral status not on something the late-gestation fetus has potentially, but on its actual possession of interests. The sentience criterion is thus better able than the brain-birth criterion to explain why late fetuses, but not embryos, count. It can explain why even severely mentally handicapped newborns, who may never acquire the ability to reason, are entitled to our protection and concern. As long as they are sentient, and capable of suffering or enjoying their lives, they have a claim to our moral attention. For these reasons, I believe that it is sentience rather than "brain birth" that marks a qualitative difference in the life of the unborn. However, sentience appears roughly to coincide with brain birth, and both occur during late gestation. From a practical standpoint, it does not matter whether we pick sentience, brain birth, or some notion of late gestation as the time at which the state may intervene to protect fetal life. The basic idea is that there are morally relevant similarities between late-gestation fetuses and newborn babies that justify, and perhaps require, that the state protect late fetuses.

At the same time, there are good reasons not to extend *equal* protection to even fully developed fetuses. Those reasons stem from the fact that the fetus is inside a pregnant woman. The question, therefore, is not simply whether the fetus counts, but how much the state can require of the pregnant woman. Some take the position that the state is never justified in requiring a woman to complete a pregnancy, regardless of the stage of fetal development. In the next section, I argue that some time limits on abortion are reasonable once the fetus is conscious and sentient.

Late Abortions

Postviability abortions are extremely rare. Ninety percent of all abortions take place in the first trimester. Ninety-nine percent are performed in the first 20 weeks. After 24 weeks, only 0.01 percent are performed.[97] Most very late abortions occur in two situations. First, teenagers tend to have later abortions than adult women, because of the greater difficulties they face in obtaining the procedure. Teenagers account for 28 percent of all abortions, but 43 percent of abortions performed after 20 weeks of gestation. The youngest teenagers tend to have the latest abortions. Abortions after 20 weeks comprise 3.7 percent of all abortions performed for girls fourteen and younger, contrasted to the national average of 1 percent of all abortions.[98]

A second reason for very late abortions is the detection of fetal anomalies. Amniocentesis is best performed at around 15 to 16 weeks of gestation. It may take two or three weeks to get the results back from the laboratory. Thus, fetal diagnosis of chromosomal, biochemical, or DNA abnormalities can rarely be established prior to 18 weeks, and possibly later. In addition, if gestation is miscalculated, the fetus may be 20 weeks old.

Nan Hunter, of the American Civil Liberties Union, argues that there should be no time limits on abortion. If the state does not have the right to impose the burdens of pregnancy on women during early gestation, why does it acquire that right later on in pregnancy? Hunter says, "The burden to a woman of continuing a pregnancy against her will is stupefying."[99]

Instead of imposing time limits on abortion, society should adopt measures that will reduce the number of late abortions, such as contraceptive education and services, restoring Medicaid funding for abortions, and repeal of parental-consent laws.

While I agree with Hunter that all of these things should be done, it does not seem unfair for society to require women to decide within a reasonable period of time whether or not they will continue the pregnancy. Twenty-four weeks should ordinarily be enough time for a woman to learn that she is pregnant and to gain access to the health-care system. (Some women do not have access at any time because of poverty. This injustice should be corrected, but allowing late abortions will not remedy this fault.) Imposing a time limit acknowledges the claims of the late-gestation fetus to social protection, while also recognizing the right of the woman to decide not to become a mother. As Robert Goldstein says, restrictions on abortion should depend not on fetal survivability, "but on the reasonable period of time a woman needs to act on behalf of the dyadic unit as its representative, and to choose whether to make her constitutive commitment to it of mother-love."[100] Moreover, if a woman is close to giving birth, she has already gone through many of the burdens of pregnancy, and therefore prohibiting abortion at that point does not impose excessive burdens.[101]

Although abortion has occupied center stage in the debate over "fetal rights," it is only one area where the status of the fetus is an issue. Other issues include whether there can be civil or criminal liability for killing a fetus, whether fetuses are included in family insurance policies, and whether severely impaired children whose existence is the result of a physician's negligence can recover in a civil suit for "wrongful life." These and other questions are addressed in the next chapter, where I consider the legal status of the unborn beyond abortion.

3

Beyond Abortion: The Legal Status of the Fetus

Apart from criminal abortion, the law has been reluctant to accord legal rights to the unborn "except in narrowly defined situations and except when the rights are *contingent upon live birth.*"[1] For centuries, the common law has held that a fetus, viable or otherwise, could not be the subject of homicide. Most states continue to follow this common law rule. In 1989, the Supreme Court of North Carolina held that the unlawful, willful, and felonious killing of a viable fetus is not murder under North Carolina law.[2] A Connecticut Superior Court judge reached the same conclusion in 1986. He rejected the first formal request for a murder warrant in the shooting death of a six-month-old fetus, finding that under state law a fetus—even a viable one—is not considered a human being.[3] In other areas of the law, however, the fetus appears to have a different status. The majority of jurisdictions allow recovery for the stillbirth of a viable fetus, even though the wrongful-death acts of most states allow recovery only in the death of a "person." For example, the Supreme Court of Missouri ruled in 1983 that a stillborn fetus is a person within the meaning of the state's wrongful death statute.[4]

Other examples of so-called "fetal rights" abound.

89

In Minnesota, a person who assaults a pregnant woman and causes the death of the unborn may be guilty of murder.[5] In 1984, supreme courts in South Carolina and Massachusetts, reversing case law, ruled that a fetus is a person in criminal and vehicular homicide cases. The Supreme Court of Iowa has held that the parents of a viable fetus killed in an automobile accident may recover for loss of consortium under the uninsured-motorist provisions of their auto insurance. The court held that an unborn child is a "family member" and a "person" within the scope of the insurance policy.[6]

It appears, then, that not only do jurisdictions differ on the status of the fetus, but also that the fetus can be a "person" for one purpose but not for another. Many have found these discrepancies intellectually unsatisfying. Once again, the interest view can help to resolve apparent contradictions and avoid a purely ad hoc approach to the legal status of the unborn. The interest view maintains that there is an important distinction between the fetus per se and the surviving child. Prior to becoming conscious and sentient, fetuses have no interests at all. However, surviving children clearly do have interests: in life, in health, in avoiding injury or disability. They are entitled to be compensated when these interests are wrongfully infringed. Allowing *surviving children* to recover for injuries inflicted prior to birth in no way implies that preconscious fetuses have interests, rights, or moral or legal status.

Prenatal wrongful-death actions pose a different problem. Recovery for the wrongful death of a fetus should be seen, on the interest view, not as according personhood, interests, or rights to the unborn, but as compensating prospective parents for the loss of an expected child. Laws that permit a charge of murder in the destruction of a fetus through an attack on the pregnant woman can be similarly rationalized. The aim is to protect pregnant women from physical attack and from the harm of losing a wanted pregnancy. As Dawn Johnsen notes, "Holding third parties responsible for the negligent or criminal destruction of fetuses is therefore consistent with, and even enhances, the protection of pregnant women's interests."[7] Such laws thus do not conflict with the Supreme Court's abortion decisions, and do not ascribe an independent status to the unborn.

Section I discusses recovery in torts for prenatal injury and preconception torts, against third parties and mothers, and for purposes of insurance coverage. Prenatal wrongful death is covered in Section II. Section III considers the criminal law relating to fetuses, including prenatal neglect, murder, and vehicular homicide. Wrongful life suits are the topic of Section IV.

I. RECOVERY FOR PRENATAL INJURY IN TORTS

Against Third Parties

Prior to 1946, there was no recovery for prenatal injuries, not even on the part of surviving children. Then, in the landmark case of *Bonbrest* v. *Kotz*,[8] the District Court for the District of Columbia allowed recovery against an attending physician for injuries inflicted *in utero* on a child who was subsequently born alive. Within a few years after *Bonbrest,* most American jurisdictions followed suit.[9] Today, virtually all American jurisdictions allow tort claims for prenatal injuries if the child is subsequently born alive.[10]

What explains the refusal of American courts until relatively recently to allow a cause of action for prenatal torts? The judicial stance toward the unborn was based on a decision of the Massachusetts Supreme Court in *Dietrich* v. *Northampton.*[11] Justice Oliver Wendell Holmes held that no duty of care was owed to the unborn child. Until live birth, it was not *in esse,* but part of the mother. Any damage to it that was not too remote to be recovered for at all was recoverable by her.

Although Holmes's decision concerned the *death* of a *nonviable* fetus, the Illinois Supreme Court appealed to *Dietrich* in its decision in *Allaire* v. *St. Luke's Hospital*[12] when it held that there was no cause of action for a *child born seriously and permanently disabled* from injuries to his mother just prior to delivery. The case was significant not only because it was relied on for the next forty-six years, but also because of the cogent dissent of Justice Boggs.

Boggs argued that the fact that the injuries were inflicted prior to birth should not operate to deny a cause of action. "The appellee corporation owed it as a duty of care to the plaintiff, though unborn, to bestow due and ordinary care and skill to the matter of his preservation and safety before and at the time of his birth."[13] To regard the fetus, once it is viable, as merely a part of its mother is to deny a palpable fact, "for her body may die in all of its parts and the child remain alive, and capable of maintaining life, when separated from the dead body of the mother."[14] If the viable fetus is a separate existence, and not merely a part of its mother, then negligence that causes him to be born maimed and crippled is an injury to him, and not to his mother. Boggs concluded that once the fetus had reached the stage where it could live separable from the mother, and is afterwards born, the child "has a right of action for any injuries wantonly or negligently inflicted upon his or her person at such age of viability, though then in the womb of the mother."[15]

The Irrelevance of Viability

The implicit rationale for the viability requirement, as regards a surviving child, is that, prior to viability, there is no independent being to whom the defendant owes a duty of care.[16] In his effort to refute Holmes's mistaken notion that the unborn was merely a part of the mother's body, Justice Boggs focused on viability as the basis for separate existence. It is true that, prior to viability, the fetus cannot *exist separately*. However, the fetus is a separate entity, biologically distinct from its mother, throughout pregnancy. This led the New York Supreme Court in *Kelly* v. *Gregory* to allow recovery by a surviving child for injuries sustained by its mother in her third month of pregnancy. The court held that the legal entity of a child "begins at conception and hence a child, born alive, may recover for prenatal injury tortiously inflicted at any time at or after conception, regardless of whether [the] fetus was viable at [the] time of injury."[17]

This ruling reaches the right result for the wrong reason. The reason that viability at the time of the injury is not a prerequisite for recovery by a surviving child is not that separate existence begins prior to viability, at conception. It is rather that the separate existence of the fetus *at the time of the injury* is irrelevant to the merits of the *surviving infant's* cause of action. As Justice Proctor pointed out in *Smith* v. *Brennan*, ". . . whether viable or not at the time of the injury, the child sustains the same harm after birth . . ." and therefore "should be given the same opportunity for redress."[18] In other words, it is the *surviving child,* not the fetus, who has the cause of action, although the injury was sustained prior to birth. Indeed, once it is understood that it is the surviving child who has the cause of action, there is no philosophical or logical reason to restrict recovery to injuries incurred after conception.

Preconception Torts

Not only can there be a duty of care prior to viability, but the duty of care can exist even before the conception of the individual injured by the negligence. Wrongful acts today can harm future people who have not yet been born or conceived. Professor James puts the point well: ". . . the improper canning of baby food today is negligent to a child born next week or next year, who consumes it to his injury. The limitation of the *Palsgraf* case contains no requirement that the interests within the range of peril be known or identified in the actor's mind, or *even in existence at the time of the negligence.*"[19] The relevant factor is causation, and there is no reason to bar as a matter of principle the possibility of injury caused before birth, or even conception. The first American court to recognize this was the U.S. Court of Appeals for the Tenth Circuit in *Jorgensen* v. *Meade Johnson Laboratories*.[20] In that case, the father of twin girls with Down syndrome alleged that, prior to the twins' conception, their mother's genetic structure had been altered through her ingestion of birth-control pills. The district court found that the plaintiffs failed to state a cause of action under Oklahoma law and dismissed the suit. On appeal, the Tenth Circuit reversed, holding that the timing of the tortious conduct should not be determinative in allowing or denying the child's right of action. Assuming that causation could be established, the fact that the injury resulted from preconception conduct was no reason for denying recovery.

Other jurisdictions have reached the same result.[21] Despite these precedents, the New York Court of Appeals rejected a cause of action based on preconception negligence in *Albala* v. *City of New York*.[22] An infant sought recovery for congenital brain damage, allegedly due to his mother's uterus having been perforated during an abortion more than three years before his conception. Judge Wachtler, writing for the majority, held that to allow such a cause of action would stretch traditional tort concepts beyond manageable bounds. If this is interpreted to mean that traditional tort concepts cannot accommodate preconception torts, the claim is simply false. The operative tort concept is that a person is responsible for all damage resulting from, and as a natural consequence of, a wrongful act. It might be impossible for Mrs. Albala to prove that the negligently performed abortion was in fact the cause of her son's brain damage, but the difficulty of proof is no reason to deny a cause of action. Moreover, remoteness of the cause from the time of injury is not always a problem in establishing the cause of injury, as is shown by Professor James's example of improperly canned baby food.

It seems likely that the court's decision was based largely on the fear that recognition of preconception torts would create limitless liability and a flood of cases. This is understandable, particularly in light of the factual situation in *Albala*. However, it seems grossly unfair to deny compensation to someone who has been seriously injured by another's negligence, simply because there are many others in the same boat.

Preconception tort liability has arisen in connection with diethylstilbestrol (DES). The drug, which was given to as many as two million women from 1941 to 1970, in order to prevent miscarriage, was eventually found to be ineffective. However, the drug caused some adverse effects, including a rare vaginal and cervical cancer known as clear-cell adenocarcinoma in a few of the daughters of the women who took it. DES daughters are also more likely to have miscarriages or stillbirths. In 1990, an Appellate Division court ruled that the *granddaughters* of women who took DES, who were not even conceived at the time, could sue for the drug's alleged harmful effects.[23] The plaintiff was Karen Enright, who was born in 1981 with cerebral palsy. The complaint alleged that Karen's mother, Patricia, was exposed *in utero* to DES, resulting in certain anatomical abnormalities and deformities in her reproductive system that prevented her from carrying a baby to full term. Karen's disabilities were allegedly caused by her premature birth, which was attributed to her mother's exposure to DES. The lower court (which in New York is the Supreme Court) had dismissed all causes of action seeking to recover damages for Karen's injuries. The appellate court reversed, saying, "Although plaintiff is not a 'DES daughter'—one who was exposed to DES while *in utero*—she may be no less a victim of the devastation wrought by DES than her mother, who is a DES daughter, and we see no sound basis for denying plaintiff her day in court along with her mother."[24] The court maintained that its decision did not conflict with the Court of Appeals' rejection of preconception torts in *Albala,* because the necessity of establishing manageable bounds for liability—the rationale for denying a cause of action in *Albala*—is "conspicuously absent" under a strict products-liability theory. Moreover, while restriction of liability is an important policy consideration, it is balanced in this case by a competing consideration—namely, the need for a remedy for those who have suffered the devastation caused by DES. The court noted that both the Court of Appeals and the New York State Legislature had made it easier for DES victims to sue the manufacturers of the drug,[25] demonstrating "deep concern for those injured by toxic substances in general and DES in particular."[26] The economic incentive of manufacturers to turn out safe products would only be diluted by creating "an arbitrary generational limitation on the legal responsibility for birth defects caused by DES . . ."[27] The court stressed that DES is a "singular case," which does not have implications for preconception torts in general.

On February 19, 1991, the Court of Appeals, New York's highest court, decided against Karen Enright.[28] The court held in accord with their decision in *Albala* that no cause of action accrues in favor of a "third generation" plaintiff against the drug manufacturers. As in *Albala,* the reason for the decision was fear of limitless liability. The court said, "For all we know, the rippling effects of DES exposure may extend for generations. It is our duty to confine liability within manageable limits. Limiting liability to those who ingested the drug or were exposed to it in utero serves this purpose."[29] On October 7, 1991, the United States Supreme Court declined to hear *Enright* v. *Lilly,* thereby blocking the first suit that has come before the Court that sought to establish preconception torts.[30]

Because the *Albala* and *Enright* decisions were based on a concern to limit liability, rather than a principled objection to preconception torts, it is possible that a case that did not raise the possibility of rippling effects through several generations could succeed in New York. This would be in accord with the position of the interest view that someone who has been injured by another's negligence should be able to recover damages, regardless of when the wrongful act occurred.

The right of surviving children to sue third parties for prenatal injuries is well established. Some commentators have urged the states to expand the conception of fetal rights to permit the fetus to sue its mother in tort for prenatal injuries.[31] Such an extension raises questions about the parent–child tort immunity doctrine and the infringement of the mother's rights to privacy and bodily self-determination.

Against the Mother

Parental Immunity

The doctrine of parental immunity is that a child cannot sue his parent in tort for personal injuries resulting from a negligent or intentional act. The doctrine is relatively new in American common law. It was created by the Mississippi Supreme Court in 1891 in *Hewellette* v. *George*.[32] Without citing any prior case law or statutory authority, the court simply held that a child's personal tort action against a parent would disturb the peace of society and be contrary to public policy. Within a few years, most states had adopted the doctrine of parental tort immunity, relying on three primary justifications: that allowing a child to sue a parent for a personal tort would (1) disrupt family harmony, (2) encourage collusion, perjury, and fraud between family members, and (3) impair parental authority and discipline.[33]

For the next thirty years, courts continued to uphold the doctrine of parental immunity, while creating numerous exceptions to it. Then, in 1963, in the landmark case of *Goller* v. *White,* the Wisconsin Supreme Court abolished the general rule of nonliability, with immunity in two areas: parental authority and ordinary discretion in providing food, clothing, housing, and medical care.[34] Today, states that remain loyal to the parental immunity doctrine are in the minority.[35]

The ability of a surviving child to sue for prenatal injuries, combined with the abrogation of the common-law doctrine of parental immunity, has resulted in the potential for lawsuits by surviving children against their mothers. According to Ron Beal, the majority of jurisdictions should recognize a duty on the part of a woman to her fetus in order to remain "consistent with their policy justifications as set forth in their decisions abolishing parental immunity and recognizing the right of a child born alive to recover for prenatal injuries.''[36] In other words, if surviving children can recover for their prenatally inflicted injuries from *third parties,* and if parents are no longer immune from liability simply because they are *parents,* injured children should be able to sue their mothers for injuries negligently inflicted during pregnancy.

The Woman's Right of Privacy

In deciding whether such suits should be allowed, we cannot ignore the ''geography of pregnancy.''[37] The fetus is inside its mother's body. Whatever she is required to do to benefit or avoid harming the fetus will also have an impact on her own body. So the issue is not simply the extent of the duty a parent owes to a child, but also what risks and costs a pregnant woman is required to bear for the sake of her not-yet-born child. Some have argued that a woman could be obligated to undergo surgery if necessary to sustain the life or health of the fetus. This imposes an obligation on pregnant women that is not imposed on anyone else, and so violates equal protection. In addition, it ignores the woman's rights to privacy and bodily self-determination, rights that do not arise in the case of third party lawsuits.

In response, it might be said that the woman's legitimate interests could be considered in determining the duty owed to the child. A woman would not have a duty to do *whatever was necessary* to protect the not-yet-born child, but only a duty to behave *reasonably* during pregnancy. This was the finding of the Court of Appeals of Michigan in *Grodin* v. *Grodin,*[38] the first case explicitly to consider the right of a surviving child to sue its mother for injuries resulting from the mother's negligence during pregnancy. The case concerned a child born with tooth discoloration caused by his mother's taking tetracycline during pregnancy. The child, Randy Grodin, sued his mother for negligence in failing to seek proper prenatal care, for her failure to request that her doctor perform a pregnancy test, and for her failure to inform her doctor that she was taking a medication that might be contraindicated for pregnant women.

The child also sued his mother's doctor. The suit against the physician alleged that he was guilty of malpractice in not administering a pregnancy test to Mrs. Grodin after symptoms of pregnancy were brought to his attention. Indeed, the doctor allegedly assured Mrs. Grodin that it was impossible for her to become pregnant. Only after consulting a different doctor who told her she was seven or eight months pregnant did Mrs. Grodin stop taking the medication that caused the discoloration of her son's teeth.

John Robertson provides the background to the case:

> The child originally filed suit against the physician alone for his injury. During discovery the physician claimed that he had warned the mother to stop taking tetracycline. To guard against the possibility that the jury might ascribe the child's injury to the mother and refuse to award damages, the attorney advised amending the complaint to include the mother as a defendant, because a homeowner's policy insured the mother against tort liability. But for the existence of a homeowner's insurance policy, the suit against the mother would not have been filed.[39]

The main issue in the case was whether the parental tort immunity doctrine protected the mother from liability. Michigan overruled the doctrine of intrafamily tort immunity in the early 1970s, using the *Goller* approach, which creates two immunity exceptions. The trial court granted Mrs. Grodin's motion for summary judgment, based on the second exception, parental discretion in the provision of ordinary care. The summary judgment precluded testimony on either the necessity of the use of tetracycline to maintain the mother's health, or the risk created for her child. The Michigan Court of Appeals reversed and remanded the case to determine whether the mother had acted *reasonably*.

Some commentators have viewed *Grodin* as alarming in that it sanctions monitoring the behavior of women during pregnancy. "Reasonable" behavior might include regular prenatal checkups, a balanced diet with vitamin supplements, judicious use of medications and caffeine, and abstention from tobacco, alcohol, and narcotics. It might require women to abstain from too much exercise, sexual intercourse, or working. Virtually every area of a woman's life could come under scrutiny, seriously threatening women's rights to privacy and bodily self-determination. As Dawn Johnsen notes, "If the current trend in fetal rights continues, pregnant women would live in constant fear that any accident or 'error' in judgment could be deemed 'unacceptable' and become the basis for a criminal prosecution by the state or a civil suit by a disenchanted husband or relative."[40]

Concern for privacy distinguishes third-party lawsuits from lawsuits against mothers, and should make us extremely reluctant to extend civil liability to women for their behavior during pregnancy. However, the privacy argument does not apply to the circumstances in *Grodin*. Mrs. Grodin's privacy was not threatened by allowing her son to recover damages under the family's insurance coverage. Recognition of such causes of action will not make women live in fear of civil suits resulting from some accident or error of judgment, because the woman herself benefits if the insurance company compensates her child for his injuries. It is unlikely that any suits would be filed in the absence of an insurance policy. On the other hand, having allowed a child to sue his mother where there was a family insurance policy, the Michigan courts might find it difficult to deny a cause of action where there was no insurance. In that case, fears about exposing virtually every area of a woman's life to judicial scrutiny would be justified. Imposing an open-ended duty of reasonable care in pregnancy sets a dangerous precedent, and threatens women's liberty and privacy interests. However, as I will argue in the next section, the situation is different in the case of automobile liability.

Automobile Liability

Seven states have abolished the parental-immunity doctrine in the area of automobile liability, because of the prevalence of insurance coverage. This type of suit is not a truly adversarial situation, but rather one in which *both* parties are seeking to recover from the insurance carrier to provide for the child so as not to deplete the family assets.[41]

This approach has been criticized as legally weak and untidy. The mere presence of insurance without additional justification has never been the basis for recognizing a cause of action. However, the claim is not that the parent is liable because there is insurance. Liability stems from the principle that an injured party has the right to compensation for negligently inflicted injuries. It is *immunity* from liability that must be justified. The primary justification for parental immunity is the preservation of family harmony. The harmony of the family is not threatened when an injured child recovers damages from an insurance company. Thus, there is no justification for exempting parents from liability in this situation.

This was the reasoning of the Appellate Court of Illinois in *Stallman* v. *Youngquist*.[42] Bari Stallman was five months pregnant in 1981 when her auto collided with another, driven by Clarence Youngquist. Her subsequently born daughter, Lindsay, filed suit against both her mother and Youngquist, alleging that their negligent driving resulted in serious prenatal injuries that became apparent at birth. Because the plaintiff sought to recover damages from Mrs. Stallman's automobile-insurance policy, Mrs. Stallman's insurer controlled her trial.

The trial court dismissed Lindsay's complaint against her mother, on grounds of the state's parent–child tort immunity doctrine. The Illinois Appellate Court reversed, holding that Lindsay should have the opportunity to show that her mother's actions fell outside the doctrine. On remand, the trial court found that the immunity doctrine did apply to the case and granted the mother's motion for summary judgment. Once again, the court of appeals reversed, holding that, as the Illinois Supreme Court had never adopted the parent–child tort immunity rule, it was subject to abrogation by the Appellate Court. The court announced that it was joining the many states that have abrogated the doctrine, saying, "We agree with the Massachusetts Supreme Judicial Court that '[c]hildren enjoy the same right to protection and to legal redress for wrongs done them as others enjoy. Only the strongest reasons, grounded in public policy, can justify limitation or abolition of those rights.' "[43] The court concluded that an unemancipated minor child may recover damages against a parent for personal injuries caused by the negligence of the parent in the operation of a motor vehicle, and an infant who is born alive can maintain a tort action to recover for prenatal injuries.

The Supreme Court of Illinois reversed. Declining to address the issue of parental immunity, the court held that a fetus has no cause of action against its mother for unintentional infliction of prenatal injuries. The court distinguished such suits from suits against third parties on three grounds. First, such causes of action would establish a legal duty on the part of the mother to create the best prenatal environment possible. They would make the mother and fetus legal adversaries from conception until birth, and would require the mother to guarantee the health of that potential adversary.

Second, holding a third party liable for prenatal injuries doesn't interfere with the defendant's right to control his or her own life, whereas imposing such liability on a mother subjects to state scrutiny all the decisions a woman must make during her pregnancy and thus infringes on her right to privacy and bodily autonomy. Third, the absence of any clear, objective standard of due care during pregnancy would create the danger that prejudicial and stereotypical beliefs about the reproductive abilities of women might skew jury determinations of liability. Finally, the court suggested that disparities in wealth, education, and access to health care would prevent a fair application of any legal standard of prenatal care. The best way to achieve healthy newborns, the court argued, is not through after-the-fact civil liability in tort for individual mothers, but rather through before-the-fact education of all women and families about prenatal development.

These are all good arguments against the creation of broadly construed duties of pregnant women to their not-yet-born children (see Chapter 4). But none of these arguments applies where a surviving child seeks to recover under a parent's automobile-insurance policy. The duty to drive carefully and avoid injuring others is not a duty of prenatal care. It is a duty of care imposed on all drivers to everyone who might be injured by the failure to drive carefully. Allowing surviving children to sue their mothers for prenatal injuries caused by negligent driving does not imply a legal duty on the part of the mother to create the best prenatal environment possible. Nor does it subject the entire lives of pregnant women to State scrutiny, or infringe on their rights to privacy. If there is automobile insurance, allowing such suits does not make the mother and fetus—or, rather, subsequently born child—genuine adversaries, since the whole family benefits by allowing the child to recover. If Mrs. Stallman had had a pregnant passenger in her car, that woman's subsequently born child would have a cause of action against Mrs. Stallman, and would be able to collect damages under her insurance policy. Why should Mrs. Stallman's own child be denied the benefit of insurance that would be available to a stranger? Finally, even if the best way in general to achieve healthy newborns is through prenatal education and care, this has no relevance for the compensation of infants injured in car accidents. The best prenatal care in the world would not have protected Lindsay from being injured in a car accident. Concern for women's autonomy and privacy should not lead us to deny Lindsay Stallman her right to recover for her injuries. If she is entitled to make a case against Clarence Youngquist, she should also have been permitted to make her case against Bari Stallman.

II. PRENATAL WRONGFUL DEATH

So far we have been discussing suits in which the fetus survives and seeks to recover damages for injuries negligently inflicted before birth. What if the negligence results in the *death* of the fetus? Can there be a cause of action for the wrongful death of a fetus?

In order to understand the special case of prenatal wrongful-death actions, it is necessary to understand the nature of wrongful-death actions in general.

Wrongful-Death Actions

Until the middle of the nineteenth century, there was no right of recovery for the death of a human being killed by the negligence or wrongful act of another.[44] This common-law rule left the bereaved, and often destitute, family of the victim without a remedy. This intolerable result was changed in England by the passage of the Fatal Accidents Act of 1846, otherwise known as Lord Campbell's Act. The Act provides that whenever the death of a person is caused by the wrongful act or negligence of another, in such manner as would have entitled the party injured to have sued if he had survived, an action may be brought in the name of his executor for the benefit of certain relatives, such as husband, wife, parent, or child.

In wrongful-death actions, the duty of care is *to the deceased,* but the damages are measured by the loss suffered *by the survivors.* This feature, unique (so far as I know) in tort law, means that the basis for recovery is not the loss suffered by the one who is tortiously killed, but rather the loss suffered by his or her survivors. As we will see, this has particular importance for prenatal death.

In general, common-law countries do not allow the relatives of a wrongful-death victim compensation for mental anguish. Where there is no pecuniary loss, as is likely in the death of a minor child or aged parent, there can be no recovery. Financial loss may be prospective, but must be likely, and not merely possible. This obviously rules out recovery for the loss of an unborn child. The pecuniary-loss rule has been vigorously criticized, and has been rejected by a number of common-law jurisdictions.[45] In a number of American states, some form of mental distress damages is explicitly recognized.

Most states now permit prenatal wrongful-death actions, at least after viability. Some commentators regard this as part of the trend toward recognizing the separate existence of the fetus, which led to allowing recovery on the part of surviving children for injuries inflicted prenatally. On the interest view, however, there is an important difference between prenatal torts and prenatal wrongful death. A child who is injured before her birth, and must go through life crippled or maimed, has had her most basic interests set back; she has been harmed. By contrast, when a fetus is killed before it acquires any interests, it is not harmed. Permitting recovery on the part of surviving children for injuries inflicted prenatally does not imply a right of recovery if the fetus is tortiously killed.

In Chapter 2, I argued that death can be a harm to conscious fetuses. For this reason, it might be thought that prenatal wrongful-death actions should be permitted for, but limited to, late-gestation (viable) fetuses. This seems to me to misconceive the nature and purpose of wrongful-death actions. Despite a persistent tendency on the part of some courts to view prenatal wrongful-death actions as redressing the wrong to the unborn,[46] their real function is to redress the wrong *to the parents.* The correct basis for allowing recovery for prenatal wrongful-death was expressed by the Supreme Court of Washington, when it held that damages for anguish at the loss of an eight-month-old fetus were recoverable under the state's wrongful-death statute, because a parent's mental anguish would not be dependent on whether the child survived to full term.[47] The court offered no conclusion as to whether there could be recovery for a nonviable fetus.

In 1967, the Supreme Judicial Court of Massachusetts held that nonviability of a fetus should not bar recovery. In *Torigian* v. *Watertown News Co.,*[48] an action for wrongful-death arose when a woman who was three and a half months pregnant was struck by the defendant's motor vehicle. A little more than two months after the accident, the child was born and lived about two and a half hours. Since the child survived birth, even for a limited time, the fact that it was a nonviable fetus at the time of the injury did not bar recovery.

However, if parental anguish is the basis for recovery, *neither live birth nor viability at the time of the injury* should be a condition of recovery. Admittedly, the grief occasioned by losing a baby during labor or delivery is likely to be greater than the grief caused by an early miscarriage, and this might properly affect the *amount of damages*. Nevertheless, it is likely that the expectant parents will experience emotional distress whenever a pregnancy is negligently terminated, regardless of the fetus's stage of development. The viability requirement is as unwarranted here as it is regarding prenatal injury, although for entirely different reasons. In the case of prenatal injury, it is the born child who is harmed by the negligence that occurred when she was a fetus. Her characteristics at the time of the injury are irrelevant. What matters is that there now exists a harmed individual whose suffering is the result of another's negligence, and who deserves to be compensated. In the case of prenatal death, the previable fetus is not harmed by being killed, but this is irrelevant because the wrong is not to the fetus anyway, but to its parents. They should be compensated for their grief and anguish at the loss of a wanted and expected child. Their distress is not contingent on the unborn's having attained a certain developmental stage.

The Implications for Abortion

Several judges have expressed the view that recognition of prenatal wrongful-death suits conflicts with the right to abortion. One court maintained that it is "incongruous" to allow a woman the constitutional right to abort and yet hold a third party liable to the fetus for merely negligent acts.[49] Another held that "There would be an inherent conflict in giving the mother the right to terminate the pregnancy yet holding that an action may be brought on behalf of the same fetus under the wrongful death act."[50]

The suggestion that recovery for prenatal wrongful death conflicts with the right to abortion is incorrect. Acknowledging the woman's right to have an abortion, stemming from her right to privacy, is entirely consistent with recognizing her right to be compensated when a wanted pregnancy is negligently terminated. Indeed, both prenatal wrongful-death actions and legal abortion can be seen as aspects of reproductive liberty. The perception of inconsistency stems, I think, from the error of regarding prenatal wrongful-death actions as primarily intended to protect the lives of the unborn. Why, it may be asked, should such protection be extended to some fetuses and not others? The corrective is to realize that prenatal wrongful-death suits are not premised on entitlement of the fetus to the protection of law, but rather on the right of its prospective parents to compensation for their loss.

The fact remains that the Supreme Court held in *Roe* that the unborn is *not* a person, while the death statutes of most states restrict recovery to the death of a person. Some judges have regarded this as an insurmountable obstacle to prenatal wrongful-death actions. In response, it has been noted that *Roe* is a federal constitutional decision rather than a tort or death-statute decision, and so its interpretation of "person" does not compel for these decisions.[51] However, deeming fetuses persons for the purposes of wrongful-death actions could be the first step toward recognizing fetal personhood generally, with ominous consequences, and not just for women. The economic implications of treating the unborn as legal persons are staggering. If fetuses were counted as dependents for purposes of federal income tax, a total revenue loss in excess of $1 billion per year is possible.[52] The law of estates, property, and trusts could be dramatically affected. A host of legislative provisions use age to measure the time for receipt of benefits. If age is measured from conception, the fiscal consequences could be severe. Discussing the implications of *Webster,* which upheld the constitutionality of a Missouri law proclaiming that human life begins at conception, columnist James Kilpatrick noted, "If the 40,000 or so Missourians who are 61 years old today were allowed to add nine months to their ages, about 30,000 of them would suddenly become eligible for Social Security, at a total potential cost of $150 million a year." Finally, endowing fetuses with legal personhood might have unforeseen effects on the legal system. Four weeks after the Supreme Court's decision in *Webster,* Kansas City lawyer Michael Box filed a lawsuit against the state's governor and attorney general for jailing the fetus of a pregnant prison inmate without due process of law.

Fortunately, recognition of the fetus as a person is not necessary to achieve the desirable aim of redressing the injury of the loss of an expected child. Prospective parents have a right that others refrain from tortiously killing their unborn children, and a right to compensation for emotional distress when this right is abridged. Recognition of prenatal wrongful-death actions compensates prospective parents, but it also extends legal personhood to the unborn. The emotional-distress approach focuses on the wrong done to the parents, without implying that a person has been killed.

III. THE CRIMINAL LAW

In the above two sections, I have argued that there should be civil liability for tortiously injuring or killing a fetus. What about criminal liability? In some states, it is manslaughter to kill a fetus in the course of an attack on a pregnant woman. In California, the unlawful killing of a fetus "with malice aforethought" is murder. In a few states, drunk drivers who cause the death of a viable fetus may be charged with vehicular homicide. In one case, the driver was the pregnant woman herself.

A range of issues are raised in conjunction with criminal liability for injuring or killing a fetus. These include the interpretation of statutes, the evolution of the common law, and the proper functions of the judiciary and the legislature. We will need to consider the distinction between civil and criminal law, and how much consistency is possible or desirable in these two areas of law. We will also need to consider the social and political impact of treating feticide as a form of homicide.

Prenatal Neglect

A number of commentators advocate subjecting women to criminal penalties for behavior during pregnancy that harms a viable fetus.[53] In Chapter 4, I will argue that such an approach is not warranted on public-policy grounds; that it is unlikely to protect any babies, while being certain to infringe women's rights to privacy and bodily self-determination. In this section, I would like to stress that such an approach is not legally warranted either.

It is sometimes claimed that the imposition of criminal liability follows from the existence of civil liability. In a Comment in the *Whittier Law Journal,* the authors note that the court in *Grodin* imposed civil liability on a woman for damage to her fetus, and conclude, "Therefore, if both a third person and a pregnant woman can be held equally culpable for negligent harm to a viable fetus, then it logically follows that the prospective mother should be subject to criminal sanctions resulting from identical conduct."[54] Nothing of the kind follows. From the fact that someone is civilly liable for injuring another, it doesn't follow that he or she is criminally liable. The degree of culpability for criminal liability is much higher than it is for civil liability, because the penalty imposed by the criminal law (imprisonment) is so much more serious than that imposed by the civil law (payment of damages). In general, criminal wrongs are those that merit moral condemnation by the community.[55] *Grodin,* cited in the above-quoted Comment as a "perfect example" of maternal obligation, carries no implication of moral wrong. The harm to the child (discolored teeth) was hardly egregious, the mother did not act recklessly or wantonly in taking a prescribed medicine, and the "penalty" was imposed, not on the mother, but on the insurance company. It is ludicrous to imagine that *criminal* sanctions might be imposed against Mrs. Grodin. Even where the culpability is much greater, and the mother's actions morally condemnable, there are compelling policy reasons not to impose criminal liability on women for their behavior during pregnancy (see Chapter 4).

Homicide

The Born Alive Rule

Since at least the fourteenth century, common law has held that the destruction of a fetus *in utero* is not a homicide.[56] Only someone who has been born alive can be the victim of a homicide. This is known as the "born alive rule" (BAR). A number of commentators have criticized the rule,[57] calling it arbitrary and illogical because it permits a conviction for homicide if the fetus survives birth, however briefly. If the same fetus is stillborn, however, it cannot be the victim of a homicide.

Clarke Forsythe, Staff Counsel for Americans United for Life Legal Defense Fund, argues that the BAR is obsolete. He maintains that if we examine the origins of the rule, we will see that it was "entirely an evidentiary standard, mandated by the primitive medical knowledge and technology of the era . . ."[58] Before the twentieth century, it was difficult to determine whether the fetus died as the result of an attack on the mother, or from natural causes. Live birth was required to prove that the fetus was alive in the womb at the time of the attack, since obviously there can be no homicide if the "victim" was already dead. Today, medical technological advances, such as fetal heart monitoring, ultrasound examinations, and fetal autopsies, make it possible to know whether the fetus was living at the time of the material acts, what gestational stage it had attained, and the cause of its death. According to Forsythe, the problems of proof that led to the formulation of the BAR no longer exist, and therefore the rule should be dropped.

I think that Forsythe is wrong about the purely evidentiary nature of the BAR. It seems rather that there are three reasons why the common law insisted on live birth for a homicide conviction, only one of which is evidentiary. That is the reason Forsythe gives—namely, that in the past it was not possible to be sure that a miscarriage or stillbirth was the result of the attack on the pregnant woman, or whether the fetus was dead before the attack. Indeed, in the past, it was not always clear if the woman was even pregnant. However, in addition to this evidentiary reason, there are two other reasons why live birth traditionally has been considered significant. First, prior to live birth, the fetus was considered to be a part of the pregnant woman, and not a separate existence. In Holmes's words, it was not *in esse* until it was born alive. Second, a fetus is not yet a fully developed human being, a person like the rest of us. This was expressed by the great common-law authority, Sir Edward Coke, who held that the killing of a fetus is a "great misprision, and no murder." But if the child is born alive and then dies from the attack on its mother, this is murder, "for in law it is accounted a reasonable creature, *in rerum natura,* when it is born alive."[59] Blackstone, in his *Commentaries,* closely followed Coke. "[T]he person killed must be a 'reasonable creature in being and under the king's peace,' at the time of the killing . . ."[60]

Forsythe argues that the "reasonable creature" requirement is itself based on evidentiary considerations. He points out that in his section on the "law of persons," Blackstone says that the right to life—the most basic right of persons—begins as soon as the infant is able to stir in the mother's womb—i.e., at quickening, when the fetus was considered to be alive. Yet although Blackstone ascribes a right to life to the quick fetus, he nevertheless maintains that the killing of a quick fetus is not murder. This sounds contradictory, Forsythe says, but only if the born alive rule is taken to be substantive. "There is no contradiction when the born alive rule is recognized to be an evidentiary principle that was required by the state of medical science of the day. Thus, Blackstone held that the unborn child was a 'person' with a right to life at quickening, but recognized that proof of the denial of that right at common law could not be obtained without live birth."[61]

Blackstone may have been influenced by evidentiary considerations. However, this explanation does not cohere with the fact that the common law did not allow recovery for prenatally inflicted wounds by a child who survived live birth. The reason for refusing to allow such suits was not the evidentiary problem of proving that the plaintiff's injuries were caused by the defendant's negligence. Rather, it was universally held that the defendant owed no duty of care to a being that was not *in esse* at the time of the negligence.

It seems, then, that neither the requirement of separate existence, nor that of being a reasonable creature, is based solely on the difficulties of proving that the attack on the pregnant woman killed the fetus. If the born alive rule is properly interpreted as a substantive definition of a legal person, and is not merely evidentiary, it is not made obsolete by advances in medical technology.

It could be argued that even if the BAR was not formulated entirely because of problems of proof, nevertheless only such considerations support the rule. For example, it might be argued that it is simply untrue that the fetus is only a part of its mother, like a limb or an organ. From conception onward, it has its own unique genetic code, and, unlike any mere bodily part of the pregnant woman, is developing into a being capable of independent existence. As a matter of biological fact, the separate existence of the fetus throughout pregnancy must be conceded. It is not a mere body part. On the other hand, neither is the pregnant woman a mere fetal container. The geography of pregnancy—the fact that the fetus is inside the mother and capable of being affected only through her body—provides very strong reasons for refusing to treat the fetus as a separate legal entity prior to live birth.

However, it may be argued that the differences between a newly born infant and a nearly born infant are so minimal that the grounds for protecting newborns extend to late-gestation fetuses (see Chapter 2). If late-gestation fetuses are, for the most part, protected from being aborted, shouldn't they also be protected from being killed by third parties? Punishing individuals who attack pregnant women, killing their fetuses, does not raise the issues of privacy and bodily self-determination that are central to the abortion debate. Moreover, sometimes the behavior is so egregious that prosecution for murder seems not only warranted, but called for.

Murder

The "born alive rule" was applied by many state courts during the 1980s to prohibit homicide convictions for the deaths of viable fetuses, even in the face of gruesome facts and a high degree of culpability of some defendants.[62] For example, Robert Lee Hollis told his estranged wife that he did not want a baby, then forced his hand up her vagina, manually aborting her fetus, alleged to be 28 to 30 weeks old. In separate indictments, Hollis was charged with murder "of the unborn infant child" and assault in the first degree on his estranged wife. The Kentucky Supreme Court held that until the fetus was born alive, it was not a "person," as that word is used in the context of criminal-homicide statutes, and could not be the victim of criminal homicide.[63] Another defendant repeatedly struck and kicked his eight-and-a-half-months-pregnant girlfriend, killing both her and the fetus.[64] The

Illinois Supreme Court held that, although the killing of the woman was murder, the killing of the fetus was not. In *Keeler* v. *Superior Court of Amdaor County,*[65] an estranged husband, upon learning that his former wife was pregnant by another man, told her, "I'm going to stomp it out of you," and shoved his knee into her abdomen. She later delivered a stillborn fetus of up to 36 weeks gestation. The California Supreme Court held that an unborn but viable fetus is not a human being within the meaning of the statute defining murder.[66] Its ruling was based partly on the fact that the California legislature had declined to create a crime of feticide. Nor had the California Code Commission, which was supposed to revise all statutes, correct errors and omissions, and recommend enactments to remedy defects, proposed any feticide laws for California. Thus, the *Keeler* court was persuaded that the legislative intent was to exclude fetuses from the homicide statute. To include fetuses as subjects of murder would be rewriting the murder statute, not interpreting it. To create a new common-law crime would violate the due-process rights of the defendant.[67]

Not all courts have agreed. In South Carolina, a man stabbed his former wife, who was pregnant with a full-term fetus. The South Carolina Supreme Court prospectively applied the state homicide statute to fetuses that could be proved viable at the time of the injury to the mother.[68] The court declared that it had a right and a duty to develop the common law to better serve a changing society, and that it would be grossly inconsistent to classify a fetus as a human being for the purpose of imposing civil liability, but as a nonhuman for the imposition of criminal liability.

Several states have enacted feticide statutes.[69] In others, the homicide statute has been amended so that it applies to fetuses. This was the approach taken by the California legislature in reaction to *Keeler.*[70] California courts have interpreted the statute as applying only to the intentional killing (murder) of a fetus.[71] It is less clear whether the statute applies only to *viable* fetuses. This has been the ruling in some cases;[72] however, the ruling in *People* v. *Apodaca* indicates that even the killing of a *nonviable* fetus "with malice aforethought" can be murder in California. In that case, the defendant told his former wife, who was 22 to 24 weeks pregnant, that he intended to kill the fetus. He tied her up, repeatedly struck her in the stomach, and raped her. As a result of this attack, she gave birth to a dead fetus. The defendant argued that his conviction for murder violated his right to due process of law because section 187 did not notify him as to exactly what stage of development the term "fetus" was intended to cover. The court reasoned that the statute, as written, was sufficient to give "all persons of common intelligence ample warning that an assault on a pregnant woman without her consent for the purpose of unlawfully killing her unborn child can constitute the crime of murder."[73]

The sheer viciousness of the attacks in *Greer, Apodaca, Keeler,* and *Hollis* led many people to support a conviction for murder. A different approach treats the fact that the attack causes the death of a fetus as an aggravating factor, making the assault a more serious crime.[74] The fact that the woman has lost an expected child compounds the suffering the attack has caused her. This approach has the advantage of focusing on the assault on the pregnant woman. The convicted person is punished for what he did to her—namely, forcibly and violently cause her to miscarry. On this approach, fetal viability should not be a condition for conviction, since losing a pregnancy at any stage would be an additional trauma, aggravating the seriousness of the assault. However, the punishment for causing a woman to lose a baby late in her pregnancy should be more severe, as her suffering will be greater the closer she is to giving birth. Similarly, a specific intent to kill the fetus should not be necessary to convict someone of aggravated assault. It would be enough that the defendant knew, or should have known, that the woman was pregnant when he attacked her.

A few states have adopted the aggravated-assault approach.[75] Which approach is dictated by the interest view? The interest view acknowledges that late gestation fetuses, who are capable of experiencing and valuing their lives, have an interest in continued existence. There is therefore no conceptual bar to ascribing to them a right to life, and to acknowledging them as homicide victims. The aggravated-assault approach may seem to leave out an essential element—namely, that an innocent victim has been deprived of his or her life. As the Supreme Court of Massachusetts said in *Commonwealth* v. *Cass,* a case concerning vehicular homicide, "If a person were to commit violence against a pregnant woman and destroy the fetus within her, we would not want *the death of the fetus* to go unpunished."[76]

However, punishing individuals who commit violence against pregnant women is unlikely to be the only result of changing the common law to allow fetuses to be homicide victims. It seems clear that those who advocate this change have a larger agenda: the ultimate abolition of abortion and the coercion of pregnant women to protect the fetus.

This was made clear in the case of Sean Patrick Merrill, who was charged in Minnesota with murder for killing his girlfriend and the 28–day embryo she was carrying at the time of her death. Mr. Merrill is widely believed to be the first person charged with homicide of a fetus in such an early stage of development. His lawyers say there is no evidence that either the defendant or the woman, Gail Anderson, knew she was pregnant when Mr. Merrill was alleged to have killed her with a shotgun blast to the chest in November 1988. Apparently, that is irrelevant under Minnesota's fetal-homicide statute, which is described as the most sweeping of its kind in the nation. It defines an embryo or fetus as a person from the point of conception onward. Arguing that the law has "profound implications" that go beyond the arena of criminal homicide, the Minnesota Civil Liberties Union wrote in a brief that "if fetuses are persons within the meaning of the 14th Amendment, it is difficult to imagine how a state could constitutionally permit abortion." Pro-life advocates agree. Laurie Anne Ramsey, director of public affairs for Americans United for Life, said fetal-homicide statutes "sensitize the public to the fact that the unborn child—at any stage of his or her development—deserves protection and does have rights." Ms. Ramsey went on to say, "Such laws will make people think about the humanity of the unborn child; to understand that abortion—like murder—is violence against a member of our society."[77]

We need to keep the threat to abortion rights in mind when considering the merits of the born alive rule. The aggravated-assault approach does not threaten women's rights to privacy and autonomy. As long as assaults against pregnant women that cause them to miscarry can be punished sufficiently severely, the aggravated-assault approach may be preferable to abrogating the born alive rule.

Vehicular Homicide

Most vehicular homicide statutes make it a felony to cause the death of "another person" by driving recklessly or driving while intoxicated. In recent years, a number of courts have considered the question of whether a fetus should be considered a "person" for the purposes of vehicular homicide. To date, the highest courts of twenty-four states have refused to uphold vehicular-homicide convictions involving the demise of a fetus.[78]

A notable exception is the Supreme Judicial Court of Massachusetts in *Commonwealth* v. *Cass*. The case involved a female pedestrian, eight and a half months pregnant, who was struck by a car. The fetus died in the womb and was delivered by cesarean section. The autopsy revealed that the fetus was viable at the time of the incident and that it died of internal injuries caused by the impact of the vehicle operated by the defendant. The court had to decide whether a viable fetus is a "person" within the meaning of the vehicular-homicide statute. The court ruled that it was, although it applied this prospectively. On due-process grounds, its decision was not applied to the instant case, saying that the decision may not have been foreseeable.

The court's decision was based on two arguments. The first concerned legislative intent. The court held that it was reasonable to assume that the legislature intended the statute to include viable fetuses. This assumption was based in part on the "ordinary" meaning of the word "person," which the court took to be synonymous with "human being": "An offspring of human parents cannot reasonably be considered to be other than a human being, and therefore a person, first within, and then in normal course outside, the womb."[79] In addition, the Supreme Judicial Court had already ruled, in *Mone* v. *Greyhound Lines, Inc.*,[80] that a viable fetus would be considered a person for purposes of the state's wrongful-death statute: "Despite the fact that *Mone* was a civil case, we can reasonably infer that, in enacting Sect. 24G, the Legislature contemplated that the term 'person' would be construed to include viable fetuses."[81]

The court's second argument was that the "born alive rule" was based on evidentiary considerations that have been made obsolete by advances in medical technology. It decided to formulate a "better rule": "that infliction of prenatal injuries resulting in the death of a viable fetus, before or after it is born, is homicide."[82]

Justice Wilkins dissented, joined by Justices Liacos and Abrams. The dissenters dismissed as totally implausible the majority's claim that the legislature intended to include fetuses in the vehicular-homicide statute. "Nowhere does the court explain why the Legislature should be assumed to have disregarded hundreds of years of the common law nor why this court should ignore the commendable judicial restraint of every other court that has considered the point." Justice Wilkins characterized the decision as "an inappropriate exercise of raw judicial power."[83]

Cass has been widely criticized as a usurpation of legislative power, both by scholars[84] and judges, who have held that the matter "must be left to the good judgment of the legislature, which has the primary authority to create crimes."[85] Should legislatures amend vehicular-homicide statutes so as to explicitly include fetuses? Once again, the benefits of such statutes must be weighed against the dangers they pose to women. Statutes that treat fetuses as persons, even for a rather narrow purpose, might serve as a wedge, opening the door to legislation that protects fetuses at the expense of women's rights of privacy and self-determination. A better solution might be a statute along the lines discussed above, of "aggravated vehicular assault."

A novel twist in the debate over the protection of fetuses by vehicular-homicide statutes occurred when the driver who was charged with killing the fetus was also its mother.[86] On the evening of July 14, 1989, Beth

Levey, eight and a half months pregnant, was alleged to have driven while intoxicated, and to have struck a telephone pole. Her fetus was stillborn, the imprint of the steering wheel in its head. Ms. Levey was indicted for several charges, including operating a motor vehicle under the influence of alcohol, but she was also charged with felony motor-vehicle homicide. It was the first time anyone had been prosecuted in a comparable situation anywhere in the United States.

The prosecutor brought the homicide charge against Ms. Levey for two reasons. First, he considered this to be an egregious drunk-driving case, as her blood alcohol content was very high and she had had previous convictions for drunk driving. As it happened, she hurt herself and lost her own baby, but she could very well have injured someone else.

Second, the prosecutor felt bound by *Cass,* which held that the vehicular-homicide statute includes viable fetuses. If Ms. Levey had had a pregnant friend in her car, who lost her viable unborn child as a result of the accident, Ms. Levey would undoubtedly have been charged with vehicular homicide. So why should the fact that the dead fetus was her own be a reason not to charge her? It would not be a reason if the victim was Ms. Levey's own born child. Drunk drivers often kill the people they love most. Sympathy for their loss may be relevant at the sentencing stage, on the ground that the person has already suffered enough, but it is not considered a reason for not prosecuting.

The defense argued that *Cass* was not a relevant precedent, as it addressed only the case in which a pregnant woman was herself the victim of violence. The cases cited by the Court in *Cass* were exclusively cases in which a third party intentionally and brutally harmed a woman. "The Court did not—nor could it—cite a single civil case in which a mother was held liable for wrongful death, much less a single criminal case in which a mother was prosecuted for vehicular homicide."[87] The defense called the application of the vehicular-homicide statute to this case "a grotesque extension of the criminal law."[88]

The defense acknowledged that the common law of torts has evolved to allow recovery for prenatal injuries; however, with very few exceptions, this has been limited to third parties. The defense argued that the rationale for the extension of liability was not to protect the fetus, but "to vindicate the mother's interest in having a live, uninjured child."[89] It interpreted *Bonbrest* v. *Kotz,* the first case allowing a surviving child to recover for injuries inflicted *in utero,* as vindicating the interests of the parents, not the child, nor the fetus.

It seems to me that this reading of *Bonbrest* is mistaken. While permitting recovery for prenatal torts is not aimed at vindicating the interests of the *fetus,* neither is it aimed at vindicating the interests of the *parents.* Rather, it is the *surviving child* who has been injured and who deserves compensation. It is very important to distinguish actions brought by surviving children for prenatally inflicted injuries from prenatal wrongful-death suits. The interests of the parents are vindicated in prenatal wrongful-death suits, but it is the interests of the surviving child that are vindicated in prenatal-injury cases. It may be wise social policy not to allow children to sue their mothers for prenatally caused injuries, but we should not pretend that the justification is that the only interests involved are those of the mother.

The fundamental question raised by *Levey* is the rationale for punishing someone whose negligent or reckless driving causes the death of a fetus. If the rationale focuses on the harm done to the pregnant woman, as the defense argued, then it is absurd to press charges when the pregnant woman herself is the driver. On the other hand, if the rationale is that a viable fetus is entitled to the protection of the state or commonwealth, then it is irrelevant that the person responsible for causing the death is the mother.

This issue was never resolved because the prosecution entered a nolle prosequi. This is an entry on the record of a legal action denoting that the prosecutor will proceed no further with the action. The district attorney decided not to prosecute further for several reasons. First, Ms. Levey had already pleaded guilty to several lesser charges, including operating under the influence of alcohol. As part of her sentence, she was ordered to complete a fourteen-day residential alcoholism-treatment program, and was prohibited from driving during her period of five years probation. Finally, a review of confidential medical records regarding the diagnosis and treatment of the defendant and her fetus indicated that the fetus was alive for a long time after Ms. Levey was hospitalized. Certain standard medical procedures had not been performed; for example, she was not put on a fetal monitor and her placenta was not checked for damage. If these procedures had been done, the fetus's death (which the autopsy indicated was due to placental abruption, not the trauma to the head) could have been prevented.

The entry of a nolle prosequi in the *Levey* case left open the question of whether other pregnant women could be prosecuted for vehicular homicide in Massachusetts. The defense lawyers argued that the implications of such prosecutions would be ominous:

> . . . if it is appropriate for the courts to interpret "personhood" for the vehicular homicide statutes, then it could be no less appropriate for the courts to reinterpret "personhood" for all offenses under the criminal law. If *Cass* is seen as announcing the principle that a viable fetus is a person for purposes of the criminal law, then pregnant women will be at risk of prosecution for a host of offenses deriving from what they did or did not

do during pregnancy—from negligent driving to delivering alcohol or controlled substances to a minor.[90]

As we will see in the next chapter, these are not farfetched predictions. Such prosecutions have taken place. While they are not ruled out by the interest view, I will argue in Chapter 4 that there are substantial policy reasons not to use the criminal law against pregnant women as a means for protecting ''not-yet-born'' children.

IV. WRONGFUL LIFE[91]

''Wrongful-life'' suits are suits in which infants with birth defects seek to recover damages from allegedly negligent physicians. These suits differ in important ways from ordinary medical malpractice suits, and they raise special legal and philosophical questions. To date, only California, Washington, and New Jersey have recognized such suits as stating a legally cognizable cause of action.

The claim in a wrongful-life suit is not that the negligence of the physician was the cause of the impairment. It is, rather, that the physician, by failing to inform the parents adequately, is responsible for the birth of an impaired child who otherwise would not have been born and therefore would not have experienced the suffering caused by the impairment. The plaintiff in a wrongful-life suit is the child; typically, such suits are brought by the parents on behalf of the infant plaintiff. By contrast, in ''wrongful-birth'' suits, the plaintiffs are the *parents,* who claim that because of negligence on the part of health care providers or laboratories (either in performing incomplete sterilizations or abortions or in giving improper advice about the risk of having handicapped children), they have been wrongfully deprived of the option to abort. As the result of a growing recognition of the responsibilities of medical workers to meet ordinary standards of care in advising parents about the risk of genetic abnormalities, and a corresponding recognition of the rights of parents to collect damages when these standards are not met, wrongful-birth suits have met with increasing success in the courts.[92] There has been considerably more resistance to wrongful-life suits.

The infant plaintiffs in wrongful-life cases have severe handicaps: they may be blind or deaf or mentally retarded. They may suffer from such crippling or fatal ailments as cystic fibrosis, neurofibromatosis, or Tay-Sachs disease. They typically require expensive medical care and often need special education and training. It seems only fair that such children, whose impaired existence is allegedly due to the negligence of others, should have a legal remedy. At the same time, it is acknowledged that the negligent parties are not responsible for the children's handicaps. Nothing the physician did, or failed to do, caused the child to be born blind or mentally retarded or sick. Had the physician acted properly and non-negligently, the child would not have been born healthy—the usual claim in a tort action. Rather, he or she would not have been born at all. In essence, these suits allege that the infants would be better off never having been born, that they have been harmed or wronged by being born. Some find this claim morally offensive; others regard it as metaphysically puzzling.

The term "wrongful life" was used first in 1963 in *Zepeda* v. *Zepeda*,[93] in which a healthy infant plaintiff claimed that his father had injured him by causing him to be born illegitimately. The Illinois appellate court declined to permit recovery, fearing that it would be flooded with suits for wrongful life brought by parties born under adverse conditions. Subsequent courts have distinguished between being born under adverse conditions and being born with a severe handicap or fatal disease. Presiding Justice Jefferson wrote for the majority in *Curlender* v. *Bio-Science Laboratories* (1980):

> [A] cause of action based upon impairment of status—illegitimacy contrasted with legitimacy—should not be recognizable at law because a necessary element for the establishment of any cause of action in tort is missing, *injury* and damages consequential to that injury. A child born with severe impairment, however, presents an entirely different situation because the necessary element of *injury* is present.[94]

Nevertheless, even if wrongful-life suits are limited to cases involving severe impairment, they pose difficult problems. To see why, let us examine the reasons why courts have rejected wrongful-life suits.

Gleitman v. *Cosgrove*[95] was an early wrongful-life suit, decided by the New Jersey Supreme Court on March 6, 1967. The Gleitmans contended that the defendant doctors had erroneously assured Mrs. Gleitman that the rubella she had contracted early in her pregnancy posed no risk to her unborn child, who was born deaf, mute, probably retarded, and nearly blind. The Gleitmans claimed that they would have chosen abortion had they been accurately advised. The New Jersey Supreme Court barred recovery by either the parents or the infant, Jeffrey, holding that there were no damages cognizable at law and also, in the case of his parents, that public policy precluded recovery.

The court rejected Jeffrey's suit on the ground that it was "logically impossible" to measure the infant's alleged damages. The court asserted that since nonexistence is beyond the experience of juries, there is no reasoned way to calculate the difference in value between nonexistence and the child's impaired life. It is an established principle of tort law that damages that are uncertain, contingent, or speculative in nature cannot be made the basis of a recovery. However, the comparison of existence and nonexistence is not unique to wrongful-life cases. In wrongful-death suits, juries must measure damages by comparing the value of the deceased's existence, healthy or impaired, with the value of nonexistence. As one commentator has noted, "If the jury is capable of making this comparison in wrongful-death suits, there is no reason to doubt their ability to make the same comparison in wrongful life suits."[96]

A different argument against wrongful-life suits is based on the value of human life. In *Berman* v. *Allan*[97] (1979), the New Jersey Supreme Court explicitly rejected its earlier rationale offered in *Gleitman* for dismissing the infant plaintiff's cause of action—namely, the difficulty of ascertaining damages. Instead, it based its dismissal on the premise that life, however handicapped, cannot be an injury. The court held that the infant, Sharon Berman, who was born with Down syndrome, would be able to love and be loved and to experience happiness and pleasure, and therefore it could not be said that she would be better off had she never been born.

The *Berman* court was no doubt right that Sharon's life was not an injury to her. It is increasingly recognized that the lives of children with Down syndrome can be happy, even if they cannot be normal. However, this decision provides no guidance with respect to the lives of more seriously impaired children. Consider, for example, the child born with Tay-Sachs disease. The Tay-Sachs child is doomed to a short and increasingly handicapped existence. The child appears well at birth and develops normally for six to eight months, when progressive psychomotor degeneration slowly begins. By eighteen months the child is likely to be paralyzed and blind, unable to take food by mouth, and to suffer from constipation and bedsores. There are increasingly frequent convulsions that cannot be controlled by medication. The last few years of the child's life are spent in a vegetative state. Death typically occurs between the ages of three and five years, usually from infection.

There is no comparison between the life of a child with Down syndrome and the life of a child with Tay-Sachs. The Down syndrome child can have relationships with other people, can learn, can enjoy life, however limited that life may appear from the perspective of normality. By contrast, the life of a Tay-Sachs baby cannot be seen as a good to that child. The infant cannot see, eat, sit up, or even hold up his head, much less crawl around. What possible pleasure can there be in such an existence? The best that can be said is that once the child enters a vegetative state, he or she no longer suffers. But the mere absence of suffering is not sufficient to make life a good.

Some people reject the notion of a life not worth living. They maintain that life, no matter how severely defective, no matter how filled with suffering or devoid of pleasure, must be a good. This seems simply false. A life devoid of any of the things that give meaning to human life—pleasure, the ability to love, to learn, to have relationships—is not a life worth living.

A third argument against wrongful-life suits is that they are logically incoherent. This argument maintains that it is impossible for a person to be better off never having been born. For if I had never been born, then I never was; if I never was, then I cannot be said to have been better off. The problem can be put another way. To be harmed is to be made worse off; but no individual is made worse off by coming to exist, for that suggests that we can compare the person before he existed with the person after he existed, which is absurd. Therefore, it is logically impossible that anyone is harmed by coming to exist and wrongful-life suits are both illogical and unfair in that they require the defendant to compensate someone he has not harmed. As Justice Schreiber noted in his dissent in *Procanik* v. *Cillo:* ". . . sympathy for a handicapped child and his parents should not lead us to ignore the notions of responsibility, causation and damage that underlie the entire philosophy of our system of justice. It would be unwise—and, what is more, unjust—to permit the plaintiff to recover damages from persons who caused him no injury."[98] The challenge, then, for the advocates of the infant plaintiff is to express precisely the nature of the injury or wrong done to the infant.

One formulation was given by the New York Supreme Court (a lower division court) when it upheld a claim for wrongful life in *Park* v. *Chessin* in 1977. That case concerned an infant born with polycystic kidney disease. The parents already had one child with the condition, and were not warned of the risk that a second child would also be afflicted. In holding that the infant could recover for injuries and conscious pain and suffering, the court cited "the fundamental right of a child to be born as a whole, functioning human being." This sweeping claim has been universally rejected by other courts and commentators, and was overruled the following year when the New York Court of Appeals (New York's highest court) expressly denied in *Becker* v. *Schwartz* (1978) that there is a right to be born as a whole, functional human being.

Another approach is to express the injury to the child in terms of the wrong done to the parents.[99] Alexander Capron argues that the impaired infant has the right to have his or her parents determine whether birth would be in the infant's best interests. Thus, the deprivation of the parents' right to choose abortion is not only a wrong to the parents (as is claimed in a wrongful-birth suit), but also a direct wrong to the infant.

The interpretation is ingenious because it neatly avoids the logical puzzles associated with claiming that the infant was harmed by being born, while it strengthens the infant's cause of action by basing it on the increasingly accepted right of the parents to choose not to have a handicapped child. Despite these advantages, I reject Capron's interpretation, because it suggests, implausibly, that the *child* has been wronged whenever, because of the negligence of health-care providers, the *parents* are deprived of the choice of abortion.

The implausibility of this view is revealed if we think of an infant born with a relatively minor impairment, something that can be corrected, but not completely, such as a clubfoot. There may be individuals who would choose abortion rather than have a child with a clubfoot, because they consider life with even a minor disability, such as a limp, to be not worth living. If the doctor negligently fails to inform the parents that the child will have a club foot, he or she wrongs the parents, since they were deprived of the chance to terminate the pregnancy. Yet, according to Capron, the infant has the right to have his parents decide whether birth would be in his best interests. It follows that, by depriving the parents of the chance to decide whether life with a club foot is in the child's best interests, the doctor wrongs both the parents and the child. However, it is scarcely plausible that the negligent doctor wrongs the child by allowing him or her to be born, despite what the parents unreasonably believe. This suggests that the wrong done to the infant cannot be understood solely in terms of violating the parents' right to decide whether or not to terminate a pregnancy. The notion of wrongful life cannot be divorced from the welfare of the infant plaintiff.

We cannot either ignore the logical puzzles in wrongful-life suits, or sidestep them by construing the infant plaintiffs' right as a right to have their parents decide whether birth is in their best interests. The infant plaintiff's claim makes sense only if we recognize that existence itself can sometimes be an injury and that a child who will be forced to live under such conditions has a right not to be born.

To understand the claim that there can be a right not to be born, we must explain how someone can have an interest in not being born. Fetuses, for most of gestation, do not have interests. So if there is an interest in not being born, it must belong to the born child. A child can be said to have an interest in not being born if his or her existence is inexorably and irreparably such that life is not worth living. Joel Feinberg explains the right not to be born this way: "Talk of a 'right not to be born' is a compendious way of referring to the plausible moral requirement that no child be brought into the world unless certain very minimal conditions of wellbeing are assured. When a child is brought into existence even though those requirements have not been observed, he has been wronged thereby . . ."[100] The crucial idea is that the condition of the infant at birth can doom the child's future interests to total defeat. Feinberg argues that the advance dooming of a child's most basic interests—that is, those that are essential to the existence and advancement of any ulterior interests—deprives the child of what can be called his birthrights. And if you cannot have that to which you have a birthright, you are wronged if you are brought to birth.

In *Harm to Others,* Feinberg concedes that the infant plaintiff in a wrongful-life suit has not been, strictly speaking, harmed. For to harm someone is to make that person "worse off"; coming into existence cannot make someone worse off than he or she would otherwise have been. If the physician in these cases had acted properly, the parents would have chosen abortion, and the child would never have existed. Nonexistence is not a *better* condition to be in; *it is no condition at all.* In *Harm to Others,* Feinberg concludes that the negligent physician in a wrongful-life case cannot be said to have *harmed* the child, because the physician's negligence did not make the child worse off than he was. However, the physician can be said to have *wronged* the child by depriving him of his birthright: the right not to be brought into the world if all of one's most basic interests are doomed. In a more recent article,[101] Feinberg has come to the conclusion that it is possible to harm someone by being responsible for his being brought into existence, and that his failure to see this in *Harm to Others* stemmed from the failure to clarify what it means to say that someone has been made "worse off." This phrase is ambiguous. It could be interpreted to mean "worse off than he was *before* the wrongdoer acted." Feinberg dubs this interpretation "the worsening condition." Clearly, the worsening condition cannot be satisfied in the wrongful-life situation. That is, no one can be worse off than he was before he existed, since this suggests comparing the individual before he existed with the individual after he existed, which is absurd. In some cases, however, the individual who has been harmed is not worse off than he *was;* rather, he is worse off than he *would have been,* had the wrongdoer not acted as he did. This expresses a *counterfactual condition.* Expressed intuitively, the counterfactual claim is that the individual would have been better off not coming into existence, or "better off unborn." Once we distinguish the counterfactual test from the worsening test, Feinberg suggests, the logical problem posed by coming into existence disappears. For although, as we have seen, the worsening condition cannot be satisfied in wrongful-life suits, the possibility remains that the counter-factual condition can be satisfied. And if the counterfactual condition is satisfied, and the plaintiff is "worse off" because of something the defendant did, then the defendant can be said to have harmed the plaintiff. This enables us to place wrongful-life suits squarely within traditional tort concepts. The challenge is to explain what it means to say that someone is "worse off" for coming into existence, or "better off unborn."

It may help to start with the expression "better off dead." To say that someone is better off dead is not to compare his condition while alive with his condition after he is dead. That would be absurd, since after someone ceases to exist, he is in no condition at all. Instead, the phrase "better off dead" simply means that life is so terrible that it is no longer a benefit or a good to the one who lives. In the case of a competent adult, the criterion by which we judge whether a person is better off dead is ordinarily whether the person himself considers life not worth living.[102] This test, however, cannot be applied in the case of infants. It isn't just that infants cannot *express* their preferences; they do not yet have the intellectual equipment necessary for *having* the relevant preferences. Infants cannot understand the choice between severely handicapped existence and no existence at all. They cannot weigh up benefits and harms to reach a decision as to whether life is, on balance, worth living. Therefore, it doesn't make any sense to ask what the infant would want, if he could only tell us. The test of "substituted judgment" is simply inapplicable in the case of never-competent individuals.[103]

What sense, then, can be given to the judgment that the infant would be better off not existing? It might be thought that if we cannot consult the infant's own preferences, then life is necessarily a benefit and a good to the child. The implausibility of this is seen if we consider the example of an infant who is severely physically and mentally handicapped, and who suffers from chronic and unrelievable pain. The child's physical handicaps prevent him from the ordinary pleasures of infancy and childhood, while his mental handicaps prevent him from acquiring compensating interests. At the same time, he suffers without comprehension. Even if we cannot ascribe a *preference* for nonexistence to the child, surely we can say that this is a life so awful that no one could possibly wish it for the child. In saying this, we are not making a "substituted judgment," since this is not possible in the case of infants, but rather offering the judgment of a "proxy chooser," someone who acts as the infant's advocate, concerned to promote his or her welfare.

Parents often play this role in deciding whether to continue invasive and painful treatment on their extremely premature or severely impaired newborns. Sometimes they decide that saving or prolonging the baby's life is not in the baby's own best interest. If such a decision can be made regarding treatment, it would seem that it can be made regarding wrongful life. The danger in both situations is that the proxy chooser will be biased against the sort of life available to a severely handicapped person. It should be remembered that being born deaf, blind, unable to walk, or mentally retarded is not necessarily incompatible with having a life worth living. A life that a normal individual might find intolerable might not be so awful for an infant who has known nothing else. Handicaps, even severe ones, do not necessarily make a child better off dead, or better off unborn.[104]

The proxy chooser is therefore neither to express the child's own preferences, nor to ascribe his own values, goals, ideals, or aspirations to the child. Rather, the proxy is to represent the child's best interests. Feinberg explains his choice as follows:

> [The proxy chooser] . . . exercises his judgment that *whatever* interests the impaired party might have, or come to have, they would already be doomed to defeat by his present incurable condition. Thus, it would be irrational—contrary to what reason decrees—for a representative and protector of those interests to prefer the continuance of that condition to nonexistence. The proxy might also express the retroactive preference, on the incompetent's behalf, not to have been born at all.[105]

There are two important features of the proxy's choice. First, the choice of nonexistence is not merely rational in the weak sense of being in accordance with reason, but in the strong sense of being required by reason. Second, his nonexistence is rationally preferable in the strong sense only if all of his interests, present and future, are "doomed to defeat."

The "doomed-to-defeat" test works best where there is chronic pain, combined with such severe mental retardation that the child will not be able to develop any compensating interests. This was the prognosis given to the parents of "Baby Jane Doe." They were told that she would never know happiness, only pain. She'd be so retarded that she would never talk, never learn, never even recognize her parents. In addition, she'd be bedridden, paralyzed, and subject to constant bladder and urinary-tract infections. Her parents decided that such a life would not be in her best interest, and so they decided against life-prolonging treatment.[106]

However, cases falling under this description are rare.[107] Relatively few impaired newborns, even those with the severest anomalies, have lives filled with severe, chronic, and intractable pain. Far more common are cases in which the infant's condition precludes the ability to develop or to do any of the things that human beings characteristically develop. This would include children like Jeffrey Gleitman and Peter Procanik, who, because of congenital rubella syndrome, were born deaf, blind, and severely mentally retarded. Is nonexistence clearly preferable for such infants?

John Robertson argues that life-prolonging treatment is almost always in the best interest of even severely handicapped babies. He considers the case of a profoundly retarded, nonambulatory, blind, and deaf infant who will spend his few years in a crib in the back wards of a state institution, and writes:

> One who has never known the pleasures of mental operation, ambulation, and social interaction surely does not suffer from the loss as much as one who has. While one who has known these capacities may prefer death to a life without them, we have no assurance that the handicapped person, with no point of comparison, would agree. Life and life alone, whatever its limitations, might be of sufficient worth to him.[108]

John Arras agrees.[109] Such a child suffers no pain. He is neither horrified by his plight, nor depressed by his neglect in the state institution. He just lies there. *We* may consider such a life totally miserable, but can we be sure it appears so to the infant? If we confine ourselves to the infant's own perspective, it does not seem that we can say with confidence that the child is "better off dead" or "better off unborn." It is not even clear that the most radically impaired infant *suffers* from, or has interests *of his own* that are defeated by, his impaired condition.

We are left with two possibilities. We can restrict ourselves to the child's own interests (a "best-interests" standard) and acknowledge that an infant is clearly "better off dead" only in cases that combine severe physical and mental handicaps with chronic, severe, and intractable pain. Alternately, we can broaden the criteria to encompass a more objective, or intersubjective, notion, that of a "minimally decent existence." Arras says that if we are honest with ourselves, we will acknowledge that in most cases where it is thought best to stop life-prolonging treatment, death is not necessarily in the child's "best interest." (Indeed, in some of these cases, the infants barely have any interests.) Rather, we support letting the child die because we do not believe that a life of little more than biological existence constitutes a minimally decent existence. We do not think that such a life is worth sustaining.

The intuitive idea is that mere biological existence is not a good or a benefit. It is the ability to experience life, to partake in human experience, that makes life worthwhile, including such capacities as conscious awareness, the ability to experience pleasure, to give and receive love, to think, to learn. If all or most of these capacities are missing, then the child does not have a minimally decent existence. The suggestion here is that a child who does not have even a minimally decent existence is "better off unborn"—that is, worse off for having been brought into existence. And if the child can be said to be "worse off" for having been born, then the child can be said to have been harmed by being brought to birth.[110]

I have suggested that we will have a more plausible analysis of both "better off dead" and "better off unborn" if we allow the proxy chooser to apply either the "doomed-to-defeat" or the "minimally decent existence" criterion. However, even if we broaden the criteria in this way, "wrongful life" may still be a null—or virtually null—set, on Feinberg's analysis. The reason is that Feinberg insists that the choice for nonexistence must be rational, not merely in the weak sense of consistent with reason, where this means that the choice is one that a rational person *could* make, but in the strong sense of *required by reason,* where this means that the choice is one that a rational person would *have to* make. According to Feinberg, a child can be said to have been harmed by being brought into existence *only if* it would be *irrational* for a proxy chooser, acting out of concern for the child's best interest, to choose existence for that child. It is unlikely that this extremely restrictive standard could be met in most cases. Perhaps it could be met in the case of Tay-Sachs disease or Lesch-Nyhan syndrome. (This is an X-linked recessive condition that involves a process of neurological and physiological deterioration from approximately the sixth month of life; the most striking feature of the syndrome is compulsive self-mutilation.) However, in the majority of cases, there seems room for rational people to disagree about whether life is worth living. In relatively few cases, if any, can a proxy chooser who opts for the child's existence be said to be acting "contrary to reason."

It seems to me that Feinberg sets too stringent a standard of rationality for his proxy chooser. It is a much more stringent standard than is required of parents deciding on life-prolonging care for their severely impaired newborns. No one demands that their decision be one that *could not be rejected by a rational decision-maker.* It is acknowledged that different parents, with different values, may arrive at different decisions. So long as their decision is not clearly contrary to the child's best interests, parents are allowed to make medical decisions for their children, including decisions to stop life-prolonging treatment. Moreover, much less is at stake in the wrongful-life context than in the medical decision-making context. If a mistake is made in the medical context, a child who could have had a life worth living may be denied care and die. If a comparable mistake is made in the wrongful-life context, a negligent physician may be required to compensate a severely handicapped child who was not in fact "better off unborn." That is hardly a tragedy, and for that reason, it is hard to understand why so stringent a standard of rationality should be required in the wrongful-life context, when it is not required in the medical decision-making context.

I conclude that Feinberg's analysis of wrongful life could be improved in two ways: first, broaden the criterion for determining that an infant is "better off unborn" to include a "minimally decent existence" test. Second, weaken the rationality criterion; that is, permit the proxy chooser to make choices that are rational in the weak sense of "consistent with reason," or *reasonable,* instead of insisting that the choice for nonexistence be one that a rational person would perforce make. So long as the choice for nonexistence is a reasonable one, the child can be said to have been harmed by being brought into existence. It should be pointed out that, even if we modify Feinberg's analysis in this way, relatively few wrongful-life suits would succeed. Someone playing the role of advocate for the infant could not reasonably choose nonexistence over life with such impairments as deafness, blindness, confinement to a wheelchair, or mild mental retardation. These conditions do not entail a life that falls below a decent minimum. Many handicapped people have lives that are well worth living. The irony is that it is just these children who would be most able to benefit from recovery in a wrongful-life suit. There is not a lot that can be done for children so severely impaired that their lives can be plausibly said to be "not worth living." By contrast, money awarded to a child with Down syndrome or spina bifida, to a child born deaf or blind, can be used for medical treatment and education.

A solution might be to suspend traditional tort rules. Feinberg suggests this, saying:

> This would be a "victimless tort," that is, not a tort at all in the traditional sense, but perhaps justice would support it anyway, as it supports various kinds of strict and vicarious liability. It might not be fair to make a person pay damages to another whom she has not directly wronged, but it may be more unfair still to make the miserable impaired party pay, or do without the aid he needs.[111]

A separate issue is whether wrongful-life suits are the best way to ensure that the needs of disabled people for medical treatment and special education are met. This seems unlikely. Ideally, all handicapped people should receive the treatment they need, regardless of whether their handicap or their existence is someone's fault.[112] However, denying recovery to wrongful-life plaintiffs is not going to improve the situation of other impaired children. Until the interests of all disabled people are met through universal access to health care, litigation may be the only way for some infants to get the services they need.

In the next chapter, I consider the problem of behavior during pregnancy that exposes the fetus to serious health risks. Increasingly, there have been calls for coercive measures to protect the "not-yet-born" child. Such recommendations are consistent with the interest view. Whether they are wise public policy is a separate matter. Feminists and civil libertarians caution against the threat of a "pregnancy police" that would intrude into every aspect of a woman's life and decision-making. These are valid concerns. Coercive measures are neither necessary nor likely to safeguard the health of future children, while they threaten women's rights to privacy and self-determination.

4 | Maternal-Fetal Conflict

A newborn baby whose urine shows traces of an illegal drug is taken from the custody of its mother. A woman whose baby is born with severe brain damage is jailed for prenatal child abuse. A pregnant drug user who commits a minor crime is jailed in order to protect her fetus from addiction. A company that has potentially embryotoxic substances in the workplace refuses to hire fertile women under its "fetal protection policy." A court order compels a pregnant Jehovah's Witness to have a blood transfusion, contrary to the tenets of her religion, to protect the life of her fetus. Another woman is forced to undergo an emergency cesarean section. Each of these situations raises the question of the resolution of conflict between the interests of the expectant mother and those of her unborn child.

In Chapter 2, I used the interest view to defend abortion. I argued that, before becoming conscious and sentient, the fetus has no interests at all, and so no interest in continued existence. Without an interest in continued existence, the preconscious fetus is not harmed or wronged by being killed. Since abortion is not a wrong to the preconscious fetus, and the preconscious fetus has no right to life, the state should stay out of abortion decisions.

127

I. MORAL OBLIGATIONS TO THE NOT-YET-BORN

The moral situation changes when a woman decides not to abort, but to carry her baby to term. For once this decision is made, the fetus is not simply a potential child, but a child-who-will-be-born. Once born, that child will have interests, including an interest in a healthy and painless existence. That interest can be adversely affected by his or her mother's behavior during pregnancy. If she neglects her own health, if she has an inferior diet, if she smokes or drinks too much or uses illegal drugs, she takes risks with the health of her future child. Insofar as these risks are unnecessary or unreasonable, taking them is morally wrong, a violation of parental duty. So there are things that pregnant women ought to do, or refrain from doing, not only for their own health, but for the sake of the baby. As the sign in the obstetrician's office says, "Now you have two reasons to quit smoking."

For the vast majority of women, the decision not to abort, but to carry to term, is made early in the pregnancy. As we saw in Chapter 2, ninety percent of all abortions in the United States take place in the first trimester; most women know very quickly whether the pregnancy is welcome. In the case of a planned pregnancy, the decision to become a mother is made even before conception. Changes in life-style, then, may be required as soon as pregnancy is determined, or even earlier. Women who are trying to become pregnant are told that they should improve their diets, as well as those of their husbands (the better his nutrition, the healthier his sperm). They may be advised to take vitamin-mineral supplements that have been shown to prevent certain birth defects. They are told to lose excessive weight and get into shape. It is recommended that they cut down on caffeine and alcohol, to quit smoking, to avoid marijuana and other "recreational" drugs, and to take only those medicines that their doctors prescribe. Having been told to do all these things, they are told that, above all, they should relax![1] These recommendations are aimed at giving the baby the best possible odds of being born alive and well. They reflect the idea that the decision to have a baby brings with it moral obligations to the child who will be born.

The idea that mothers-to-be have moral obligations to their not-yet-born children is relatively uncontroversial. Disagreement occurs when we try to say precisely what these moral obligations are. Behavior that is protective of the fetus may impose sacrifices or even risks on the pregnant woman. How much sacrifice or risk is an expectant mother morally required to undergo? And even if we could agree on that, it would be a further, and much more complex question, whether these moral obligations should be made into legal ones. For some people, the very idea of the state telling women how to act because they are pregnant is "a paranoid fantasy," while others think that the need to protect fetuses is "absolutely self-evident."[2]

The interest view does not by itself provide a resolution to this dispute. The interest view simply acknowledges that, once born, children have interests in healthy existence, and that these interests can be damaged before the children are born, or even conceived. Thus, the interest view acknowledges the intelligibility of obligations to future as-yet-unborn children. Although the obligation is to the born child, and it is the born child who has the right not to be injured, there is a sense in which the interest view can accommodate "fetal rights" since the fulfillment of these obligations occurs while the child is still a fetus. But it is one thing to say that the notion of fetal rights is conceptually possible, quite another to say that our legal system ought to recognize fetal rights. That is a complex substantive normative issue, not merely a conceptual one. In this chapter, I argue that there are compelling policy reasons not to recognize fetal rights, as the use of legal coercion will do little to protect the not-yet-born while seriously endangering women's rights to privacy and self-determination.

Risks to the Fetus

Part of the motivation for increased intervention to protect fetuses stems from increased, and relatively recent, awareness of the dangers to fetal health from maternal behavior during pregnancy. It used to be thought that the womb provided a shielded environment, which protected the fetus from external factors. It wasn't until the 1940s that experiments using animals demonstrated that maternal dietary deficiency and X-ray exposure could adversely affect intrauterine mammalian development. About the same time, the association between rubella infection and abnormal fetal development was recognized.[3] The thalidomide tragedy in the 1960s, which resulted in the births of thousands of severely malformed infants, demonstrated the potential danger to the fetus of an apparently innocuous tranquilizer.

In the late 1960s and early 1970s, fetal alcohol syndrome (FAS), characteristic of offspring of chronic alcoholic mothers, was described. There are an estimated 1,800 to 2,400 cases of children born with FAS each year in the United States. Full-blown FAS exists when the patient has signs in each of three categories: prenatal or postnatal growth retardation, central nervous system damage (neurological abnormality, developmental delay, or learning disabilities), and characteristic facial dysmorphology, such as microcephaly and a flattened nose.[4] Some children do not show the full FAS but have some manifestations of the syndrome. In such cases, the term "possible fetal alcohol effects" (FAE) is used. The most commonly observed anomaly in FAE is growth retardation. FAE is far more common than FAS, with an estimated incidence of 36,000 cases per year in the United States.[5]

Tobacco is another legal substance that can cause serious damage to the unborn. Smokers' offspring are at higher risk for miscarriage, stillbirth, prematurity, and low birthweight.[6] The best-documented adverse effect of smoking during pregnancy is fetal growth retardation. Studies conducted during the 1980s found that from 21 to 39 percent of the incidence of low birthweight (under 2,500 grams or $5\frac{1}{2}$ pounds at birth) was attributable to maternal cigarette smoking. Low-birthweight babies have a significantly higher mortality rate than full-birthweight infants; for example, they are ten times more likely to die from intrapartum asphyxia (lack of oxygen during labor).[7]

New evidence is emerging about the danger that cocaine—once popularly believed relatively harmless—can pose both to fetal health and to the health of born children. According to one commentator, "If cocaine use during pregnancy were a disease, its impact on children would be considered a national health care crisis."[8] Seventy-three percent of the deaths in abuse and neglect cases in New York City in 1987 resulted from parents abusing drugs, up from 11 percent in 1985.[9] Between 1985 and 1990, the number of babies born to cocaine-addicted mothers in New York City more than quadrupled.

Nor is the problem of drug use during pregnancy confined to large urban areas like New York City. A 1988 survey of thirty-six hospitals across America indicated that 11 percent of women were using drugs during pregnancy, with cocaine the most common, resulting in 375,000 drug-exposed infants annually.[10] Other surveys placed the number as high as 15 percent. Use is not confined to particular racial or socioeconomic groups, although most women *prosecuted* for using illegal drugs while pregnant have been poor members of racial minorities.[11]

Fortunately, there are signs that the crack epidemic is beginning to abate. Recently, the *New York Times* reported that a decline in the use of cocaine by pregnant women, combined with improved prenatal care, helped significantly reduce infant mortality in New York City in 1990 for the first time in four years.[12] The crack epidemic appears to have peaked in 1988, though it continues to ravage many families.

The effects of fetal exposure to cocaine include retarded growth in the womb and subtle neurological abnormalities, leading to extraordinary irritability during infancy and learning disorders later. In more extreme cases, cocaine can cause loss of the small intestine and brain-damaging strokes. Cocaine-exposed babies face a tenfold increase in the risk of crib death.

Studies conducted at Northwestern Memorial Hospital in Chicago have shown that some of the worst effects occur during the first three months of pregnancy, when the fetal organs are forming, often before the woman knows she is pregnant. Damage may occur even if the woman stops using the drug, once pregnancy is diagnosed.

> In fact, the research suggests that a single cocaine "hit" during pregnancy can cause lasting fetal damage. . . . Cocaine, which is soluble in fat, readily crosses the placenta, where the baby's body converts a significant portion of it to norcocaine, a water-soluble substance that does not leave the womb and that is even more potent than cocaine. Norcocaine is excreted into the amniotic fluid, which the fetus swallows, re-exposing itself to the drug. As a result, the researchers believe, almost no cocaine-exposed baby fully escapes its damaging effects.[13]

Not all researchers have found such clear evidence of harmful effects on the fetus from cocaine use.[14] It is often difficult to tell whether the symptoms in the child are specifically due to cocaine use or to other features of poverty: poor nutrition, poor maternal health, and little or no prenatal care. It may be that using cocaine during pregnancy is comparable to drinking alcohol or smoking cigarettes: certainly not recommended, but not something that is certain to cause damage to the fetus.

With respect to alcohol, there is no consensus regarding the amount of alcohol intake by the pregnant woman and the likelihood of adverse effects on the fetus. According to Elias and Annas, a clear relationship between alcohol use and adverse pregnancy outcome has been demonstrated only for heavy and prolonged maternal alcohol abuse of at least 5.0 ounces of absolute alcohol per day.[15] Other researchers claim that maternal consumption of over three drinks per day (1.5 oz. of alcohol) triples the risk of subnormal IQ.[16] They report that children born to women who had as little as one to two drinks a day in the first months of pregnancy had a slower reaction time in their early school years and difficulty in paying attention.[17] Experts agree that there is no known minimum "safe" level of alcohol consumption. It is possible that any consumption of alcohol produces some risk to the fetus.

In light of this information, what are the moral obligations of pregnant women regarding alcohol consumption? Certainly, heavy and prolonged alcohol use during pregnancy runs an unjustifiable risk of harming the not-yet-born child. These days, many people apparently regard *any* consumption of alcohol by pregnant women as equally wrong. Some even take it upon themselves to influence the behavior of pregnant women. In March 1991, a bartender and a waitress attempted to dissuade a pregnant woman in Seattle from ordering a rum daiquiri. First they asked her whether she wouldn't prefer a nonalcoholic drink. When she said she would not, the bartender removed the warning label from a bottle of beer, which says that the Surgeon General has determined that pregnant women should not drink alcohol because of the risk of birth defects, and placed it before her. She complained to the management, and the waitress and bartender were fired for harassing a customer.

In my view, the waitress and the bartender, though well-meaning, were out of line. It is one thing to *inform* pregnant women of the risks posed by alcohol, through warning labels, and quite another for bartenders and wait-resses to assume the role of enforcers.[18] Ironically, the greatest risk to the unborn occurs during the first trimester, when the pregnancy is unlikely to be evident and outside intervention therefore impractical. In this case, as it turned out, the woman was past her due date and had been very careful to avoid liquor throughout her pregnancy. She had decided that one drink was unlikely to do any harm, a perfectly reasonable assessment of the available evidence.

Admittedly, total abstinence is the safest course for the not-yet-born child, but are people morally obligated to follow the *safest* course? We do not require this standard of parents regarding their already-born children. If we did, we could not justify leaving children with baby-sitters to go out to dinner. What if something should happen? It seems to me that having a single drink occasionally in pregnancy falls into the area of individual dis-cretion, both because the risk of causing harm is very low (perhaps non-existent) and the nature of the harm (loss of a few IQ points) hardly dev-astating.

Although heavy use of alcohol is not good for anyone, pregnant or not, light to moderate alcohol consumption has been connected to a reduced risk of heart disease. The moderate use of alcohol may therefore be a healthful habit. By contrast, smoking has nothing at all to recommend it from a health perspective. The risk it poses to the baby imposes on the expectant mother an obligation to make a good-faith effort to stop, or at least cut down on, smoking. However, we now know that nicotine is an addictive drug. A woman who is addicted to cigarettes may be unable to do what she ought to do for the sake of her baby.

Similarly, it is the heavy and chronic drinker, whose drinking is most detrimental to the unborn, who is least likely to be able to modify her behavior to protect her baby. Is she nevertheless obligated to stop drinking during pregnancy? On the one hand, people cannot have obligations they cannot fulfill. I cannot have an obligation to save your life if it is literally impossible for me to save you. The "ought implies can" principle may incline some people to say that pregnant drug addicts and alcoholics are not under a moral obligation to stop using drugs and alcohol. However, the fact that they cannot stop *at will* does not mean that they are literally incapable of stopping. We can recognize that it may be very difficult for some women to fulfill their moral obligations to the babies they plan to bear, and acknowledge that they will need help to do so, without denying that they have such obligations.

The argument so far recognizes that women have moral obligations to the children they plan to bear, obligations to consider the impact of their behavior on the developing fetus and to avoid taking unreasonable risks with their health and well-being. In the following sections, I argue that there are compelling reasons not to make these obligations legal.

II. LEGAL OBLIGATIONS TO THE NOT-YET-BORN
Extending Child-Abuse Laws

Emergency Custody of the Newborn

Parents have legal obligations to care for their children. Failure to meet these obligations can result in having their children taken away. Should existing laws on child abuse and neglect apply to the fetus as well? This is in effect the policy in New York's Nassau County, where the Department of Social Services has a twenty-year-old policy of automatically removing newborns from the custody of their mothers if illegal drug use of any kind during pregnancy is discovered. When drug-related distress is suspected, babies can be given a toxicology test, without their parents' consent. The presence of illegal drugs in the baby's urine is treated as evidence of fetal abuse. And fetal abuse, the agency says, is tantamount to child abuse, requiring immediate removal of an infant from the mother's care. According to Marvin Rachlin, an attorney for Nassau County's Department of Social Services, "The fact that she . . . [fed drugs] to this baby in utero rather than in the crib doesn't make a difference. It does the same thing to the baby."[19] Of course, a woman who fed her baby alcohol would also be guilty of child abuse, but no one has suggested taking newborns away from mothers who are discovered to have used alcohol during pregnancy. For social and cultural reasons, we have enormous tolerance of alcohol, despite the objective risks it poses to life and health, and an irrational overreaction to other drug use. In the fall of 1988, the Legal Aid Society filed a suit on behalf of seven Nassau County mothers, arguing that a single positive drug test is not enough evidence that a woman will be an unfit mother.[20]

In most states, it is still an open question whether a pregnant woman's drug abuse constitutes child neglect or abuse. As the issues are raised more frequently in courts, different judges reach different conclusions, even in the same state. A Nassau County Family Court judge ruled in December 1988 that a pregnant woman's use of cocaine and failure to obtain prenatal care were acts of neglect. While acknowledging the woman's right to abort in early pregnancy, the judge, Joseph DeMaro, said, "There is no reason to treat a child in utero any differently from a child ex utero where the mother has decided not to destroy the fetus or where the time allowed for such destruction is past."[21] But, in the Bronx, Judge Jeffrey H. Gallet of Family Court disagrees. In October 1988, he wrote a decision rejecting the state's claim that a woman who admitted using cocaine in pregnancy, and whose newborn tested positive for cocaine, could therefore be found guilty of child neglect. Judge Gallet said:

> I see no authority for the state to regulate women's bodies merely because they are pregnant. . . . By becoming pregnant, women do not waive the constitutional protections afforded to other citizens. To carry the law guardian's argument to its logical extension, a state would be able to supersede a mother's custody right to her child if she smoked cigarettes during her pregnancy or ate junk food, or did too much physical labor or did not exercise enough.[22]

There is, as Judge Gallet recognizes, a reason for treating the fetus *in utero* differently from the fetus *ex utero:* namely, that the fetus *in utero* is inside the body of the pregnant woman. Any attempt to protect it, without her consent, involves an invasion of the woman's rights to bodily integrity and self-determination. These rights simply are not involved in abuse and neglect cases involving born children. Judge Gallet is concerned that allowing any intrusion into the pregnant woman's private life will ultimately result in legal regulation of every aspect of pregnant women's behavior. Why should the state stop at illegal drug use? As we have seen, perfectly legal activities may also result in fetal damage, and thus would also come under state scrutiny, if child-abuse and child-neglect statutes were applied to the unborn.

In response, it might be pointed out that taking some steps to protect not-yet-born children does not commit us to taking all such steps. We may wish to make distinctions based on the nature of the risk. Cocaine appears to be more dangerous to the developing fetus than tobacco or alcohol; at least some researchers have found that much smaller amounts can cause more serious damage. Moreover, no one is a "recreational" crack user for long, as crack is highly addictive. Crack also has far worse effects on behavior than virtually any other drug. Drug abuse has always disrupted families, but many Family Court judges believe that crack introduced something even more sinister into the equation, producing an epidemic of children being beaten, raped, and murdered within their own families. Judge Leah Ruth Marks of Manhattan Family Court remarks, "I look back on the good old days of heroin. Heroin didn't destroy their ability to be human the way crack does."[23] Someone who engages in prolonged and heavy use of crack is almost certain to be a neglectful or abusive parent,[24] something that is just not true of cigarette smokers or junk-food addicts. Removing newborns from the custody of crack addicts is not an unreasonable or excessive step. It does not commit us to intervening in every aspect of a pregnant woman's life.

At the same time, we should be extremely wary of giving officials the power to take children away from their parents, because such power can be misused, with tragic results. It has been recommended that parental substance abuse be considered *prima facie* evidence of inadequate parenting.[25] Unfortunately, many officials regard *any* use of illegal drugs as "substance abuse." Such officials may take children from homes, where this is *not* necessary to protect the children, as a way of punishing the parents for their drug use or life-style. This happened in Nassau County, when a child was taken from its mother, who used marijuana to relax in the latter part of her pregnancy. The removal was based solely on the mother's use of marijuana during pregnancy. There was no other evidence of child abuse, or even evidence that the woman continued to use marijuana after the baby was born.[26] We are not told whether the mother's use of marijuana during pregnancy actually injured the baby, but if it did, that damage is already done. To remove the infant after birth cannot protect him or her from prenatal injury, but instead inflicts further physical and emotional harm by depriving a baby of his or her mother. This would be justified only if continued care by the mother posed an imminent risk of danger to the child, something that was not proved, or apparently even seriously considered.

In a recent Illinois case, a baby was removed from its mother's custody after it was learned that she had used cocaine during her pregnancy. The baby did not appear to be cocaine-addicted at birth, but the woman apparently had revealed her drug use to medical personnel during labor. (Such information might seem to be privileged and confidential, but evidently it was not so treated.) The baby's urine was tested, and it was found that the child had indeed been exposed to cocaine. This was enough to enable the removal of the child, despite the fact that the baby had not developed any signs of addiction or other serious health problems. Judge Frederick J. Kapala regarded this as insignificant, saying, "It's the same as if a mother gave a child a pack of razor blades to play with in the crib. The child might drop the blades out of the crib and not get hurt, but the exposure to danger is the same."[27]

The mother has been in a drug-treatment program, and could conceivably regain custody if she is able to provide a drug-free environment for the baby and acquire parenting skills. According to Paul Logli, the Winnebago County state's attorney, the woman has three other children, all in foster care. However, according to Mr. Logli, it is likely that the baby would have been removed even if there were no other indications that she was incapable of adequately caring for it.[28] The policy in Winnebago County appears to be like that of Nassau County. Prenatal drug use is itself sufficient evidence of child abuse and neglect. As I have argued, that policy is unlikely to be in the best interests of children.

Mr. Logli says that there were twenty-seven "cocaine babies" between the summer of 1988 and the spring of 1989, nine more than in the previous year. In response, on May 8, 1989, Melanie Green, the mother of a baby whose death was linked to her cocaine abuse during pregnancy, was charged with involuntary manslaughter and delivery of a controlled substance to a minor. Mr. Logli was quoted as saying, ". . . the actions of this office reflect the concern, sometimes the outrage, of this community that children are born [at risk]."[29] However, a grand jury refused to indict, citing concern for the mother's privacy rights. Medical and social services officials fear that if such prosecutions become common, they could simply drive addicted mothers underground, making them afraid to give birth in hospitals. Mr. Logli responds to such concerns, saying, "I don't know how else to protect babies."[30]

In the next section, I will examine the issue of criminal penalties for women whose behavior during pregnancy causes serious injury to their newborns.

Criminal Penalties for Fetal Abuse

The Case of Pamela Rae Stewart

Some district attorneys have attempted to use the criminal law to punish women whose behavior during pregnancy allegedly caused the death of their subsequently born children. The first of these cases involved Pamela Rae Stewart, a California woman who was charged with failing to provide her fetus with necessary medical care. In November 1985, Ms. Stewart gave birth by emergency cesarean section to a baby with severe brain damage, who died a few months later.

Ms. Stewart had been diagnosed as having a breech presentation and a complete placenta previa. Placenta previa is a serious condition that can result in the detachment of the placenta from the uterus, causing hemorrhaging and endangering the lives of both the mother and fetus. She was told to take a prescribed medication daily to delay labor, to stay off her feet, to refrain from sexual intercourse, and to get to the hospital immediately should she begin bleeding heavily. According to the district attorney, she failed to follow these instructions. On the day of delivery she allegedly stopped taking her medication, used amphetamines, engaged in sexual intercourse with her husband, and refused to go to the hospital when she began bleeding. In a letter to Child Protective Services, Dr. Paul Zlotnik, head of the Neonatal Intensive Care Unit at Grossmont District Hospital where Thomas, Jr., was born, blamed Ms. Stewart for the outcome of her pregnancy, saying, "Overall, the mother was extremely negligent in her care of herself and subsequently her infant. She created the outcome that is so evident in the infant now."[31]

Ms. Stewart offers a different version. She says that she did not know about the placenta previa, that she knew only that she had a breech presentation. She maintains that she did her best to stay off her feet, but found it difficult with two little girls, aged three and five, to care for. She claims she took her pills, although they made her feel quite ill. She admits having used marijuana on the day Thomas, Jr., was born, but not amphetamines.

These factual discrepancies were never resolved, because the charges against her were dropped on legal grounds. The prosecutor had wanted to charge her with child abuse, but could not because California courts had earlier ruled that fetuses were not covered by child-abuse statutes.[32] So the district attorney, in what the defense characterized as a "fishing expedition,"[33] found a child-support statute that had been amended specifically to include the unborn. The reason for the amendment was to enable pregnant women to collect for their prenatal care from the men who had impregnated them. Later the statute was changed again, on grounds of gender equality, to apply to both parents. In its 114–year history, the statute had never been used to prosecute a woman for alleged deficiencies in prenatal care.

In dismissing the charges, the judge ruled that the statute was never intended to apply to the behavior of pregnant women, but was intended to compel parents to pay child support. It would violate due process, he said, to use a law intended and always interpreted for one purpose for a completely different purpose. He recommended that the state legislature pass a more appropriate bill "protecting the life of the unborn child under certain narrowly defined conditions." Shortly thereafter, such a bill was introduced in the California legislature, but it died in committee.

Because the charge against Ms. Stewart was dropped, the court did not reach the issue of the constitutionality of criminalizing maternal prenatal conduct. Most courts have so far refused to utilize child-abuse laws to criminalize fetal abuse, although some commentators have called for interpreting such statutes as providing protection for the unborn.[34]

Some states are entering child-abuse statutes that explicitly cover fetuses.[35] It has been argued that broad fetal-abuse statutes patterned on child-abuse statutes—those that make neglecting or abusing a fetus a crime without specifying what constitutes neglect or abuse—would be unconstitutionally vague.[36] Virtually everything a pregnant woman does could have an effect on her fetus. Unless prohibited activities were specified in advance, a woman would have no way of knowing if ordinarily perfectly legal activities were criminal. Perhaps it might be specified that only behavior explicitly ruled out by the woman's doctor would be prohibited. But failing to follow doctor's orders is not a crime, and it would be very dangerous if it were. It would give doctors the power to place whatever restrictions upon pregnant patients they thought desirable. It would deprive women of the right to make their own decisions about the management of their pregnancy, a right for which women have fought very hard in recent years.

Delivering Drugs through the Umbilical Cord

Statutes most likely to pass constitutional muster would be ones that specifically prohibited the use of illegal drugs likely to harm the fetus. Since these drugs are already illegal, their prohibition during pregnancy does not violate a right to privacy. As of this writing, no laws that would make drug use during pregnancy a felony have been passed, although efforts to impose additional criminal penalties for using drugs during pregnancy have been made in several states, including Idaho, Illinois, Oregon, Michigan, and Montana.[37] Since 1987, about 180 criminal proceedings against women for drug use during pregnancy have been instigated in various states and the District of Columbia.[38] The charges include criminal child abuse, assault with a deadly weapon, manslaughter, and criminal delivery of drugs. In most cases the charges were ultimately dismissed or dropped, sometimes before indictment.[39] In July 1989, Jennifer Johnson of Florida became the first woman to be convicted of delivering cocaine to her newborn child through the umbilical cord.[40] She was sentenced to one year in a rehabilitation program and fourteen years probation. The conviction was upheld by a Florida appeals court. At this writing, the case is before the State Supreme Court (*State* v. *Johnson*, 77831).

"The important thing to remember about the Jennifer Johnson case is that this is a woman who tried to get treatment and was turned away," says Dr. Wendy Chavkin, who did a survey of drug treatment programs in New

York City.[41] She found that 54 percent of treatment programs categorically excluded the pregnant. Sixty-seven percent rejected pregnant Medicaid patients and only 13 percent accepted pregnant Medicaid patients addicted to crack.[42] And even in areas where there are treatment programs for pregnant addicts, there are not enough spaces for everyone who wants help. For example, in 1988 the waiting list for a bed in L.A. County's rehabilitation program for pregnant women was seven months long, according to a study by the county.[43]

By charging Johnson with delivering a drug to her newborn, not her fetus, the prosecution avoided the issue of the legal status of the unborn. Even so, the legal basis for these prosecutions is shaky. Applying existing drug laws to the prenatal cases ignores very real differences between the two situations. For one thing, the intent ordinarily necessary for a criminal charge is missing. A woman who uses drugs during pregnancy does not intend to give her child drugs. It is absurd to treat her like a pusher in a schoolyard. The absence of criminal intent is seen in the case of Kimberly Hardy, a Michigan woman who smoked crack the night before her baby was born. Reportedly, Ms. Hardy thought that smoking crack would help her relax and go into labor. She was quoted as saying, "The baby was so far along that a couple of hits couldn't possibly hurt."[44] As it turned out, she was wrong. The underweight baby was jaundiced and couldn't keep his formula down. Ms. Hardy was charged with criminal delivery of drugs, a charge usually reserved for drug dealers. Whereas drug use itself is typically a misdemeanor punishable by probation, especially in a first-offense case, delivering drugs is a felony in most jurisdictions in the United States, which can be punished with a hefty jail term. On April 2, 1991, a Michigan appeals court ruled that Ms. Hardy should not stand trial. The court unanimously rejected the state's argument that Ms. Hardy passed cocaine to her baby in a way that constituted criminal delivery of drugs. The prosecutor plans to appeal to the Michigan Supreme Court.[45]

Most experts who have studied the problem of pregnant drug users believe that rehabilitation programs are a more effective way of protecting the unborn than criminal prosecutions.[46] Marie Y. Bockwindel, general counsel for the Legal Aid Foundation of Los Angeles, points out an additional irony in the spending of public funds to prosecute pregnant drug users: "We are unwilling to invest the necessary funds to provide proper prenatal care for poor women; we don't have sufficient drug treatment programs for drug and alcohol abusers of any type, much less pregnant women . . ." She concludes:

> We know what the problems are; we know what works in resolving them; but we'd rather pay for more police and prisons than engage in a long-

term plan with adequate funding to solve them. Let's get our priorities where they need to be—by providing adequate prenatal care, medical and psychological services to children and families, family planning, safe and affordable child care, and drug treatment for drug and alcohol abusers, instead of incarcerating pregnant women.[47]

It may be objected that the same considerations against "fetal abuse" laws could be used against postnatal child abuse statutes. Arguably, laws against child abuse do little to protect children. It is unlikely that such laws have much deterrent effect, because most abuse is not deliberate or planned, but stems from inability to control frustration and anger. So why punish anyone who harms a child through abuse and neglect? And if we do think that some abusers *deserve* to be punished, whether or not punishing them has a deterrent effect, why can't we say that *some* women who inflict prenatal abuse deserve to be punished? This may not be the only or the best way to protect babies, but it could be argued that criminal sanctions are, in some cases, fully justified. They are justified when a woman is aware that her *voluntary* and *noncompulsive* behavior poses serious risks to the health of her not-yet-born child, yet she disregards these risks, causing the baby to be born seriously damaged. Perhaps a yuppie recreational cocaine user would come into this category. Surely we would all agree that her behavior is immoral. Why shouldn't she be prosecuted?

In response, I would concede that prosecution in such a case could be justified. My fear is that it is unlikely that prosecution would be confined to such cases—if they exist at all. There is a real danger that statutes that punish women for drug use during pregnancy would be used primarily to prosecute uneducated, low-income addicts: women who are likely to be less than fully responsible for their harmful behavior.

What about jailing pregnant addicts to prevent them from taking drugs? The rationale here is neither retributive nor based on deterrence. Rather, the aim is to protect specific not-yet-born babies. How successful is it likely to be, and how should we balance the protection gained against the infringement of privacy and liberty?

Jailing the Pregnant Addict

In the spring of 1988, Brenda Vaughan, a twenty-nine-year-old Washington, D.C., woman, pleaded guilty to forging about $700 worth of checks. It was her first offense, and one that normally would have brought probation. But because Ms. Vaughan was pregnant, and tests showed she had used cocaine, the judge sent her to jail until the date her baby was due. There were no treatment programs available, and he wanted to protect the fetus from cocaine addiction. In defending his decision, Judge Peter H. Wolf said many of his judicial colleagues have told him they incarcerate pregnant drug abusers for the same reason.[48]

Is it fair to give a more severe sentence than one ordinarily would to protect the unborn? Feminists and civil libertarians argue that it is not. Women do not lose their civil rights when they become pregnant. Pregnancy should not be used as an excuse for depriving a woman of liberty. Pregnancy is not relevant to desert, and therefore should not be considered in determining the sentence.

My own view is different. My opposition to the jailing of pregnant drug users is based on pragmatic grounds. Jailing pregnant offenders is unlikely to benefit the future child, while it clearly imposes great hardship on the woman. For these reasons, pregnancy rarely, if ever, justifies imposing a jail sentence. However, if a jail sentence *could* prevent a child from being born addicted, sparing him or her a great deal of pain and the possibility of irreparable neurological damage, then I do not think that a judge is *obligated* to offer probation as opposed to prison, not even if probation is routinely given to nonpregnant first offenders. No one has a right to be given probation, rather than punishment. In giving probation, a judge is being lenient, and while leniency may be justified and appropriate, it is not something to which anyone has a right. It is not, therefore, unfair for a judge to decide against probation if there are compelling consequentialist considerations in favor of giving the penalty allowed by law.

The strongest argument against jailing pregnant addicts is that this is extremely unlikely to protect the health of future children, for two reasons. First, in many prisons, it is not difficult to obtain illegal drugs. Second, the standard of prenatal care in jail is frequently seriously inadequate. In the spring of 1985, a series of incidents at the California Institute for Women led to a class-action lawsuit filed by Legal Services for Prisoners with Children on behalf of pregnant and postpartum women prisoners.[49] One woman suffered severe abdominal cramping and bleeding for seventeen days without being allowed to receive treatment from an obstetrician. Her son was born in the ambulance on the way to an outside hospital, and lived only two hours. Another woman was seated upright and shackled while she was in active labor, as she was being transported to an outside hospital. By the time she arrived at the hospital, the baby was in severe distress and required more than thirty days in neonatal intensive care, with some degree of permanent disability a likely result. A third woman had gained over a hundred pounds by her eighth month of pregnancy and had protein in her urine. Despite these critical high-risk factors, she was seen only twice at the high-risk OB/GYN clinic in an outside hospital. Prison officials flatly refused to issue her the special diet recommended by the clinic.[50] It is clear that jailing women cannot ensure medical screening, regular monitoring, and other such minimum-care requirements to protect the fetus. Incarcerating pregnant women to ensure healthy children is an improbable venture.

Congress has mandated that states spend 10 percent of their federal Alcohol, Drug Abuse and Mental Health Services block-grant funds on the development and expansion of prevention and treatment programs for alcoholic and drug-dependent women, with special emphasis to be given to services for pregnant women. Yet most states have failed to comply with this mandate.[51] As a matter of public policy, it makes more sense to fund drug-treatment programs than to incarcerate pregnant drug addicts. Protection of the unborn will be best accomplished not by jailing pregnant offenders, but by attacking drug addiction directly, and by securing adequate prenatal care for all women.

Fetal-Protection Policies in the Workplace

Growing numbers of companies are adopting policies designed to protect unborn children by excluding women of childbearing age from exposure to certain workplace hazards. Rigorous implementation of fetal-protection policies could close more than 20 million jobs to women.[52] Although such policies are ostensibly intended to prevent the birth of children with severe and avoidable birth defects, I will argue that they are scientifically unjustifiable and they discriminate unfairly against women workers.

The Scientific Evidence

The scientific case for excluding women is ambiguous at best. It rests partly on the unexamined assumption that the fetus is uniquely susceptible to injury from hazardous workplace exposures, or that it is susceptible at lower exposure levels than those that would threaten adult workers. Review of the scientific literature, however, suggests that adverse health effects of toxic chemicals are rarely confined to the fetus.[53] Substances that are teratogenic (causing defects in the developing fetus) are also often mutagenic (causing mutations in cells, including sperm and ova) and carcinogenic. It is likely that workplace exposures will be as harmful to adults as to a fetus. Banning or severely limiting substances found to be teratogenic would protect all workers, instead of denying employment to one class of workers—namely, women.

Interestingly enough, precisely this approach *has* been taken—when the substance has been found to be harmful to men. For example, in 1977, male workers at an Occidental Chemical Company plant in California reported an unusually low birth rate in their familes. Subsequent testing showed that fourteen of twenty-five tested men were either sterile or had extremely low sperm counts. All of the affected men had worked with the pesticide dibromochloropropane (DBCP). Subsequently, DBCP was banned for almost all uses, based on the human data regarding low and zero sperm counts, on animal test data showing that DBCP was carcinogenic, and on laboratory studies showing that DBCP caused heritable genetic damage.

It is instructive to contrast the response to DBCP with the approach to lead. Lead has been connected with increased frequency of spontaneous abortions and stillbirths, neurologic defects, intrauterine growth retardation, and postnatal failure to thrive.[54] As a result, the Lead Industries Association has publicly opposed the employment of fertile women since 1974.[55] However, exposure to lead by *both* men and women workers can pose a risk to the fetus. In 1978, the Occupational Safety and Health Administration (OSHA) examined the health effects of workplace exposure to lead. It concluded that exposure to lead can cause genetic damage in the egg *or* sperm cells prior to conception. The result of this genetic damage could be failure to implant, miscarriage, stillbirth, or birth defects. The singling out of women workers in fetal-protection policies seems to reflect unconscious sexism, rather than a rational attempt to protect the unborn.[56] Joan Bertin notes:

> These and other examples reveal starkly the problem of selective vision in acknowledging workplace health hazards: hazards are often ignored or minimized, except when they involve female aspects of reproduction. . . . [C]hemicals that are particularly harmful to men (i.e., DBCP, kepone) have been banned, while women have been barred from working around chemicals suspected to cause fetal harm. These patterns once again reinforce the notion that the workplace must accommodate the needs of men, but not women, and that society requires and benefits from the paid labor of men, but not that of women.[57]

Discrimination

Exclusionary policies are subject to Title VII of the Civil Rights Act of 1964 that prohibits employment discrimination on the basis of sex. The Pregnancy Discrimination Act of 1978, an amendment to Title VII, specifically forbids discrimination on the basis of pregnancy, childbirth, or related medical conditions. Policies that overtly discriminate between the sexes are known as "disparate-treatment" cases. Such policies are permissible only if gender is a "bona fide occupational qualification" (BFOQ). This very strict standard acknowledges that there are a few jobs that can be done only by men (e.g., male stripper) and a few that can be done only by women (e.g., wet nurse).

Sometimes the requirements for a job, while not directly based on gender, nevertheless exclude most women. These are known as "disparate-impact" cases. For example, few women would qualify for a job that required one to be over five feet ten inches. Such a requirement would be discriminatory, under Title VII, unless required by "business necessity," a less stringent standard than the BFOQ. Three tests must be met for a job requirement to count as a business necessity: the reason for the rule must be compelling; it must carry out a business purpose effectively; and there must be no acceptable alternative.[58]

Recently, a fetal-protection policy came before the courts in *UAW* v. *Johnson Controls, Inc.*[59] In 1982, Johnson Controls, Inc., a Milwaukee-based producer of automotive and specialty batteries, adopted a policy excluding "women with childbearing capacity" from high-lead-exposure positions in its battery division. It applied the policy to exclude all women under the age of seventy, unless they could produce medical documentation of infertility. The UAW and several other unions brought suit in the United States District Court for the Eastern District of Wisconsin, alleging that Johnson Controls' fetal-protection policy violated Title VII. The District Court granted summary judgment for the employer. (Summary judgment is a judgment granted without a formal trial, when it appears to the court that there is no genuine issue of fact, and the moving party is entitled to judgment as a matter of law.)

In a 7-to-4 decision, the Court of Appeals for the Seventh Circuit affirmed the judgment of the District Court. Adopting a "business necessity" standard, the court held that a fetal-protection policy will survive a Title VII challenge where there is substantial risk of harm to the fetus, the risk is transmitted only through women, and the plaintiff fails to present evidence of an equally effective, less discriminatory alternative. Since the first two conditions are both factual matters about which there is considerable dispute, it is astonishing that the majority disposed of the matter by summary judgment.

The most critical dissent was filed by Judge Frank Easterbrook. He argued that Johnson Controls' policy constituted disparate treatment, necessitating a BFOQ defense. However, their policy could not satisfy the BFOQ standard, partly because the employer's concern for the welfare of unborn children was "unrelated to its ability to make batteries."[60] Furthermore, he noted that a BFOQ defense fails unless the employer shows that all or substantially all of the excluded women would be unable to perform their jobs safely and efficiently; but most women employees will not become pregnant or have children with birth defects caused by lead exposure.

Noting that many substances and activities pose potential hazards to the unborn, Judge Easterbrook argued that assessments of acceptable risk should be made by women themselves: "No legal or ethical principle compels or allows Johnson to assume that women are less able than men to make intelligent decisions about the welfare of the next generation, that the interests of the next generation always trump the interests of the living woman, and that the only acceptable level of risk is zero."[61]

On March 20, 1991, the Supreme Court ruled that Johnson's policy violated the Federal Civil Rights Act of 1964.[62] All nine justices agreed that fetal-protection policies would have to meet the BFOQ standard, and that the Court of Appeals was mistaken in permitting the less rigorous defense of "business necessity." The Court was divided over whether fetal-protection policies could ever be justified under the law, with three justices suggesting that a more narrowly tailored version of the Johnson Controls policy could be upheld. However, the majority, in a strongly worded opinion by Justice Harry A. Blackmun, declared that the Civil Rights Act prohibits all fetal-protection policies. Echoing Judge Easterbrook, Justice Blackmun said, "Decisions about the welfare of future children must be left to the parents who conceive, bear, support, and raise them rather than to the employers who hire those parents."

The objection may be made that companies adopt fetal-protection policies not primarily to protect future children, but to avoid liability. Certainly, it would be unfair both to require companies to hire fertile women, and to expose them to liability for doing so. Justice Blackmun dismissed this risk, saying that as long as an employer fully informs a woman of a given risk, "the basis for holding an employer liable seems remote at best." It may be responded that it is expensive for companies to have to defend themselves in court, even if they are not ultimately held liable. However, when challenged, companies that have exclusionary policies are frequently unable to cite a single instance in which a lawsuit has been brought by a damaged child against its mother's employer. This may be because it is extremely difficult to prove that the damage to the child was caused by exposure to toxins in the workplace, and not by any other environmental or genetic factor.[63] In any event, most suits to date alleging reproductive damage have been brought by *men,* who are virtually never the targets of exclusionary policies.[64]

The threat of potential liability does not justify discrimination. Joan Bertin gives the following advice to employers:

... an employer's best protection is to prevent foreseeable injury. The employer who conscientiously monitors the workplace environment, informs employees fully, abates known hazards, and when necessary offers voluntary transfer without loss of pay or benefits will be best insured against an adverse judgment. The law does not require an employer to have a crystal ball—only to be prudent and diligent. No less should be expected from those whose profit-making activities expose others to potential hazards.[65]

Compulsory Medical Treatment of Pregnant Women

Advances in medical technology have enabled doctors to diagnose fetal disorders and sometimes even treat the fetus while still *in utero*. Doctors have treated fetuses with medications, given blood transfusions, implanted shunts, and removed fetuses for minor surgery on their bladders.[66] A dramatic breakthrough occurred in June 1989, when the first successful major surgery on a fetus was performed.[67] The fetus had a diaphragmatic hernia, a fairly common and usually fatal congenital malformation. His stomach, spleen, and large and small intestines had migrated through a hole in the diaphragm, taking up so much space that his lungs could not grow, making it impossible for him to breathe. His parents, Rick and Beth Schultz, were told by a specialist in Detroit that they had three options: end the pregnancy, attempt surgery after birth (which is successful in only about 25 percent of cases), or try experimental fetal surgery. They were referred to Dr. Michael R. Harrison, head of a team of surgeons at the University of California at San Francisco that had successfully performed the operation on baby lambs and fetal monkeys but had never been successful with human fetuses. After talking to Dr. Harrison on the phone and learning of the risks, the Schultzes opted for the prenatal surgery.[68]

With mother and fetus both under anesthesia, Dr. Harrison made an incision in the uterus, drained the amniotic fluid, and exposed the fetus's left arm and side. He cut into the fetus's abdomen and moved the stomach and intestines back into the abdominal cavity. Then he stitched a patch of synthetic Gore-Tex fabric over the hole in the diaphragm. A second patch was placed on the outside of the abdomen to relieve any pressure on the developing organs, and the fetus was returned to the womb. Beth spent the next six weeks in bed, to minimize the danger of a miscarriage. On August 5, 1989, Blake Schultz was delivered by cesarean section, through the same incision made for the surgery. He had to spend three weeks on a respirator in the hospital, but is now at home, growing and developing normally.[69]

The Schultzes are full of gratitude toward Dr. Harrison. Nevertheless, the surgery raises ethical questions. The risks to the mother—two cesarean operations, daily ingestion of a drug to prevent labor, and the danger of uterine rupture—are considerable, while there was no guarantee of a successful outcome for the fetus. Before Dr. Harrison's success with Blake Schultz, he had had six failures.

Less dramatic, but equally ethically problematic, are situations when the lifesaving procedure is standard medical practice. Surgeons are unlikely to pressure a patient to consent to experimental surgery; quite the reverse. However, when a commonly performed procedure (such as cesarean section) poses little risk to the woman (or even reduces maternal mortality or morbidity), and may be the only way to secure live birth, physicians may feel an obligation to the fetus to act as its advocate, and to get the woman to consent to lifesaving surgery. Admittedly, refusal in such circumstances is rare. Most women, faced with the possibility of fetal damage or death, readily consent to the treatment their doctors recommend. Nancy Rhoden comments, "The vast majority of women will accept significant risk, pain, and inconvenience to give their babies the best chance possible. One obstetrician who performs innovative fetal surgery stated that most of the women he sees 'would cut off their heads to save their babies.' "[70] Occasionally, however, a woman rejects a physician's recommendation, perhaps on religious grounds, perhaps because she does not think that surgery is necessary, or perhaps because she is afraid of surgery. The courts have long held that competent adults may refuse lifesaving medical treatment. But does the right to refuse treatment for oneself include a right to refuse treatment necessary to save another's life? These cases pose agonizing dilemmas for physicians. Rhoden says, "They pit a woman's right to privacy and bodily integrity . . . against the possibility of a lifetime of devastating disability to a being who is within days or even hours of independent existence."[71]

With a few notable exceptions,[72] most commentators have argued that pregnant women should not be forced to undergo medical treatment for the sake of preserving the life or health of their fetuses.[73] Attitudes among practicing physicians seem to be more split. A study published in 1987 found considerable support among heads of fellowship programs in maternal-fetal medicine for legal intervention of various kinds into the management of pregnancy. Almost half of those surveyed supported involuntary detention of pregnant women whose behavior endangers their fetuses. About the same number thought that the precedents set by the courts for emergency cesareans should be expanded to include other procedures, such as intrauterine tranfusion, as these become part of standard medical care.[74]

Sometimes doctors, faced with a refusal, do not resort to the courts, but simply treat without consent. In one case, the placenta of a woman in labor detached prematurely from the inner wall of the uterus (a condition known as abruptio placentae), presenting an imminent threat to fetal survival. The mother repeatedly refused to give consent to a cesarean section, and the attending physicians felt that there was no time to attempt to secure a court order. Despite her refusal of consent, she did not actively resist when given general anesthesia. The physicians then delivered a severely stressed but otherwise healthy infant by cesarean section.[75]

The temptation simply to ignore the mother's refusal is understandable. Doctors are naturally reluctant to stand by and watch a baby who would be fine if delivered surgically die, or perhaps worse, suffer profound neurological damage. If they turn out to be right—the baby's life is saved and it is clear that the baby would have died if they had not operated—it seems harsh to blame them. If the woman herself is later glad that the doctors ignored her refusal, if she is *grateful* to them for having saved her life and that of her child, it does not seem that anyone else can say that they acted wrongly. Nevertheless, I will argue that these conditions cannot be guaranteed in advance, and therefore doctors are not morally justified in ignoring the refusals of competent patients.

It may seem that getting a court order puts doctors in a better ethical and legal position. The rights to privacy and bodily self-determination are not absolute. So it may be argued that doctors who take a patient to court act properly. They do not "take the law into their own hands," but instead give a judge the chance to decide whether there are compelling state interests that justify forced treatment. This ignores the reality of emergency decision-making in a medical setting. George Annas comments:

> Physicians should know what most lawyers and almost all judges know: When a judge arrives at the hospital in response to an emergency call, he or she is acting much more like a lay person than a jurist. Without time to analyze the issues, without representation for the pregnant woman, without briefing or thoughtful reflection on the situation, in almost total ignorance of the relevant law, and in an unfamiliar setting faced by a relatively calm physician and a woman who can easily be labeled "hysterical," the judge will almost always order whatever the doctor advises.[76]

A court order gives the misleading impression of a fair resolution, one that takes seriously the interests of both the woman and the fetus. In reality, the decision to summon a judge simply gives a legal veneer to the decision the doctors have already made.

Emergency cesarean sections

The justification for compelling a woman to have a surgical delivery is premised on the assumption that such a delivery is necessary to protect the health of the baby (and perhaps that of the mother as well). We may be skeptical of the claim of necessity in light of the skyrocketing rate of cesarean deliveries: from approximately 5 percent in the mid-1960s to more than 25 percent by 1988.[77] Experts estimate that more than half of the one million cesarean operations performed each year in the United States are unnecessary.[78] This means that there is a substantial chance that a woman compelled to accept a cesarean for the sake of the fetus will have been forced to undergo an unnecessary operation. And, in fact, in three of the first five cases in which court-ordered cesarean sections were sought, the women ultimately delivered vaginally—uneventfully.

In two cases, the women were diagnosed as having complete placenta previa. The facts in the only case officially reported[79] are these. Jessie Mae Jefferson was due to deliver in about four days when the hospital sought a court order authorizing physicians to perform a cesarean section and any necessary blood transfusions should she enter the hospital and refuse. She had previously notified the hospital that it was her religious belief that the Lord had healed her body and that whatever happened to the child was the Lord's will. At an emergency hearing at the hospital, her examining physician testified that she had complete placenta previa, with a 99 percent certainty that her child would not survive vaginal delivery and a 50 percent chance that she herself would not survive it. On this basis, the court decided that the unborn child merited legal protection and authorized the administration of all medical procedures deemed necessary by the attending physician to preserve the life of the defendant unborn child. The parents immediately petitioned the Georgia State Court to stay the order. The court denied their motion. A few days later, Mrs. Jefferson delivered a healthy baby without surgical intervention.[80]

In re *Baby Jeffries,* a Michigan case, also involved a woman diagnosed as having complete placenta previa. The police were sent to locate Mrs. Jeffries and bring her forcibly to the hospital. She went into hiding, and the police search for her was unsuccessful. She reportedly had a normal vaginal delivery without complications.[81]

In the third case, which occurred in New York City in 1982, the umbilical cord was wrapped around the fetus's neck. Judge Margaret Taylor went to visit the patient in the hospital to hear her side of the story. The woman's refusal of surgery was based on fear for her own health, a belief in "natural childbirth," and an intuition that the delivery (her tenth) would turn out fine. Unlike virtually all other judges in similar situations, Judge Taylor refused to grant the order, then spent "the worst two hours of my life," waiting for the child to be born. To the doctors', but not the mother's, surprise, the vaginal birth resulted in a healthy baby.[82]

Physician fallibility is only one reason why we should be reluctant to take the management of a pregnancy out of the woman's hands. Another reason is the increased risk to the woman from surgical delivery. Admittedly, cesarean sections are now relatively safe. Maternal mortality after cesarean section is extremely low, less than one per thousand, and usually is due to blood clots, infections, or the complications of anesthesia.[83] Nevertheless, cesarean section is major surgery, and, as such, is associated with higher rates of maternal mortality, morbidity, and increased pain than vaginal delivery. Overall, the risk of death from a cesarean is about four times that from vaginal delivery.[84] The question, then, is not simply whether the interests of the fetus should be considered, but how to weigh its interests against those of the pregnant woman. How much of a risk is she ethically and legally required to take with her own life and health to safeguard the life and health of her fetus?

In *Jefferson,* the Georgia Supreme Court cited *Roe* v. *Wade* as authority for a court-ordered cesarean.[85] This betrays a misunderstanding of *Roe* v. *Wade,* and subsequent abortion cases.

The Implications of Roe *v.* Wade

In *Roe* v. *Wade,* the Supreme Court held that the constitutional right of privacy, which protects a woman's decision to terminate a pregnancy, is not absolute. It can be balanced against other state interests, including the interest in protecting potential life. That "important and legitimate" state interest becomes "compelling" at viability, permitting states, if they choose, to prohibit abortions after viability, except when necessary to preserve the life or health of the mother. One commentator, noting that *Roe* v. *Wade* gives to the state "substantial authority to protect fetal life," concludes that this authority extends to non-abortion cases. John Myers writes:

> The state's interest in viable fetal life permits it to forbid abortion, an act designed to extinguish life. It follows from this that the state is empowered to proscribe other acts calculated or likely to lead to the same result. Furthermore, since the interest in preservation of fetal life authorizes intervention to prevent destructive acts, it should also authorize limited compulsion of action which is necessary to preserve fetal life.[86]

On this basis, Myers argues that the Georgia Supreme Court was correct in ordering a cesarean delivery in *Jefferson.* "The evidence was clear that fetal death would result unless the surgery was ordered. While maternal risk in cesarean delivery is not inconsequential, the certainty of fetal death outweighed that risk. . ."[87]

Ironically, in this case, there was no "certainty of fetal death." The surgery was not performed, the placenta previa corrected itself, and Mrs. Jefferson gave birth vaginally to a healthy baby girl. I am not suggesting that doctors should ignore clinical indications for cesarean deliveries because they *might* be wrong. Rather, the number of times the doctors who have sought compulsory cesareans *have* been wrong should make us examine more carefully their claims of knowledge. How accurate are their instruments for predicting that a cesarean is necessary for fetal well-being? Generally, diagnoses of placenta previa by ultrasonagraphy are exceptionally uncontroversial and accurate. Yet doctors can mistake a more benign partial placenta previa for a complete one, or the placental position may change between the time the sonogram was taken and delivery.

The most common fetal indication for surgical delivery is prediction of fetal distress, based upon electronic fetal monitoring (EFM). But fetal monitors have an astonishingly high false positive rate, due in part to the fact that the problem screened for—fetal hypoxia during labor of sufficient severity to cause fetal damage—occurs only rarely in a population of healthy, normal women. As the incidence of a condition decreases in frequency, it becomes increasingly likely that positive diagnoses are really false positives. Professor Rhoden comments:

> Given the low prevalence of the problems EFM seeks to detect, it is not surprising that randomized controlled trials of the effectiveness of universal use of EFM show either no impact on perinatal mortality or an extremely small impact . . . In studies assessing the correlation between abnormal fetal heart rate patterns and low Apgar scores, the rate of false positives from EFM has ranged from 18.5% to almost 80% . . . According to the Office of Technology Assessment, even when EFM and fetal scalp blood sampling are used together, the false positive rate is 44%.[88]

Rhoden adds that EFM requires sophisticated and knowledgeable interpretation, and that doctors do not always agree about the interpretation of abnormal heart patterns. Finally, the risk of a brain-damaged child and a multimillion-dollar lawsuit may incline doctors to opt for surgery even when the need for it is questionable.

The upshot of a policy of allowing doctors to take whatever steps they believe to be necessary to protect the fetus is an increase in maternal risk. Myers thinks that this is justified so long as the risk to the fetus from not performing the operation is greater than the risk to the woman from performing it. Several commentators[89] have argued that this sort of "trade-off" between maternal and fetal health is precisely what *Roe* v. *Wade* and subsequent abortion decisions do not permit. For example, in *Colautti* v. *Franklin*,[90] the Supreme Court invalidated a Pennsylvania statute requiring that after viability doctors use the method least likely to harm the fetus unless an alternative was necessary to preserve the woman's life or health. The Court held that by using the word "necessary," Pennsylvania impermissibly implied that a different technique must be *indispensable* for the woman's health. This flaw was compounded by the failure to "clearly specify . . . that the woman's life and health must always prevail over the fetus's life and health when they conflict."[91] Rhoden observes that this means that a woman cannot be compelled to undergo an even slightly greater risk for the sake of the viable fetus. The Court again upheld this principle in *Thornburgh*.[92] The Court struck down Pennsylvania's amended statute on the ground that it, like the old statute, "failed to require that maternal health be the paramount consideration."[93] Nelson, Buggy, and Weil summarize the Court's position: "Even though the state's interest in protecting fetal life becomes compelling at viability, this interest is *not* sufficiently compelling under the Constitution to support a statutory requirement that the mother bear *any* increased risk to her health in order to save her viable fetus."[94]

McFall *v.* Shimp and the Duty to Rescue

The principle that pregnant women should not be compelled to undergo any additional risks for the sake of the unborn, even after viability, can be given an equal protection basis. Outside pregnancy, there are virtually no circumstances in which the body of one person could be required to save the life of another. One famous case is *McFall* v. *Shimp*,[95] in which Robert McFall, who was dying of aplastic anemia, asked the court to order his cousin, David Shimp, the only family member with potentially compatible bone marrow, to donate bone marrow to him. Bone-marrow extraction is not an especially risky procedure—far less risky than major surgery—but it is painful and invasive. Shimp apparently believed that the medical risk to him was greater than his cousin's doctors assessed it. On a balancing-interests approach, McFall's interest in survival might well outweigh Shimp's interests in avoiding pain and minimal risk. The court rejected this approach. Although the court found Shimp's behavior to be morally reprehensible, it refused to order him to donate. The court emphasized that there was no legal duty to rescue others, and stated that to require this would change every concept and principle upon which our society is founded. The court said:

> For a society which respects the rights of *one* individual, to sink its teeth into the jugular vein or neck of one of its members and suck from it

sustenance for *another* member, is revolting to our hard-wrought concepts of jurisprudence. Forceable extraction of living body tissue causes revulsion to the judicial mind. Such would raise the spectre of the swastika and the Inquisition, reminiscent of the horrors this portends.[96]

McFall and Shimp were only cousins, but there is no doubt that the outcome would have been the same even had they been father and child. Angela Holder states, "In no case is an adult ever ordered to surrender a kidney, bone marrow, or any other part of his body for donation to his child, to another relative, or to anyone else."[97] In fact, it is doubtful that a parent could be legally compelled to donate a pint of blood necessary to save his or her child's life.

The case of minor children is slightly different, since they are often not capable of giving consent. This is not necessarily a bar to donation, since some courts have allowed parents to authorize an incompetent sibling to donate a kidney to a sibling suffering from renal failure, using a substituted judgment basis.[98] Other courts have rejected the claim that the test is whether the incompetent would consent to donate if he could do so, and have simply refused to authorize the transplant on the grounds that it is not in the best interest of the incompetent.[99] While courts have disagreed about whether parents may *authorize* donation on behalf of minor children, there is agreement that such authorization cannot be *compelled*. In a recent case, Tamas Bosze, a Chicago bar owner, was told that only a marrow transplant could save his son, Jean-Pierre, from dying of leukemia. The boy's only potential donors were twin half-siblings born out of wedlock to the father's former girlfriend. Bosze sued the woman in an attempt to compel her to have the children tested for tissue compatibility. She refused, on the ground that this would not be in the twins' best interest. A court upheld her decision. In so doing, the court upheld the principle that no one is legally required to donate a body part to another, not even when this is needed to save a life. (Shortly thereafter Jean-Pierre Bosze died.[100]) As we saw in Chapter 2, individuals may not be legally compelled to be "good Samaritans." This principle of our legal system must be remembered in assessing compulsory cesareans. To force women to undergo major surgery, even relatively safe major surgery, is to impose an unequal and unjustified burden on pregnant women. Even if we accept—as I do— the premise that women have *moral* obligations to the children they plan to bear, and even if these moral obligations include undergoing risks and making sacrifices to secure the health and well-being of the children they have decided to bear, it is quite another matter to think that these moral obligations should be legally coerced. I think we can agree that it would be appallingly selfish for a woman to expose her nearly born baby to the risk of an irreversible handicap simply to avoid an abdominal scar. But even in such a case, the woman should not be legally compelled to undergo surgery.

The above argument is based on the injustice of imposing burdens on pregnant women that are not imposed on other people. But what if the burdens were not unequally imposed? Would the state be justified in legally compelling all citizens, men and women, to undergo bodily risk and invasion where necessary to save a life? The answer to this question depends on one's general political outlook. Those who lean toward a more libertarian perspective will be opposed to "Good Samaritan" laws in general, and find the idea of compulsory donation of bodily parts especially repellent. Those who take a more communitarian approach may argue that all members of a community have a duty to make sacrifices for the good of the whole. For example, requiring healthy adults to make occasional blood donations might be considered justifiable. Communitarians might also argue that women should be legally compelled to undergo cesarean sections, where this is necessary to spare the child lifelong disability or death, given the relatively small objective risk to the woman and the enormous benefit to the child.

I cannot undertake a full-scale treatment of the merits of these opposing political theories. Fortunately, this is not necessary. Even communitarians should oppose compulsory cesareans, because, whether or not they could be justified in theory, there are overwhelming practical objections to them. For example, most doctors, even those who favor legal intervention in some cases, balk at using physical force to perform the surgery.[101] However, the potential for physical compulsion is implicit in legal coercion. Doctors who seek court orders should think about what they are willing to do to ensure that these are carried out. Francis Kenner, a Colorado woman who was told during labor that she needed a cesarean because of fetal distress, became more cooperative after the judge ordered a cesarean section. This was fortunate because, as her physician noted, "had the patient steadfastly refused it might not have been either safe or possible to administer anesthesia to a struggling, resistant woman who weighed in excess of 157.5 kg."[102] George Annas asks, "Do we really want to restrain, forcibly medicate, and operate on a competent, refusing adult? Such a procedure may be 'legal,' especially when viewed from the judicial perspective that the woman is irrational, hysterical, or evil-minded, but it is certainly brutish and not what one generally associates with medical care."[103]

In re *A.C.*

Perhaps the most brutish example of a forced cesarean was one performed on a dying woman in June 1987. Angela Carder (known as "A.C." in the court papers) was approximately 25 weeks pregnant, when she learned that the cancer she had had as a teenager, and had thought was in remission, had reoccurred. On Thursday, June 11, she was admitted to George Washington University Hospital. At first, the doctors were guardedly optimistic about her condition. Angela had repeatedly done better than expected in her long battle with cancer. She had been told at the age of thirteen that she had only a few years to live. So, on Friday, June 12, the possibility of participating in a new NIH chemotherapy protocol was discussed. But by the following Monday, it seemed that Angela's condition was terminal. Her long-term-care physician, Dr. Jeffrey Moscow from the National Institutes of Health, told Angela that this time she should not expect a cure or have hope for "long-term survival." Angela agreed to palliative radiation and/or chemotherapy to relieve her pain and to try to reach 28 weeks in her pregnancy, at which time the fetus's chances of viability would be greatly increased.

Angela's health rapidly deteriorated, and by Monday evening, she was transferred to the intensive-care unit and intubated (had a tube placed in her airway to help her breathe). The next morning, her condition worsened. She was in a great deal of pain. A priest was called to give the last rites. Her husband, parents, and doctors all agreed that keeping Angela comfortable while she died was what she wanted, and that her wishes should be honored.

On Tuesday morning, George Washington University, through its general counsel, Vincent Burke, asked a local trial judge to come to the hospital to decide what, if any, interventions should be performed on behalf of the fetus. Judge Emmett Sullivan of the District of Columbia Superior Court summoned volunteer lawyers, and convened an emergency hearing in the hospital. According to Nettie Stoner, Angela's mother, they were called from Angela's bedside to a "short meeting." They were not told that it was a court hearing, nor that it would take them away from their daughter all day.

Much of the hearing was an attempt to determine what Angela's wishes with regard to the pregnancy were. Angela was at that point heavily sedated in order to maintain her ventilatory function, and was unable to carry on a meaningful conversation. Angela's attending physician, Louis Hamner, testified that the night before, when Angela was alert and awake, she had agreed to have a cesarean section at 28 weeks. Her doctors did not think an earlier cesarean section would be advisable. "Much prior to that, the prognosis was poor enough that we would be extremely uncomfortable intervening."[104]

Angela's doctors did not think that her fetus was viable. This was based partly on its gestational age, but also on Angela's condition. Asked what the prognosis would be for the fetus if the court ordered intervention, Dr. Hamner replied that, generally, fetuses at 26 weeks have between 50 and 60 percent chance of survival. However, because this fetus had been exposed to multiple medication, its chances for survival were lower.[105]

Dr. Maureen Edwards, a neonatologist and Director of Nurseries at GWU Hospital, was more optimistic. Acknowledging that it was very difficult to give a prognosis for a particular neonate or fetus, Dr. Edwards nevertheless projected a 50 to 60 percent chance of survival for the fetus, and only a 20 percent chance of serious handicap. However, Dr. Edwards had not examined Angela and apparently had no specific knowledge of the condition of the fetus, nor any knowledge of the medicines to which the fetus had been exposed. Despite this, Judge Sullivan accepted her prognosis for the fetus over that of Angela's doctors.

According to Dr. Hamner, Angela understood that premature delivery has an increased risk of cerebral palsy, neurological defects, hearing loss, and blindness. It was his belief that Angela, having gone through so much illness and pain in her own life, did not want to bring a baby into the world who would have to undergo these problems. The guardian *ad litem* for the fetus, Barbara Mishkin, argued that such quality-of-life considerations were not a determining factor in deciding what medical care should be provided to the so-called Baby Does, and so "the possible disability of this particular baby ought not to be a determining factor here."[106] Ms. Mishkin argued that this case did not pose the problem of choosing between the life of the mother and the life of the fetus, because the life of the mother was already lost. At the same time, the state has an obligation as *parens patriae* to protect the life of a viable fetus: "Even in *Roe* v. *Wade* where the mother does have the possibility of making the decisions, the mother's decision-making on that score ceases at the point of viability, and we are beyond that point now, so my sense is that this is not a question of the woman's right to refuse treatment. This is the question of the state's obligation to protect this baby."[107]

Angela's lawyer, Robert Sylvester, protested that the mother's right to her choices and privacy doesn't cease with viability. He cited *Colautti* and *Thornburgh* as establishing the principle that maternal health must be the physicians' primary consideration. To perform a cesarean on Angela in her very weakened state, he said, would be in effect to terminate her life. The judge acknowledged that the performance of a cesarean might very well hasten Angela's death, but noted that she was not expected to live another twenty-four to forty-eight hours anyway. The decision was a difficult one, but, given the choices, he concluded that the fetus should be given an opportunity to live.

Dr. Hamner went to Angela's bedside, and found her arousable. He told her about the proceedings and the judge's ruling, and asked her would she consent to a cesarean section to save the baby even though it might shorten her life. Her answer was yes. This conversation was reported to the court. Dr. Hamner went back to Angela's room to verify his previous discussion with her. This time he made it clear that *he* would not perform the operation without her consent, but that it would be done in any case. Because of the tube in her windpipe, Angela was unable to speak, but she mouthed very clearly several times, "I don't want it done."[108]

Her lawyer suggested that the judge's decision should be amended to show that there was now an utterance from Angela that she did not want the procedure done. Despite testimony from Dr. Weingold that Angela was responding, understanding, and capable of making decisions, the fact that Angela had given unexplained contradictory responses within a short period of time was taken by Ms. Mishkin to indicate either that Angela was not capable of making a reasoned or competent decision, or that she had been unduly influenced by her husband and mother. It was suggested that she may have been trying to spare her mother, who is in a wheelchair, from raising a baby she did not want. Mrs. Stoner had testified that she would never put the baby up for adoption, that she would do the best she could, "but we don't want it. Angela wanted that baby. It was her baby. Let that baby die with her."[109]

Under the circumstances, Angela's change of mind does not seem evidence of "incompetence to decide." Anyone might veer back and forth, given such a terribly difficult decision. On the one hand, she wanted the baby very much, which would incline her toward taking all steps to ensure its survival. On the other hand, she had expected to give birth to a healthy baby whom she and her husband would raise. Now she was being asked whether she was willing to submit to surgery that might shorten her life, and would certainly increase her suffering, in order to give birth to an extremely premature, potentially severely handicapped infant, whom she would not survive, and whom others would have to raise. These factors might understandably have led her to change her mind regarding the cesarean.

Judge Sullivan maintained that he was unsure what Angela really wanted. Yet he never went to Angela's bedside to find out what she wanted. He said that he did not do so out of fear of worsening her condition, which is ironic, in view of his willingness to order a procedure that he recognized had the potential to shorten her life.

Despite professions of not knowing what Angela really wanted, the attorneys for the hospital, fetus, and District of Columbia said that it could be assumed that she did not want the cesarean performed. As Richard Love, assistant corporation counsel for the District of Columbia, conceded, "I don't think we would be here if she had said she wants it."[110] However, this did not matter, since they did not regard Angela's wishes as determinative anyway. The fact that her death was imminent and the fetus was viable was sufficient, they argued, to establish a compelling state interest that could override the patient's wishes.

Angela's lawyer made a last attempt to get the District of Columbia Court of Appeals to block the order as she was being wheeled into surgery. A hearing was held over the telephone, under extremely adverse conditions. All parties were not in the same room to use the phone. There was difficulty hearing because of outside noises from traffic, hospital personnel coming in and out, and so forth. In fact, the scene was precisely what George Annas had predicted would occur under such conditions in an article that appeared in the *New England Journal of Medicine* only a month before.[111] The three judges hearing the matter were unfamiliar with the relevant law, as became evident when Elizabeth Symonds, representing the American Civil Liberties Reproductive Freedom Project, cited *Thornburgh* and *Colautti* in support of the claim that the state has no authority to impose any regulations that would increase the risk to the woman's life and health.

> JUDGE NEBEKER: The authority you first rely on, is that decision in the factual context of this case?
> MS. SYMONDS: They were in abortion context. I believe the—
> JUDGE NEBEKER: It's critical we know that. I thank you for telling us. With the time constraints, we don't have the time to start reading.[112]

The court denied the request for a stay, allowing the hospital to go ahead with the operation. The baby, Lindsay Marie Carder, died approximately two and a half hours later. (Despite this, the guardian *ad litem* for the fetus continued in subsequent briefs to insist that the fetus was "viable." Apparently, she considers a fetus to be viable if it survives birth for any period of time, no matter how brief. This seems a bizarre interpretation of viability.) Two days later, Angela died. The surgery was listed as a "contributing factor."[113]

On November 10, 1987, a three-judge panel of the District of Columbia Court of Appeals upheld the emergency order. The panel said that the general principle that the state ordinarily may not infringe upon the mother's right to bodily integrity did not apply because "she had, at best, two days left of sedated life; the complications arising from the surgery would not significantly alter that prognosis. The child, on the other hand, had a chance of surviving delivery. . ."[114]

Was it certain that Angela would definitely die within a few days? Her cancer specialist, Dr. Moscow, did not agree with this extremely pessimistic prognosis. He had recommended that Angela receive radiation and chemotherapy, because he thought that she had a chance of partial remission, and possibly a few more months of life. Dr. Moscow was not even informed of the June 16 hearing, and so had no opportunity to testify as to her condition. But even if it were true that Angela had only hours to live, it was her life, and her decision. As George Annas pungently observes:

> [The judges] treated a live woman as though she were already dead, forced her to undergo an abortion, and then justified their brutal and unprincipled opinion on the basis that she was almost dead and her fetus's interests in life outweighed any interest she might have in her own life or health. This is what happens when judges (and hospital lawyers that call them) forget what judging is all about and combine rescue fantasy with dehumanization of the dying.[115]

This egregious judicial error was corrected on March 21, 1988, when in response to a request from forty organizations, including the American Civil Liberties Union, the American Medical Association, and the American College of Obstetricians and Gynecologists, a three-judge panel of the District of Columbia Court of Appeals vacated the order. Without comment, the judges announced that the full court would hear new arguments at a later hearing.

The full court issued its opinion April 26, 1990. It agreed with the vacating of the order of the trial court on the ground that the judge had improperly used a balancing analysis, weighing the rights of A.C. against the interests of the state. Instead he should have determined whether A.C. was competent to refuse the surgery. If she was, then it should not have been performed. "[T]he right to bodily integrity is not extinguished simply because someone is ill, or even at death's door."[116] If she was incompetent, or the court was unable to determine competency, then her wishes should have been determined through the substituted judgment procedure.

Citing *McFall* v. *Shimp*, Judge John A. Terry, who wrote the majority opinion for the court, stated that courts do not compel one person to permit a significant bodily intrusion upon his or her bodily integrity for the benefit of another person's health: "Even though Shimp's refusal would mean death for McFall, the court would not order Shimp to allow his body to be invaded. . . . a fetus cannot have rights in this respect superior to those of a person who has already been born."[117] The court declined to specify whether, or under what circumstances, the state's interests can ever prevail over the interests of a pregnant patient. "We do not quite foreclose the possibility that a conflicting state interest may be so compelling that the patient's wishes must yield, but we anticipate that such cases will be extremely rare and truly exceptional. This is not such a case."[118]

Less Invasive Cases

Carder makes it clear that the state cannot force a woman against her will to undergo a cesarean section, even to save a viable fetus. What about less invasive procedures, such as blood transfusions? Jehovah's Witnesses refuse transfusions, based on their religious conviction that this is forbidden by the Bible.[119] They believe that anyone who "eats" blood will be deprived of the opportunity for everlasting life and the resurrection of the body.

It is difficult for non-Witnesses to understand the opposition to blood transfusions. No other "People of the Book" interpret the relevant passages of the Bible as do Jehovah's Witnesses. However, the reasonableness of their belief is irrelevant. As Justice Warren Burger said in his dissent in *Georgetown,* the right to refuse treatment is not limited to "*sensible* beliefs, *valid* thoughts, *reasonable* emotions, or *well-founded* sensations."[120]

Does *pregnancy* change the moral and legal situation of Jehovah's Witnesses? The pregnant Witness exposes not merely herself, but also her unborn child, to the risk of death. In numerous cases, courts have held that the right to practice religion freely does not include liberty to expose children to ill health or death. The Supreme Court has said, "Parents may be free to become martyrs themselves. But it does not follow they are free . . . to make martyrs of their children."[121] There are numerous cases of court-ordered blood transfusions for children of Jehovah's Witnesses.[122] In fact, not only may courts override the decisions of parents who withhold necessary medical treatment from their children out of religious conviction, but the parents may be subject to criminal charges.[123] If courts can override parental refusal of treatment for born children, may they do the same for nearly born fetuses?

A transfusion is far less risky and invasive than a cesarean section. For this reason, some who are opposed to compulsory cesareans are willing to accept court-ordered transfusions. Neonatologist Alan Fleischman holds that

". . . it is acceptable for physicians to bring pressure to bear on the woman to accept the procedure, including the coercive step of seeking court adjudication. However, coercive measures should stop short of physically restraining or forcibly sedating a woman who continues to refuse treatment despite a court order that grants physicians permission to override her refusal."[124] Dr. Fleischman's coauthor, philosopher Ruth Macklin, would allow persuasive efforts, emotional appeals, and other noncoercive means to convince a woman to accept a low-risk medical procedure for the sake of her fetus, but she holds it unacceptable to invoke the force of law to override her refusal.

How should we decide between these two positions? One factor is the value we place on autonomy, understood here as the right of competent adults to make decisions about their own bodies and medical treatment. Macklin seems to be advocating an absolutist position on the value of autonomy, while Fleischman is willing to balance autonomy against other important values, such as the life and health of the nearly born fetus. However, it is not entirely clear that respecting a person's refusal of treatment necessarily upholds his or her autonomy. It depends on the reasons for refusing treatment. In some of the cases involving Jehovah's Witnesses, there is evidence that the patients wanted the transfusions necessary to save their lives, but felt that they could not consent to them, on religious grounds. A court order allows them to have the transfusion they fervently desire without consenting to it. Some Witnesses apparently feel that the responsibility is therefore out of their hands, and thus does not violate their religion.[125] Since their refusal is not fully autonomous, a court order overriding the refusal does not necessarily violate the patient's autonomy.[126]

A comparable situation may occur when a woman belongs to a religious sect opposed to cesarean delivery. Mary Jo O'Sullivan, professor of obstetrics and gynecology at the University of Miami School of Medicine, relates the following incident: "The baby's head was way too large. Without a c-section the only way to get the baby out would be to wait until it died and take it apart, piece by piece. I just couldn't do that. Nor was anyone else at the hospital willing to do it."[127] Dr. O'Sullivan finally got a court order authorizing a cesarean, but she was still uncomfortable about forcing surgery. "To my surprise, when I showed the patient the court order, she seemed relieved that the decision was out of her hands."

Despite the desirable outcome in this case, Dr. Nancy Milliken disagrees with Dr. O'Sullivan's decision. "Individuals can't have it both ways," she says. "We can't say: we want the right to make our own health care decisions and then turn around and expect the doctor to *make us* do what's good for us."[128] Not only does this expectation put doctors in the untenable position of having to figure out whether the patient means what she says, it also sets a dangerous precedent. Doctors, already convinced that they know what's *best* for the patient, may delude themselves as to what the patient "really wants." Less articulate and assertive patients may be forced to undergo procedures that violate their deepest religious beliefs. A woman in labor and weak from loss of blood may be in no condition physically to resist a blood transfusion. How are we to tell whether her refusal is authentic or not? What safeguards can we devise to ensure that her autonomy is not being violated? Ultimately, the criterion of interpretation will be "doctor knows best." Thus, I am led, somewhat reluctantly, to conclude that even if, in the particular case, a court order would not be coercive or violative of autonomy, physicians are not in a position to know this in general. For this reason, doctors should not be encouraged to second-guess the refusals of their competent patients.

As the degree of invasiveness decreases, the argument for intervention becomes stronger. What if the fetus can be protected from serious mental and physical handicap by simply compelling its mother to swallow a vitamin pill? Should our respect for maternal autonomy be absolute and unconditional? Can the risk to the unborn ever outweigh the woman's right to refuse treatment? In considering this question, two things should be kept in mind. First, in the vast majority of cases, the pregnant patient wants to give birth to a healthy baby, and will cooperate with her obstetrician. Where she refuses, she may have good reasons, even if they are not reasons that are acceptable to her doctor. Only rarely is noncooperation due to stubbornness or silliness or indifference to the welfare of the baby. Second, it is important to realize in such cases that legal coercion is not the only method of protecting the not-yet-born child. Other professionals may be brought in, to make sure the woman understands the full implications of her decision for her baby. Often a more creative approach on the part of health care providers will enable a resolution acceptable to all.[129]

Respect for autonomy is only one reason against a coercive approach. In addition, court orders can have a destructive effect on the physician–patient relationship.[130] Moreover, as John Robertson and Joseph Schulman point out in their discussion of pregnant women with phenylketonuria (PKU), coercive measures may offer little protection to the not-yet-born child.[131] The measures most likely to benefit the nearly born fetus, such as court-ordered cesareans, are also the most invasive and violative of the woman's right to bodily integrity. Less invasive measures, such as the restrictive PKU diet, are more easily justifiable, but difficult to impose without the consent and cooperation of the pregnant woman. Thus, although coercive measures might be justified where the risk to the woman is very low and the benefit to the baby very great, such cases are virtually non-existent. The most desirable approach, as Robertson and Schulman correctly conclude, and the one that should be taken in all but the most rare and exceptional cases, is "education, counseling, and assuring access to treatment."[132]

5 | Fetal Research

In the preceding chapters, the discussion of the embryo and fetus has been primarily in the context of *pregnancy*, where the moral and legal situation is importantly affected by the pregnant woman's interests in privacy, bodily self-determination, and autonomy. How should we think about embryos and fetuses when they are not inside anyone's body? In particular, is it morally permissible to use extrauterine embryos and aborted fetuses for scientific and medical purposes?

The interest view maintains that embryos and preconscious fetuses do not have moral status. It might be thought that this settles—or preempts—the question of the morality of fetal research. If human embryos and fetuses lack moral status, then why not use them in scientific research, or indeed, for any other purpose? Does not the denial of moral standing mean that they are mere things, to be used or discarded as we see fit? This conclusion does not follow. The interest view denies moral status to nonsentient beings because, without feelings, thoughts, or awareness of any kind, a being cannot have interests of its own. It does not matter *to it* what happens to it, nor can anything be done for *its* sake. But, as I argued in Chapter 1, it does not follow from this that it does not matter how we treat nonsentient beings. The interest view denies *moral standing* to nonsentient beings, but it allows that they may have *moral value*. Nonsentient beings can have moral value if there are moral reasons why they ought to be preserved.

There is a tendency to think that if a being ought to be protected, not for merely instrumental reasons, such as its commercial value, but because its existence has moral value, then protection must be in the interests of the being in question. However, we can recognize the value of trees, mountains, lakes, and wilderness areas without either reducing that value to their commercial worth or ascribing *to them* an interest in continuing to exist (see Chapter 1). Similarly, the interest view is compatible with the existence of moral reasons not to desecrate corpses or burn flags. The fact that *we* may have reasons for protecting them does not imply that such protection is in *their* interest.

Like human corpses, human fetuses are human. Like trees, they are alive. Like flags, they have, for many people, symbolic significance. All of these features may give rise to moral reasons for treating or not treating them in certain ways. However, in thinking about fetal research, it is important to be clear about *why* certain things may or may not be done to fetuses. Otherwise, we are likely to ascribe to embryos and fetuses interests they do not have, and to apply to them principles that are applicable only to persons or other interested beings. The failure to recognize the distinction between moral status and moral value has led to confusion in thinking about fetal research, which could be clarified by adoption of the interest view.

The term "fetal research" may be applied broadly, to quite different procedures. I will confine discussion in this chapter to research involving the fetus proper, leaving the topic of embryo research, most of which is connected to *in vitro* fertilization, to Chapter 6. A second important distinction is between "therapeutic research," or research intended to benefit the subject, and "nontherapeutic research," which has no benefit for the subject of research, but which is intended to help others. Therapeutic research on the fetus is not research in the ordinary sense at all, but rather experimental therapy on the unborn. It is intended to benefit the future child, as opposed to the fetus per se. This can be seen from the fact that it would not even be attempted unless there were a reasonable chance of the fetus surviving birth. Therapeutic research on the fetus does not raise unique ethical issues, but rather those that are raised by any experimental therapy—namely, issues of risk and benefit, and informed consent. By contrast, nontherapeutic research raises the question of whether the fetus may be used as a research tool.

Even if we restrict ourselves to nontherapeutic research, it becomes immediately clear that one cannot discuss "the ethics of fetal research" in general. Different issues arise depending on whether we are talking about using tissue from a dead fetus for transplantation, or dissecting a live abortus of 28 weeks.

Section I provides a brief history of fetal research in the United States. Section II discusses the ethics of fetal-tissue transplantation. I begin with the scientific justification for fetal-tissue transplantation research. The scientific justification is logically prior to any ethical issues, since there would be no point to pursuing the research without good reason to believe it was likely to have significant clinical benefits. The major moral debate has been over whether fetal transplantation is "tainted" by the source of the tissue, elective abortion. Some maintain that the morality of abortion can be separated from the morality of using fetal tissue derived from abortions. Anti-abortionists maintain that research with fetuses aborted electively is "ethically compromised" by the lack of authentic informed consent, its complicity with the abortion, and the possibility that such research will encourage more abortions. I argue that the complicity argument cannot be as easily dismissed as its opponents have thought, and that the morality of fetal-tissue transplants cannot be completely disassociated from the morality of abortion.

Section III considers the ethics of research on living fetuses. The basic question here is whether human fetuses should be considered to be human subjects, deserving of all the protection given to other human subjects. I argue that it is a mistake to treat presentient fetuses as human subjects, for presentient fetuses, even living ones, cannot be harmed. Nevertheless, we may have all sorts of reasons for restricting research on the fetus. The reasons will not refer to the welfare of the fetus (since it does not have a welfare of its own), but rather to commonly held fundamental values, including respect for humanity. As a potential human being, the presentient fetus is a powerful symbol of human life. This is enough of a reason not to treat it as a mere commodity or convenient tool for research. At the same time, respect for humanity is not displayed when nonsentient fetuses are protected at the expense of the vital human interests of real people.[1] Moreover, the alternative to fetal research is usually research using animals, who clearly do have interests. It is difficult to justify an absolute ban on research using living, but nonsentient, fetuses, while permitting painful and lethal experiments on sentient animals.

I. FETAL RESEARCH IN AMERICA: HISTORY AND POLITICS

Since the early 1970s, there has been a moratorium on government-sponsored fetal research in the United States. The National Research Act in

1974 (Public Law 93–348) established within the then Department of Health, Education, and Welfare (HEW) a National Commission for the Protection of Human Subjects of Biomedical and Behavioral Research.[2] The first of the Commission's mandates was to review and report on research involving living fetuses. The 1974 Act placed a moratorium on fetal research until the National Commission made its recommendations to the Secretary of HEW.[3]

On July 25, 1975, the National Commission submitted its *Report and Recommendations: Research on the Fetus* to the Secretary of HEW, Caspar Weinberger. Among its recommendations were the following: nontherapeutic research on the pregnant woman may be conducted or supported, provided it will impose minimal or no risk to the fetus, the woman's informed consent has been obtained, and the father has not objected. Nontherapeutic research on the fetus *in utero,* whether or not abortion is anticipated, may be conducted or supported, provided the purpose of such research is the development of important biomedical knowledge that cannot be obtained by alternative means, there is minimal or no risk to the fetus, the informed consent of the mother has been obtained, and the father has not objected. Under the same conditions, nontherapeutic research directed toward the fetus during the abortion procedure or toward the nonviable fetus *ex utero* may be conducted or supported, provided also that the fetus is less than 20 weeks gestational age, no significant changes are made in the abortion procedure in the interest of research alone, and no attempt is made to alter the duration of the life of the fetus. Although its mandate was primarily research on the living fetus, the Commission recommended that use of tissue from dead fetuses be permitted, "consistent with local law, the Uniform Anatomical Gift Act, and commonly held convictions about respect for the dead." Finally, the *Report* called for an immediate lift of the moratorium.[4]

The Commission's recommendations were accepted almost without change, and published as federal regulations on August 8, 1975. Since then, very little if any federally funded nontherapeutic research has taken place. The reason is that the Ethics Advisory Board (EAB), which was recommended by the Commission to interpret its guidelines, was both slow getting started and short-lived. It was not chartered until 1977 and did not convene until 1978, three years after publication of the guidelines. This delay resulted in a continuation of the moratorium on federal funds for certain fetal research. The EAB reviewed only one proposal for fetal research before it was allowed to lapse by DHEW in September 1980. With no mechanism in place for national review, researchers stopped requesting federal support for fetal research, relying upon private funding.[5]

In 1985, Congress took new action on fetal research. The Health Research Extension Act (Public Law 99–158) defines the circumstances under which living human fetuses may be subjected to research:

> In the case of living human nonviable fetuses ex utero or living human fetuses for whom viability has not yet been determined, the Secretary may support only those research projects that (1) may enhance the well-being or meet the health needs of the fetus, (2) enhance the probability of the fetus' survival to viability, or (3) whose purpose is to develop important biomedical knowledge that cannot be obtained by other means and that will pose no added risk of suffering, injury, or death to the fetus. This standard is to apply equally to fetuses that are aborted spontaneously or by induced abortion.[6]

The Act also created a Biomedical Ethics Board (BEB), made up of six representatives and six senators (evenly divided between the two major parties), and a Biomedical Ethics Advisory Committee (BEAC), made up of fourteen people from a variety of fields, to be appointed by the BEB. "These bodies were instructed to report on human genetic engineering and on the federal rules on human fetal research; a moratorium was placed on federal support for fetal research pending completion of the latter report, which was due no later than May 20, 1988."[7] The legislation also gave the BEAC a third mandate, to report by May 4, 1990, on the ethics of administering nutrition and hydration to dying patients. However, the funds necessary to conduct the three mandated studies were never appropriated.

The debate in the United States over the use of tissue from aborted fetuses for transplantation began in 1987. The Director of the National Institutes of Health (NIH), James Wyngaarden, submitted a request to the Assistant Secretary for Health, Robert Windom, seeking approval to fund the transplantation of human fetal tissue into the brain of a patient with Parkinson's disease. Windom asked the NIH to establish a special advisory panel to study ten questions about fetal tissue research, and to make recommendations about whether such research should be approved. A moratorium on the use of fetuses from elective abortions in federally funded research was announced until the panel released its conclusions. However, less than a week before the twenty-one-member Human Tissue Fetal Transplant Research Panel created by the NIH was scheduled to begin its deliberations, the press published excerpts from a White House draft order that would ban all federally financed research using human fetal tissue from elective abortions. The draft order was prepared by Gary L. Bauer, assistant to President Reagan for policy development and a conservative aide known for his antiabortion stance. This attempt to preempt the panel's recommendations was met with outrage from scientists, bioethicists and others. The

White House backed down, saying that Bauer's draft was "a very first cut" that "does not represent Administration policy or a Presidential decision in any way." Spokesman Marlin Fitzwater told reporters it was still an open question whether there would be an executive order banning fetal-tissue research.[8]

The advisory panel submitted its report on December 5, 1988. It concluded that while it is "of moral relevance" that human fetal tissue for research has been obtained from induced abortions, "in light of the fact that abortion is legal, and that the research in question is intended to achieve significant medical goals, . . . the use of such tissue is acceptable public policy."[9] This conclusion was accepted by a vote of 18 to 3, and included the following recommendations: The decision to end a pregnancy and abortion procedures should be separated from the consent to use and the retrieval of fetal tissue; proper informed consent should be obtained from the pregnant woman; the pregnant woman should be prohibited from designating the recipient of fetal tissue; payments for the procurement of fetal tissue should be prohibited, except for reasonable expenses incurred by the institution, occasioned by the actual retrieval, storage, preparation, and transportation of the tissues; potential recipients of such fetal tissues, as well as researchers and health-care personnel, should be informed about the source of tissues; fetal tissues should be accorded the same respect as other cadaveric human tissues; and regardless of research needs or convenience, health of pregnant women should remain the principal concern in changing any abortion procedures.[10]

On December 14, 1988, the Advisory Committee to the Director of NIH unanimously adopted the panel's report and recommended lifting the moratorium. According to a story in *The New York Times,* Dr. Windom was ready to approve the experiments with fetal-tissue transplants in January 1989, but he received instructions from the office of Dr. Otis R. Bowen, then Secretary of Health and Human Services, to leave the decision to the next Administration.[11] On November 1, 1989, Dr. James O. Mason, Assistant Secretary for Health in DHHS, announced that the Bush Administration had decided to extend the twenty-month-old ban on federal financing of research on fetal-tissue transplantation. The decision was approved by Secretary Louis W. Sullivan. In an interview with *The New York Times,* Dr. Mason said that his decision to extend the ban was a "matter of heart and of mind as well."

> He said the research pits the rights of fetuses against those of patients who would be helped by it, so he felt obliged to come down on the side

of the fetuses. He said he believed that women considering an abortion might be swayed by the possibility that the tissue would help medical research.[12]

Yet another attempt was made to end the moratorium when the House of Representatives voted on July 25, 1991, to overturn the ban on the use of fetal tissue in federally financed scientific research. The provision, which passed on a 274-to-144 vote, was part of a bill that would authorize financing for a host of health programs administered by the NIH.[13] On April 2, 1992, the Senate approved a similar measure, with a majority (87–10) that could override an expected presidential veto.

There is a tendency on the part of pro-choice advocates to dismiss the pro-life objections to fetal research as mere abortion politics. A number of commentators have expressed dismay that the debate over fetal-tissue transplantation has become "politicized." To some extent, this criticism is justified. It is cowardly and irresponsible for officials simply to ignore the careful deliberations of their own appointed commissions in order to avoid risking the ire of the highly vocal right-to-life lobby. However, it is certainly not illegitimate for those who believe that abortion is immoral to make the argument that the use of aborted fetuses in research compounds the moral wrong. This argument deserves to be taken seriously. Unfortunately, this cannot be done without discussing the morality of abortion, a task that various commissions and panels have understandably sought to avoid. In the interest of harmony and consensus, they have attempted to bracket the highly politicized and divisive issue of abortion. The result has been an oddly hollow and incomplete defense of fetal-tissue research. The interest view provides a much stronger defense. Indeed, on the interest view, to refrain from using tissue from aborted fetuses, when this has the potential to save and improve thousands of lives, is seriously morally wrong.

II. FETAL-TISSUE TRANSPLANTS

Before discussing the ethical issues surrounding fetal-tissue transplants, their scientific justification needs to be assessed. A major reason for proceeding with human clinical trials is the possibility of benefiting millions of people. If this expectation is unfounded, then proceeding with such trials is not only a useless exercise, but one that exposes patients to needless risks.

The Scientific Evidence

Fetal-tissue transplants are still at a very early stage of development. Nevertheless, there have been promising results from ten years of animal experimentation and three years of experiments with humans. Ultimately, fetal tissue might be used to treat a wide range of diseases, including diabetes, Parkinson's disease, Alzheimer's disease, Huntington's chorea, spinal cord injuries, leukemia, aplastic anemia, and radiation sickness.

Fetal tissue is said to have distinctive advantages for transplantation for several reasons. First, its biological plasticity, which enables it to be integrated into the physiological environment of the host. Second, its proliferative capacity, which lets it grow to the size appropriate to the recipient. Third, its angiogenetic ability, or the ability to induce blood-vessel formation, which establishes it in the new environment and assures it the nutrients it needs for survival and growth. Fourth, its immunological compatibility. The lack of antigens and passenger leukocytes means that embryonic and fetal tissue are less likely to evoke an immune reaction leading to rejection than are adult tissues. Finally, fetuses develop in a protective environment. Because of this, tissues and organs obtained before parturition are almost universally devoid of pathology and of contaminating microorganisms.[14]

Fetal-tissue transplants seem most promising in the treatment of Parkinson's disease and diabetes. Parkinson's disease is a chronic, progressive, degenerative disorder of the central nervous system. A large number of drugs are useful in the treatment of the symptoms, but the disease cannot as yet be arrested or cured. A recent study by California scientists, sponsored by Britannia Pharmaceuticals, Ltd., showed that the drug deprenyl not only helped to alleviate the tremors, slowness of motion, and instability that characterize Parkinson's disease, but also halted its progress. The findings are only preliminary, since to prove the disease had been slowed would require showing that brain cells were no longer being killed off, a feat that cannot be accomplished in living humans. If the research, which involved only fifty-four patients, is borne out in future studies on larger groups, deprenyl would become the first known drug to block Parkinson's or related diseases.[15]

Scientists believe that Parkinson's disease is due primarily to disruption of the nigrostriatal dopamine pathway and to the loss of highly specific dopamine-producing cells. In the 1970s, researchers began to explore the possibility that replacement of these dopamine cells might have useful functional effects. After successful experiments using rodents and monkeys,[16] studies on humans were undertaken in Sweden, Mexico, China, England, and Cuba. Researchers have been tremendously encouraged by the results.

According to scientists who presented their findings in November 1991 at the annual meeting of the Society for Neuroscience, held in New Orleans, nearly all of the estimated 100 patients worldwide who have been implanted with fetal brain cells over the last three years have shown at least minor improvement in their symptoms, and many have gotten dramatically better.[17] Researchers in Mexico[18] and Sweden[19] report significant improvement in patients who have received brain-tissue transplants from aborted fetuses. The first such patient in the United States, Don Nelson, fifty-three, of the Denver area, had a tiny amount of fetal brain tissue implanted in his brain in 1988. According to a report in the May 1990 issue of *Archives of Neurology,* a publication of the American Medical Association, Mr. Nelson, who suffered from Parkinson's disease for two decades, can walk better now and no longer uses a cane to walk at home. He also can speak more clearly and has regained normal functioning of both hands.

The other disease for which fetal-tissue transplants look promising is type I diabetes. Fetal-tissue-transplant research on animals with diabetes is extensive and highly successful. ''Probably more than 10,000 animals have been 'cured' of diabetes through such experimental manipulations.''[20] No results from clinical transplants of fetal pancreatic tissues to human patients with diabetes have been reported. Nevertheless, many diabetics and their families want this avenue of research fully explored. Carol Lurie of the Juvenile Diabetes Foundation International emphasized this point in her testimony before the panel:

> Like millions of Americans, I have a child who is ill and whose future is jeopardized unless we promote the research endeavor. With respect to diabetes, islet cell transplantation may not be our answer. But it *may* yield the cure which we so desperately seek.
> I do not question the sincerity of those who elevate the issue of the use of fetal tissue to an abstract and moral plane. I can only hope to make those who oppose this research understand that diabetes is very real, that the threat to my son's life is very real, and that research is the very real and *only* hope for millions of Americans afflicted with a myriad of diseases. I can only hope to help you understand that the lives of millions are truly in the balance.[21]

One of the strongest critics of fetal-tissue transplants is Peter Mc-Cullagh, an Australian immunologist.[22] Although McCullagh opposes such research on moral grounds as well, he believes that there is no scientific basis for proceeding with fetal-tissue transplants. McCullagh specifically targets the claim that fetal-tissue grafts are less likely to be subject to rejection by a host's immune system:

This claim that fetal tissue grafts are less likely to be subject to rejection by a host's immune system is probably the most pervasive, and certainly the most poorly founded, to have been made in the course of advocacy of fetal tissue usage. . . . The concept that fetal grafts in general are less "foreign" (and as a consequence, less susceptible to rejection than comparable non-fetal grafts) has not received experimental support for many years. However, it is notable that inferences based on this claim continue to receive prominence in non-scientific publications.[23]

McCullagh also says that while researchers have claimed superiority of fetal cells for transplantation, in many cases, no comparison of fetal with adult tissue was made. He suggests that it is not the *superiority* of fetal tissue to adult tissue that attracts researchers, but rather its *availability*. Indeed, he wonders, "To what extent have efforts to establish uses for fetal tissue reflected a subconscious desire to assuage unfavorable impressions, created by the ready availability of abortion, by coupling these to a beneficial outcome?"[24]

A second concern voiced by McCullagh concerns the difficulty of extrapolating from animal models to humans. Examining the literature, he finds enough differences between the morphology and function of the pancreas in fetal rats and fetal humans to make speculation about results in humans based on experimentation with rats "rather shaky." McCullagh says, "The reservations raised in the present chapter about rat to human extrapolation would cast substantial doubt on the relevance of those claims to human medicine even if the comparisons between the properties of tissues from rats of different ages had been impeccable."[25] He concludes that, in the case of fetal-pancreas transplantation, the results of animal experimentation fail to support an extensive program of clinical testing of the procedure.

The questions McCullagh raises are certainly relevant in assessing experimental protocols. It would be absurd for the government to spend large amounts of money funding research that has little hope of yielding important scientific results. Equally, it would be seriously wrong to expose potential recipients of transplanted tissue to risks, or falsely to raise their hopes, without good reason to think that such transplantation might be beneficial. But these considerations do not argue for an absolute ban on fetal-tissue transplantation, especially in light of the most recent successes in using fetal brain tissue as a therapy for Parkinson's disease. McCullagh's review of the literature is confined largely to the 1970s and early 1980s. In light of more recent animal and human experimentation, his skepticism regarding possible clinical benefit seems no longer justified.

A different kind of concern about experiments with fetal-tissue transplantation is the danger of irresponsible and uncontrolled proliferation. According to an editorial in *The Lancet,* "Surely what is needed now is not more operations, but careful long-term follow-up, with positron emission tomographic scanning and neurophysiological and clinical evaluation, of patients who have already received grafts."[26] George Annas and Sherman Elias echo this concern, pointing out that there is no current method of regulating the clinical trials of new surgical procedures (as there is of trials of new drugs) and no effective way to regulate experiments financed privately. They say:

> The NIH panel has given us an excellent beginning. But it is only a beginning, and should not be taken as a signal to proceed with trials that use fetal tissues for transplantation in patients. We have more scientific work to do, including work with animals, to help determine such things as cell survival, growth curves, and graft-host immunology.[27]

These concerns, it should be noted, are general concerns about instituting and supporting clinical trials. They are not specifically concerned with the morality of using fetal-tissue from elective abortions. Let us now turn to the claim that fetal tissue transplants are morally unacceptable, regardless of the likely benefits to be gained by such research.

The Right-to-Life Objections

Right-to-lifers start from the premise that abortion is a serious moral wrong—indeed, the murder of an innocent child. They compare the killing of a million and a half embryos and fetuses a year in the United States to the Holocaust, and predict that someday people will look back and wonder how this slaughter of the innocents could ever have been permitted. Because they believe that abortion is not merely undesirable, but an unspeakable evil, they oppose anything that appears to tolerate or condone abortion, including using fetal tissues from elective abortions. The argument has a number of related components: that there is an absence of authentic informed consent, that the research provides an incentive for future abortions, and that such research is morally complicitous with abortion.

The Lack of Informed Consent

Maternal consent to fetal research is required by existing regulations. Fetal tissues have no different legal status from that of the placenta and associated products of conception. The purpose of laws that require maternal consent for medical uses of fetal tissues is not to protect the fetus, but rather "to protect the wishes and interests of the maternal sources of those tissues."[28]

However, while a fetus is certainly a product of the pregnant woman's body, it is not just that. To treat fetal tissue as if it were like any other bodily part ignores the potential of the fetus to become a child, with two parents. For this reason, some compare donation of fetal tissue and organs to parental donation of tissues and organs from a deceased child. This seems to be the approach taken by federal research regulations and the Uniform Anatomical Gift Act. These regulations give either parent the right to donate fetal remains for research or therapy, unless there is a known objection by the other parent. The special advisory panel recommended that this be amended so that the pregnant woman's consent would be both *necessary* and *sufficient* for donation. That is, the father should not be able to authorize the donation by himself, and the pregnant woman's consent should be sufficient, except where the procurement team knows of the father's objection to such donation. There is no ethical or legal obligation to find out what the father's views are, but his wishes, if known, should be respected (unless the pregnancy resulted from rape or incest).[29]

Some have argued that the very fact that the woman has chosen to terminate the pregnancy should disqualify her from making decisions about fetal remains. James Bopp and James Burtchaell make the point this way: ". . . when a parent resolves to destroy her unborn, she has abdicated her office and duty as the guardian of her offspring, and thereby forfeits her tutelary powers. She abandons her parental capacity to authorize research on that offspring and on his or her remains."[30]

This analysis is flawed even if one grants the fetus the status of a child, because it misconceives the rationale for asking for parental consent to donation. Parents are not asked for their consent in their role as *guardians* of their dead child. Rather, the request is made in deference to their wishes and feelings about the disposal of dead bodies.[31] Legislation regulating the disposal of fetal tissue does not protect *fetal* interests, but rather the interests of persons most connected to the fetus (its parents), as well as the interests of society in general.

A surprising number of people have failed to understand this point. They have mistakenly concluded that because regulations concern the disposal of the fetus, these regulations must protect fetal interests. An example is this statement by Alan Meisel:

> A fetus does not enjoy the full legal protections of personhood. Nonetheless, a fetus does have interests which the law protects. Put another way, society has an interest in according certain protections to the fetus whether

or not it is a person, just as certain protections are accorded by law to animals, the environment, and historical and aesthetically significant buildings.[32]

However, *society's* interest in protecting fetuses is not just another way of referring to *fetal interests*. We may acknowledge society's interest in the respectful disposal of fetal remains without thinking that *fetuses* have an interest in what happens to them after death.

It might be argued that even if the rationale for seeking parental consent for organ donation is based on parental interests, it is justified only because we make certain assumptions—in particular, that the parents loved the child. Some parents may experience mental anguish at the thought of the child's body being cut open, because they identify the dead body with the child they loved. We respect such feelings because we realize their source in parental love and concern. But what if it is the parent himself who has killed the child? Would it not be grotesque to worry about the killer's sensibilities regarding the child's corpse? Should Joel Steinberg, convicted of manslaughter in the beating death of his six-year-old adopted daughter, Lisa, have been asked for his consent to use her organs for transplantation? Why on earth should his feelings about what is done to her corpse have any relevance? Respect for parental feelings makes sense, it could be argued, only in the context of parental love and concern. Furthermore, it might be maintained, a woman who terminates a pregnancy is not acting as a loving parent; indeed, she is choosing not to become a parent.

It seems to me that the above argument is valid *if* we accept the pro-life premise that the fetus is a child, and abortion the murder of a child. But if abortion is not murder, there seems to be no reason to disqualify the pregnant woman as decision-maker or to ignore her preferences, especially if the decision to donate is based on altruistic reasons.[33]

Kathleen Nolan thinks that women should not donate fetal remains to research. She claims that the woman, as the mother of the dead fetus, should "fend off the scavengers."[34] Even if she does not feel able to carry the fetus to term, nevertheless, as its mother, she should protect the dead fetus, and not let it fall prey to the needs of others. I do not dispute Nolan's suggestion that aborting women are—or should be—concerned to prevent the dead fetus from being used in disrespectful or inappropriate ways. But why is using fetal tissue for transplantation disrespectful? Even some pro-lifers disagree with this characterization. A couple who lost two children to a rare genetic disease agreed to use tissue from an aborted fetus in a desperate attempt to save their unborn son. Despite their opposition to abortion, the Waldens testified before a congressional subcommittee that the government should end its ban on federal funding for transplants using the tissue of aborted fetuses, so long as precautions are taken to assure that no one is pressured to provide the tissue. The Waldens regard the use of fetal-tissue transplants as being like any other organ transplant done at any other age, in or out of the womb.[35] Moreover, the scavenger argument would apply equally to parents asked to donate their dead child's organs for transplantation. If consenting to donation in the case of one's dead child is morally permissible—indeed, something that should be encouraged—why should it be different in the case of the dead fetus?

Women should be able to choose whether or not to donate; there should be no obligation to donate fetal remains. We do not require altruism or even rationality of other potential donors. There is no reason to treat women who choose to terminate their pregnancies differently.

An Incentive for Future Abortions?

In their statement of dissent, James Bopp and James Burtchaell argued that the institutionalized use of aborted human remains would constitute an endorsement that would effectively increase the incidence of abortion in the United States. This could happen in two ways. "First, fetal tissue transplantation would further entrench the abortion industry by the symbiotic relationship which would arise between it, the medical community, and the beneficiaries of fetal tissue transplants."[36] Right-to-lifers often speak of "the abortion industry," implying that the physicians who perform abortions are actively seeking to increase the number of abortions performed, in order to raise the bottom line. One could as fairly speak of "the coronary bypass industry" or "the plastic surgery industry." Anyone who is trained to do a certain kind of procedure, and who profits from doing it, has a motive to do that procedure. There is always the danger that physicians, of all kinds, will recommend procedures inappropriately. But to suggest that physicians who perform abortions are more susceptible to financial incentives than are other physicians is unsubstantiated and unfair.

The NIH panel recommended a number of safeguards to ensure that research needs would not influence the abortion decision. These included postponing requests to use the tissue until after the decision to abort had been made, and prohibiting money payments for fetal tissue donation. Right-to-lifers remain unconvinced that such safeguards will work in practice. Mrs. Kay C. James, of the National Right to Life Committee, voices her skepticism this way:

> It is reassuring to believe there really would be a separation of "acquisition" and "transplantation," but is it likely? Especially, in the case of

neural tissue, transplantation likely would have to take place within a matter of hours.

Does anyone seriously imagine that there would not be elaborate and necessary interaction between the abortionist and the transplanting team?[37]

Testimony regarding the way fetal tissue is collected for research use was given by a representative of Hana Biologics, a for-profit biotechnology company that has developed a process to proliferate fetal pancreatic cells for transplantation. Hana obtains fetal tissue and organs from hospitals and clinics where abortions are performed. The actual procurement is usually done by nonprofit organizations. Hana plays no part in the woman's decision to have an abortion.

We obtain permission to use fetal organs from women who, having come to the clinic or hospital for an abortion and having signed the informed consent form for that procedure, also then agree to donation of fetal organs under the UAGA. The woman receives no payment of any kind.

The timing and method of the abortion are matters left to the physicians and patient; Hana plays no part in decisions on these issues. Similarly, it is the clinic or hospital and their physicians, not Hana or its representatives, who establish and monitor compliance with appropriate medical guidelines and state laws to ensure that the fetus is dead before organs are retrieved.[38]

Given the complete separation of the abortion process and the subsequent use made of the fetal organs by Hana, it is difficult to see how the collaboration feared by right-to-lifers could occur. But what about abortions in hospitals connected with medical schools? The doctors who perform abortions might also be engaged in research using fetal tissue, and thus might influence their patients to have abortions. This fear is graphically portrayed in the novel *Mindbend,* by Robin Cook, in which an unscrupulous researcher lies to women who have amniocentesis, telling them that their fetuses have chromosomal abnormalities, to get them to have abortions in order to provide him with fetal organs. While evil doctors are the stuff of good thrillers, this scenario is extremely unlikely in real life. At the same time, a number of people have pointed out that physicians and other medical personnel may have great influence over their patients' decision concerning abortions. The Stanford University Medical Center Committee on Ethics notes, "If they have direct personal interests in the resulting fetal tissue, they may, consciously or not, encourage their patients to have abortions."[39] To avoid this, the Committee recommended that medical personnel who perform induced abortions should not be allowed any direct benefit from the subsequent use of the fetal tissue. Annas and Elias support this recommendation, and go further: ". . . to avoid any conflict of interest there should be no academic incentive (such as coauthorship of publications or grant support) or other incentive for the physician performing the abortion or anyone else involved in the woman's care, to obtain her agreement for the use of fetal tissue."[40]

Such safeguards adequately address the danger of researchers manipulating women to have abortions to provide them with fetal tissue. But what about inducements stemming from women's own altruistic motives? Bopp and Burtchaell argue that ". . . the widespread use of fetal tissue could reasonably be expected to increase abortions, since knowledge of transplantation will induce some women to have abortions, who would otherwise not do so."[41] They claim that ambivalence about abortion is a "well-documented reaction of many women confronted with a problem pregnancy." . . .[42] Bopp and Burtchaell believe that the bare knowledge of fetal-tissue transplants could play a motivating role in ambivalent women. "It is reasonable to expect that this selfless motivation, when placed in the balance with all other reasons, will tip the balance in favor of abortion for some women who are ambivalent."[43]

The argument is unpersuasive. Altruistic considerations might lead a woman to donate fetal tissue once she has decided to abort, but it is scarcely likely that such considerations could tip the balance and make her decide to abort. Can anyone seriously imagine a woman, torn between abortion and having the child, who decides to have an abortion because of the bare possibility that the fetal remains might be used for transplantation into a stranger? This is so implausible as not to merit serious consideration.

The Complicity Argument

A decisive majority of the panel (18–3) found that it was "acceptable public policy" to support transplant research with fetal tissue either because the source of the tissue posed no moral problem or because "the immorality of its source could be ethically isolated from the morality of its use in research."[44] The ethical-isolation claim is based on the following argument. Assume that abortion is seriously morally wrong—indeed, murder. It doesn't follow that it is also wrong to use the resulting fetal tissue for transplantation, any more than it would be wrong to use the organs and tissues of adult homicide victims. John Robertson writes, "If organs from murder victims may be used without complicity in the murder that makes the organs available, then fetal remains could also be used without complicity in the abortion."[45] Robertson argues that one is not complicitous in a wrongful act simply by virtue of benefiting from it. So long as the researcher does not cause the abortion, he or she is not morally responsible for or complicitous in the abortion.

However, moral complicity is more complex than Robertson is willing to acknowledge. Burtchaell compares researchers using fetal tissue to bankers laundering funds from drug transactions. The function of the banker in no way affects the drug transactions, because they have already taken place. They would have taken place even without the banker there ready to launder the funds. "Nevertheless, the banker is an accessory: he is complicit by this institutionalized arrangement of interaction and association with those in the drug industry." [46]

It seems to me that Burtchaell has a point. Suppose that "factory farming" is morally wrong because it unjustifiably causes great animal suffering. Obviously, someone who believes this cannot in good conscience engage in factory farming, but surely this is not enough. He or she would also refrain from eating the flesh of animals raised on factory farms. It would be absurd for an opponent of factory farming to say, "I completely agree that factory farming is morally wrong and should be abolished. But as the animal is already dead, the harm's been done, so I may as well eat it." Similarly, it seems hypocritical for a researcher to agree that abortion is a terrible injustice and a practice that ought to be outlawed, but to see no reason why he shouldn't make use of the tissue, so long as it's available.

It may be argued that the two situations are not analogous. Abortions will occur whether or not the fetal tissue is used for transplantation, because the purpose of abortion is not to gain tissue but to end an unwanted pregnancy. The purpose of factory farming is to produce meat and eggs for consumption. It can only exist if there's a market for the resulting products. In enabling the industry to exist, the consumer is complicitous in the institution of factory farming. But researchers who use fetal tissue, and patients who receive it, are not necessary for the continuation of abortion. Women would continue to have abortions regardless of whether fetal tissue could be used for transplant. Because of this, it might be argued, researchers who use this tissue are not complicitous with abortion.

However, the claim that only those whose participation in a practice is necessary for its existence are complicitous with that practice seems false. Consider the following example. Imagine that animals are primarily raised for food, and their skins discarded. Then someone gets the idea that these waste products could be used. The skins of the animals may be used to make clothes, the feathers to stuff pillows, and so on. Whether or not this idea is adopted, factory farming would continue, since its purpose is to produce food. Yet should not those opposed to factory farming be equally opposed to the manufacture of clothing from animal skins? There does not seem to be a way to separate the initial wrong from the subsequent side effects. Similarly, if abortion is a serious moral wrong and a grave injustice, then the appropriate response is to see that it is stopped. Attempts to extract benefit from such a practice are themselves tainted.

The Nazi Analogy

The complicity argument against the use of aborted fetuses is often based on an analogy with using the results of experiments done by Nazi doctors on concentration-camp inmates. Annas and Elias dismiss the complicity argument as "primarily an emotional appeal based on an analogy to Nazi experimentation."[47] However, I think that the argument deserves to be taken seriously. First, I will consider the claim that researchers who use Nazi data are complicitous with the original Nazi experiments. Then I will turn to the implications for fetal-tissue transplants.

Nazi doctors performed a variety of gruesome experiments on concentration-camp inmates. Most had no scientific value whatsoever, but some yielded results that might be important. In one kind of experiment, the doctors at Dachau plunged prisoners, usually naked, into tanks of ice water and left them for two to five hours to shiver and often die. They then documented the specific temperatures at which the prisoners became unconscious, had irregular heartbeats, or died. Some scientists have found the Nazi measurements of the rate of body cooling in cold water useful in the testing of cold-water survival suits. They have used the Nazi cooling curves to extrapolate how long the suits would protect people at near-fatal temperatures—information used by search-and-rescue teams to determine the likelihood that a capsized boater is still alive.[48] Assuming that the data is scientifically valid, is it morally wrong to use it? Not necessarily, says Kristine Moe. "A decision to use the data should not be made without regret or without acknowledging the incomprehensible horror that produced them. We cannot approve of the methods. Nor, however, should we let the inhumanity of the experiments blind us to the possibility that some good may be salvaged from the ashes."[49]

Let us call Moe's argument the "salvaging good from evil" argument. It is countered by an argument that using the Nazi data is wrong, regardless of the good that might be achieved, because this legitimizes what the Nazi experimenters did. To cite their data is to support their perception of themselves as ordinary scientists conducting legitimate experiments. When the data appears in reputable scientific journals, it lends respectability to those inhuman experiments. Willard Gaylin says, "We cannot cite these atrocities. To use this data is to become an onlooker, and beyond that, an accomplice. To publish this data in a scientific journal is to legitimize it."[50]

Against the legitimacy argument, it could be said that it is more important to save lives than to dissociate ourselves from evil. The significant interests of living persons should take precedence over merely symbolic importance. Similarly, it could be argued that if fetal-transplant therapy can save lives and reduce suffering, this is more important than posssible complicity in abortion, even if abortion is a serious moral wrong. However, there is an important difference between using Nazi data and using fetal tissue from elective abortions that prevents us from analogizing them. The Nazi experiments occurred in the past, and nothing can be done to prevent their occurrence. They are beyond our reach. By contrast, abortion is an ongoing practice, and one that could be made illegal. As pro-choice advocates point out, this is unlikely entirely to stop abortion, but no doubt it would stop some abortions. Moreover, outlawing abortion would express condemnation of the practice, and both reflect and influence social attitudes. If the right-to-lifers are correct in their assessment of abortion—that it is the murder of innocent children—then abortion should be illegal, and no use should be made of (illegally) aborted fetal tissue. The claim that it is morally permissible to try to salvage good out of evil is persuasive only if nothing can be done to prevent the evil. One is not justified in doing nothing to stop evil, and then trying to derive some benefit from it.

In summary, the morality of fetal-tissue transplantation is not as easily distinguished from the morality of abortion as some commentators have thought. Fetal-tissue transplantation is "acceptable public policy" only if abortion is acceptable public policy—that is, should remain a legally available option. So long as abortion should remain legal, there is nothing wrong with using fetal-tissue for medical purposes. Indeed, if using fetal-tissue can cure serious illness and prevent death, it would be wrong not to use it.

The NIH panel understandably wished to avoid the explosive question of whether abortion should be legal. Instead, it noted that abortion *is* legal, and went on from there. However, as the dissenters rightly noted, the fact that abortion is legal does not mean that it should be legal. Without resolving this underlying issue, neither the question of informed consent nor the complicity argument can be adequately addressed.

A Feminist Objection

Some feminists think that even asking women to donate fetal tissue imposes an unjustified burden on them. Dr. Janice G. Raymond, professor of women's studies at Massachusetts Institute of Technology, testified before a congressional subcommittee in favor of keeping the ban on fetal-tissue research and transplants. "Abortion is a hard enough decision for many women to make, without being burdened with another decision of whether or not to donate fetal tissue. . . . More and more it is the women who are expected to be altruistic with what issues from their bodies."[51] Dr. Raymond thinks that such research makes women into mere environments and containers for the fetus.

This position is equally unpersuasive. First, although the problem of subtle pressure to donate is a real one, safeguards, such as those already discussed, should be sufficient to protect women from such pressure. To go beyond safeguards by denying women the ability to decide for themselves whether to donate is objectionably paternalistic. Second, Dr. Raymond confuses altruistic behavior with Good Samaritanism. There is nothing wrong with encouraging altruistic behavior. It is only when this behavior imposes extra risks and burdens that an equal protection–type argument can be made (see Chapter 4). Unlike undergoing a cesarean section, donating fetal tissue after an abortion does not impose any extra risks or burdens on women. There is, therefore, no reason to refrain from asking women to consider donation, once they have decided to abort. Finally, fears about making women into "fetal containers" seem misplaced. The fact that fetal tissue can be used no more makes women into fetal containers than the fact that retinas can be used makes people into eyeball containers.

Abortion for the Purpose of Procuring Fetal Tissue

Those who support using fetal tissue in medical and scientific research point out that if the tissue is not used, it is simply incinerated. This seems a terrible waste. As one presenter noted, "It is socially and ethically reprehensible to destroy fetal cadaver tissue which can be used towards perhaps savings millions of lives."[52] The basic point is that the fetus is already dead. The only question is how to dispose of the remains. The moral situation changes, it seems, if the retrieval of tissue is the reason for the abortion decision. Is it permissible deliberately to terminate, or deliberately to create, a pregnancy for the purpose of obtaining tissue for transplant? In 1987, a California woman called medical ethics expert Arthur Caplan to ask whether she could be artificially inseminated with sperm from her father, who suffers from Alzheimer's disease, in order to obtain brain tissue from the resulting fetus to transplant into her father's brain. Caplan says, "I told her first that it was technically not possible, and second that it was ethically wrong. This is the ultimate issue of intergenerational justice. You're not just asking for the pocketbooks of the young—you're asking for body parts.''[53]

Virtually everyone who has written or spoken on the issue of fetal-tissue transplantation has agreed with Caplan. Indeed, it has been more or less taken for granted that conception and abortion for tissue procurement is so clearly unethical that the prospect hardly merits discussion. The only issue has been the creation of guidelines to prevent its occurrence. To that end, the NIH nel recommended that the pregnant woman should be prohibited from designating the recipient of fetal tissue.

One of the very few commentators to give the topic extended discussion is Professor John Robertson. Robertson notes that the issue is not, at present, a practical one. There appears to be no need for a woman to conceive and abort to help a relative, for two reasons. First, there appears to be no medical advantage in there being a genetic relation between the fetus and the recipient of the tissue. Indeed, in autoimmune diseases, such as diabetes, a family member's cells are uniquely *unsuited* for transplant.[54] Second, with about one and a half million elective abortions a year in the United States, there appears to be no shortage of fetal tissue.[55] Admittedly, this could change if the incidence of surgical abortion were reduced due to medical alternatives such as RU 486, an experimental hormonal drug that induces very early miscarriage. The demand might also exceed the supply if fetal-tissue transplants proved successful for a large class of patients, such as those suffering from Parkinson's or diabetes. However, at this stage of research, it appears likely that fetal tissue from elective abortions is more than adequate for most current research and transplant purposes.

The question of the morality of deliberately aborting to obtain fetal tissue is thus a purely hypothetical one. Indeed, Robertson calls it "a red herring," because there is little advantage to be gained from such abortions and no one is recommending them. He goes on to say, "Yet the fear that women will conceive and abort to produce tissue for transplant has figured so largely in the current controversy that the ethics of the practice deserve careful attention—in the unlikely event the need for such abortions arises."[56] Robertson argues that such a practice is ethically more complex and defensible than most commentators have assumed. Our ethical assessment depends on "the value placed on early fetuses and the reasons deemed acceptable for abortion."[57] He goes on to say:

> An ethically sound distinction may be made between fetuses that have developed to such a level of neurologic and cognitive capacity that they are sentient and thus have interests in themselves, and those which are so neurologically immature that they cannot experience harm. While aborting

fetuses at the earlier stage prevents them from achieving their potential, it does not harm or wrong them, since they are insufficiently developed to experience harm.[58]

However, even if early abortion does not harm or wrong fetuses, it might still impose "symbolic costs," such as a general reduced respect for human life. These symbolic costs are outweighed by the woman's interests in privacy and bodily autonomy, especially when the reasons for having an abortion are compelling, such as protecting the mother's life or health, avoiding the birth of a handicapped child, or avoiding the burdens of a pregnancy due to rape or incest. Robertson argues that aborting to obtain tissue to save one's own life or the life of a close relative is as compelling a reason as these. It is not something that would be done joyfully. "Yet one cannot say that the choice to abort is ethically impermissible, if early abortion of unwanted pregnancies, or abortion for more compelling reasons, is acceptable."[59]

III. RESEARCH ON THE LIVING FETUS

Benefits from Fetal Research

In the past, research on fetuses prior to, during, or after induced abortion was not uncommon. As recently as 1972, the federal government's policy was described as follows: "Scientific studies of the human fetus are an integral and necessary part of research concerned with the health of women and children."[60] What kinds of studies have been done, and what scientific and medical benefits have thereby been gained?

Growth and Development *In Utero*

The primary purpose of anatomic and physiologic investigations of the human fetus is the obtaining of information concerning normal developmental processes in order to understand abnormal situations, with the ultimate aim of providing medical services to the fetus. Anatomic studies have been mostly done on dead aborted fetuses. Physiologic and metabolic studies have used living fetuses and live fetal material. Some investigators have begun the experimentation before or during induced abortion, often recovering chemicals afterward from umbilical-cord blood or from tissues of the abortus. Similar studies have been done during cesarean section at term when a chemical is given to the mother a few hours before the operation and metabolic products are measured in fetal umbilical cord blood at the time of delivery.[61]

Diagnosis of Fetal Disease or Abnormality

A number of techniques for the detection of genetic defects in the fetus have been developed. Amniocentesis, ultrasound, maternal serum alphafetoprotein (AFP) screening, and fetoscopy are now standard techniques. Chorionic villus sampling (CVS) is a new procedure that is gaining in popularity, though still considered experimental. Genetic screening using fetal cells in maternal blood, though promising, has not yet proved successful.[62]

Some of these techniques, such as amniocentesis, could not have been developed without research on the human fetus. Animal models offer major limitations as a true model of the human situation, because of important biological, anatomical, and physiological differences between humans and other animals. ''Accordingly, amniocentesis, which was first developed in the 1930s as a technique for fetal monitoring for blood group incompatibility between fetus and mother, has been extended to the second trimester for genetic disease detection primarily through *human experimentation.*''[63]

Research on the fetus-to-be-aborted can be extremely valuable for developing proficiency in some of the techniques used for prenatal diagnosis. Most of these techniques require considerable skill, which can only be achieved by performing the procedures repeatedly. For example, fetoscopy, which introduces an endoscope transabdominally into the amniotic sac, has a risk of fetal loss of about 3 to 5 percent, considerably higher than the fetal-loss risk associated with either CVS or amniocentesis. To minimize the complication rate, it has been suggested that individuals desiring to attain proficiency in fetoscopy perform the procedure on volunteers undergoing elective midtrimester abortions. Unfortunately, this is illegal in several states, which prohibit experimentation on fetuses that are the subject of a planned abortion.[64]

Fetal Therapy and Pharmacology

A substantial amount of information regarding the pharmacology of the maternal/placental/fetal unit has been derived from studies on experimental animals, but it is extremely difficult to predict whether observations made in a particular animal species will have relevance to human beings. For example, preliminary testing of the rubella vaccine in monkeys indicated that the vaccine did not cross the placenta. Human studies were then undertaken with women requesting therapeutic abortion. Examination of tissues from dead aborted fetuses showed that the vaccine virus did cross the placenta and infect the fetus. As a result, administering rubella vaccine to pregnant women, or women who might become pregnant within sixty days, is now proscribed. Another example of the perils of extrapolating from other species comes from the thalidomide tragedy in the early 1960s. Thalidomide was extensively tested on animals. No teratogenic effects were seen in pregnant rodents, cats, dogs, or monkeys. Yet when it was used by pregnant women during early pregnancy, thousands of severely malformed infants were born. As Elias and Annas note, "Animal studies may help establish the teratogenic potential of an agent and define teratologic mechanisms, but the final proof that an agent is teratogenic in humans must be demonstrated in humans."[65]

The medical advances stemming from research on fetuses *in utero* have been significant. Many physicians and biomedical scientists agree that the legal prohibition of research on embryos and fetuses will gravely retard the advancement of medical knowledge in many areas. Yet others argue that living embryos and fetuses should be protected from all but the most innocuous forms of nontherapeutic research. What are the moral reasons offered to support severe limitations on fetal research?

Moral Objections

The Possibility of Sentience

There is on the part of many people a gut reaction against experimentation using living fetuses, stemming from the assumption, perhaps unconscious, that such experimentation inflicts suffering on a tiny, innocent, living human being. It is bad enough, they may feel, that the fetus must be aborted and not permitted to live. To experiment on live abortuses goes too far, regardless of the scientific and medical value that may be thereby obtained.

This objection has validity only on the assumption that the aborted fetuses used in these experiments can feel pain. Some experts have objected that no one knows whether a fetus feels pain. John P. Wilson, a lawyer who submitted a report to the National Commission, noted that fetuses react to stimuli at a gestational age of only a few weeks.

> This may be a reflex action not indicative of pain, but there is no clear evidence proving the validity of this assumption, nor is it apparent that conclusive evidence can be obtained in the near future. As many capacities which serve no functional purpose until after viability and birth are acquired and develop during the previable stage, there is no reason to believe that the ability to experience pain does not also begin to develop early in gestation.[66]

However, as I argued in Chapter 2, there is good reason to think that the ability to experience pain does not develop until well into the second trimester. Pain perception requires more than brain waves. It involves the development of neural pathways and particular cortical and subcortical centers, as well as neurochemical systems associated with pain transmission. In light of this, it seems extremely unlikely that a first-trimester fetus could be sentient. Surely, more than a remote possibility of sentience at this stage of fetal development is required to justify banning research that could save lives and prevent a good deal of suffering.

It is ironic that even the barest possibility that a procedure might cause pain to a fetus is considered sufficient reason to prohibit it, when millions of clearly sentient animals are routinely subjected to experiments that cause them considerable suffering. For example, in order to determine whether fetal-tissue transplants could alleviate the symptoms of Parkinson's disease, the disease was experimentally induced in monkeys. (Inducing the disease was necessary because Parkinson's disease does not exist in animals.) A major motivation for funding such research is the devastating impact of Parkinson's disease on its sufferers. Yet no one expressed any moral reservations about subjecting healthy monkeys to severe impairment from profound parkinsonism for several months and then killing them. My point is not that such research cannot be justified—I think that it can, based on the special moral status of rational agents (see Chapter 1). But even if the important interests of rational beings ultimately outweigh the equally important interests of nonrational sentient beings, that does not justify ignoring the interests of animals. In particular, it is puzzling to me why so little attention should be paid to the interests of sentient animals, who can suffer, and so much concern expressed on behalf of beings, who, we have good reason to believe, cannot experience harm or suffering at all.

Fetuses as Human Subjects

Theorists who agree on the moral status of fetuses may nevertheless disagree about the permissibility of using fetuses in research. For example, Paul Ramsey and Richard McCormick both consider fetuses to have the same moral status as children, and so to be entitled to the same protections. However, Ramsey opposes *all* nontherapeutic research on children, on the grounds that children are incapable of giving the consent necessary to justify experimental procedures.[67] Similarly, he opposes nontherapeutic research on fetuses. Experimenting on a dying, aborted fetus would be comparable to experimenting on a dying child. Ramsey views fetuses as vulnerable, helpless, and nonconsenting human subjects, precisely those whom regulations on experimentation are intended to protect.

By contrast, Richard McCormick argues that parents may give proxy consent for a child to participate in nontherapeutic experimentation where there is no discernible risk or undue discomfort.[68] Proxy consent is morally legitimate insofar as it is a reasonable construction of what the child *ought* to choose. This position is rooted in the premise that all humans have an obligation to contribute to the benefit of the human community. Applying this analysis to the fetus, McCormick concludes that research on the living fetus is justified, so long as it poses no discernible risk or discomfort, appropriate consent from the parents is obtained, and the experiments are genuinely necessary for medical knowledge calculated to be of notable benefit to fetuses or children in general.[69]

At the other extreme is the view taken by the ethicist and theologian Joseph Fletcher. In his report to the National Commission, Fletcher says, "The core question at stake in the ethics of fetal research is whether a fetus is a person."[70] Answering that question negatively, Fletcher concludes:

> Only the pregnant patient is a "human subject" to be protected in clinical experimental and research; the fetus is an object, not a subject—a nonpersonal organism.
>
> A fetus is 'precious' or 'has value' when its potentiality is wanted. This means when it is wanted by the progenitors, not by somebody else.[71]

The interest view differs from Fletcher's position in two respects. First, on the interest view, an entity need not be a person to have moral status. All that is required is that it have interests. Sentient fetuses should not be exposed to painful experiments, regardless of whether they are considered to be persons. It is not their personhood, but their capacity to suffer, that provides us with reasons for protecting them. The core issue is thus not whether the fetus is a person, but whether the fetus has moral status.[72]

Second, the interest view acknowledges that entities can have moral value or worth even if they lack interests and thus do not have moral status. Fletcher's treatment of the fetus as object implies that there would be nothing wrong with selling preserved fetuses as lucky charms, or turning aborted fetuses into lipsticks. This would be not only profoundly offensive to most people, but also morally objectionable. A human fetus, even a preconscious one, is a potential person and a powerful symbol of humanity, and, as such, should be treated with respect.

The Equality Principle

The National Commission maintained that all fetuses should be protected from potentially harmful research, regardless of whether they were going to be aborted or going to be born: ". . . the same principles apply whether or not abortion is contemplated; in both cases, only minimal risk is acceptable."[73]

Most of the Commissioners interpreted the principle of equality to mean that no procedures should be applied to a fetus-to-be-aborted that would not be applied to a fetus-going-to-term. On the interest view, such a position is indefensible. The reason for banning potentially harmful nontherapeutic research on fetuses-going-to-term is not to protect the fetus per se, but rather to protect the future child. If there will be no future child, then there is literally no one who can be harmed and no one to be protected. The woman's decision for or against abortion is thus crucial to the justification of experimental procedures on the fetus *in utero,* because her decision determines whether there will be a being with interests, who can be harmed.

Some members of the Commission felt that there was a way to acknowledge both the difference between fetuses-going-to-term and fetuses-to-be-aborted, *and* the principle of equality. They agreed with their fellow members that all fetuses, whether or not they were going to be aborted, had equal moral status, and were entitled to equal moral concern. However, they argued that what is likely *to harm* a fetus depends on whether or not it will be aborted. "For example, the injection of a drug which crosses the placenta may not injure the fetus which is aborted within two weeks of injection, where it might injure the fetus two months after injection."[74] After noting this disagreement, the Commission summarized its views by saying that its members were in "basic agreement" as to the validity of the equality principle, although they disagreed as to its "application." It recommended review at the national level to resolve such disagreements of application.

This attempt at reaching consensus obscured a real moral disagreement among the Commissioners. It is disingenuous to proclaim that all fetuses deserve equal moral concern while at the same time maintaining that some fetuses cannot be harmed. Beings who cannot be harmed cannot have claims to our moral attention and concern. It would have been more honest for those Commissioners who agree that early-gestation fetuses cannot be harmed to have rejected the principle of equality, maintaining that it is permissible to use fetuses who are going to be aborted in ways that would be impermissible if the fetus is going to be born. The difference between the Commissioners on this issue was a substantive moral one, and not simply a matter of "application."

Once again, I must stress that the rejection of the equality principle does not imply that there are *no* reasons for restricting research on fetuses-to-be-aborted, only that these reasons do not refer to the interests of the fetus. Some restrictions might protect the interests of pregnant women. For example, in the rubella-vaccine tests, women who requested abortion were asked to accept vaccination and to postpone abortion for *three to four weeks!*[75] Since any delay in having an abortion is likely to increase the medical risks to the woman, as well as create psychological stress, this strikes me as an outrageous request. Certainly, current guidelines prohibit any research that exposes pregnant women to such risks.

Other reasons for restricting scientific research on living, preconscious fetuses may refer to our own sensibilities. Experiments most likely to offend public sensibilities are not those performed on the fetus *in utero* in anticipation of abortion. Rather, they are experiments performed on the living fetus *ex utero.*[76]

Research on Living Fetuses *Ex Utero*

Consider the following experiments:

> Using movie films, the reflexes of previable fetuses outside of the uterus have been documented along with the response of the fetus to touch. These studies have shown a response to touch in a 7–week fetus, swallowing movements in a 12–week fetus, and crying expressions at 23 weeks; the fetuses were studied after hysterotomy while they were immersed in a salt solution.[77]

> To learn whether the human fetal brain could metabolize ketone bodies, brain metabolism was isolated in eight human fetuses (12 to 17 weeks gestation) after hysterotomy abortion by perfusing the isolated head (the head was separated from the rest of the body). The study demonstrated that, similar to other species, brain metabolism could be supported by ketone bodies during fetal life, suggesting avenues of therapy in some fetal disease states.[78]

> In a 1963 study done in the United States, scientists immersed fifteen fetuses in salt solution to learn if they could absorb oxygen through their skin. One fetus survived for twenty-two hours. The knowledge gained by the experiment contributed to the design of artificial life-support systems for premature infants.[79]

Experiments like these provoked public concern and outrage, and led to the current moratorium on all research with living fetuses. Are such experiments morally objectionable, and if so, on what grounds?

As we have seen, ethicists differ on whether *any* nontherapeutic research on nonconsenting subjects is permissible. However, if it is permissible to use *children* in nontherapeutic research that poses minimal risk to them, it should be equally justifiable to use viable fetuses *ex utero* in such research. Oddly enough, current federal regulations impose a *more* restrictive risk standard on research using embryos and fetuses than on research using children.[80] The reason for this is probably general opposition to abortion and therefore opposition to any research that makes use of aborted fetuses. However, for those who are not opposed to fetal research in principle, there are three possible grounds for objecting to research on living fetuses after abortion: viability, sentience, and the potential for brutalization.

Viability is important because the viable fetus *ex utero* has the same legal standing as any other premature infant, and is entitled to the same protection. As Alexander Capron explains, "The viable fetus *ex utero* is a person in the eyes of the law, and its interest in life and well-being are clearly recognized by the civil and criminal law."[81] In fact, even *nonviable* living fetuses have the same status in law as full-term live-born infants. Separation from the mother and the existence of some signs of life are "the customary indicia of birth, and hence of the creation of a new human being with full claim on society's concern and protection through the laws."[82] Nevertheless, viability makes a difference in the treatment of abortuses. For example, it is reasonable both to require that life-sustaining measures be used on viable fetuses who survive abortion (whereas this would be pointless in the case of fetuses who cannot survive) and to prohibit research that interferes with a viable fetus's chance of survival.

As we saw in Chapter 2, the limit of fetal viability at present and for the foreseeable future remains at 23 to 24 weeks. However, fetal viability cannot be determined directly, but only estimated, based on measurement of head size using ultrasound. In the best hands, this technique is accurate within ± 1 week at 20 to 26 weeks. "Relating gestational age to fetal weight, and taking into account the range of error and normal variation, an estimated gestational age of 22 weeks or less by ultrasound would virtually eliminate the possibility of fetal weight above 600 grams and actual gestational age greater than 24 weeks."[83] To avoid the risk of using a possibly viable fetus in research involving more than minimal risk, the National Commission recommended that, should research during abortion be approved by national review, the estimated gestational age should be below 20 weeks.

An earlier cutoff for using living fetuses after abortion in research might be defended on grounds of sentience. It is possible, though unlikely, that a fetus of 20 weeks g.a. is sentient; but there is virtually no chance that fetuses become sentient before the end of the first-trimester. Thus, a first-trimester cutoff on all but the most innocuous research on living fetuses *ex utero* would provide adequate protection against the possibility of inflicting pain on a sentient fetus.

Another reason for limiting research on living abortuses to the first trimester has nothing to do with the interests of the fetus, but rather with public sensibilities. By 12 to 14 weeks of gestation, a fetus *looks* human. It evokes in most people the same instinctive responses of protection that newborn babies do. It is thus not surprising that many people should be deeply distressed to learn of experiments involving the decapitation or immersion in salt solution of living second-trimester fetuses. In addition, performing such experiments is likely to take a toll on researchers, who may have to suppress their own protective responses to carry out the research. Given the social and evolutionary value of these responses, suppressing them seems a dangerous path. Such considerations argue for a ban on research using living fetuses *ex utero*. However, symbolic concerns or a speculative risk of brutalization should not be allowed to ban research using nonviable and nonsentient fetuses, if such research is likely to have important scientific and medical benefits. While societal feelings of protectiveness toward fetuses should not be ignored, neither should they be emphasized at the expense of the interests of actual interested persons. A reasonable compromise would be to require that invasive research on living fetuses have the potential for significant human benefit, and to limit such research to the first trimester.

The last chapter concerns the moral and legal status of extracorporeal embryos created in the context of *in vitro* fertilization. May such embryos be deliberately created and used in research? Who should have jurisdiction over the storage and disposal of these embryos when their "parents" disagree? How should courts regard "preimplantation embryos": as "preborn children," as property, or as something else?

6

Embryo Research and the New Reproductive Technologies

In vitro fertilization (IVF), in which fertilization takes place outside the body, is the core of the new reproductive technologies. The concept of IVF is simple. A ripe human egg is extracted from the ovary shortly before ovulation. Next, the egg is mixed with sperm in a petri dish (hence the term *in vitro,* meaning ''in glass'') so that fertilization can occur. After the fertilized egg has begun to divide, it is transferred to a uterus, normally to the uterus of the egg donor, otherwise to the uterus of a surrogate. *In vitro* fertilization and embryo transfer (IVF/ET) may be indicated for women who can produce healthy eggs but who have damaged or diseased fallopian tubes, which prevent the eggs' passing from the ovary into the uterus. IVF can also help men who have a low sperm count (oligospermia) or low motility, since sperm will not have to travel as far, nor through cervical mucus, if brought together with the egg in a dish. When used in conjunction with a surrogate, IVF/ET can enable a woman who has no uterus to have a child who is genetically related to her.

The first human baby born as a result of IVF/ET was Louise Brown, born on July 25, 1978, in Lancashire, England.[1] Today, there are IVF clinics all over the world.

195

In vitro fertilization has become an accepted treatment for some forms of infertility. It has produced more than 10,000—and perhaps as many as 12,000—births, some 2,000 of these in the United States.[2] Despite its rapid spread, IVF/ET as a treatment for infertility remains controversial. The Roman Catholic Church objects both to the method of collecting semen (masturbation), and to the severing of the unitive and procreative functions of sexual intercourse.[3] Thus, the Church objects to IVF/ET even when both gametes come from husband and wife, when the egg donor also gestates the embryo, and when all fertilized eggs are transferred to the uterus of the egg donor. A less stringent view is taken by other right-to-lifers, who do not object to IVF in itself but do object to the discarding of "surplus" embryos.

A very different sort of objection to IVF comes from some feminists. They argue that treating infertility as a serious disorder meriting expensive, invasive treatment stems from and fosters a pronatalist ideology.[4] They also object to the "technologizing" of conception and childbirth, and taking these out of the hands of women.[5] In addition, they point to the relatively low success rate of IVF,[6] and maintain that the presentation of IVF as an acceptable treatment for infertility lies to and exploits women.[7] Finally, some commentators, while not objecting to IVF intrinsically, regard funding IVF research as a low priority in a society where basic health needs of existing people are not being met.

In addition to its clinical or applied use in cases of infertility, IVF also can be used in basic or laboratory research. Such research promises significant benefit for individuals and society at large. To ban or refuse to fund embryo research thus has costs in terms of the health and well-being of members of society. However, if the embryo is considered a "human subject," then it is entitled to the same protection as any other human subject. It may not be killed or subjected to risky or harmful experimentation.

The position of the interest view on the moral status of the extracorporeal embryo is clear. Embryos have even less claim to moral status than fetuses. As we have seen in earlier chapters, biologists disagree about precisely when the capacity for conscious awareness develops during gestation. However, biologists agree that the very early embryo cannot be sentient. Prior to the development of the embryonic disc, axis, and primitive streak, which occurs at or after implantation, approximately two weeks after fertilization, there is no possibility of feeling or experience of any sort. The preimplantation embryo has not yet developed the rudimentary structures of a nervous system, and thus lacks the capacity to experience or suffer. At the same time, the absence of sentience, and thus the lack of moral status, does not entirely settle the question of what may be done to or with embryos and fetuses. Even if they lack moral status, embryos may still be a potent symbol of human life and thus deserve respect. Frivolous uses of human embryos would be as unacceptable as frivolous uses of fetuses.

Section I of this chapter discusses IVF/ET, the biological status of the extracorporeal embryo, and the moral implications for the interest view. Section II concerns the uses of embryos in pure or laboratory research. Laboratory research is generally nontherapeutic: that is, it is not aimed at promoting the health or extending the life of the individual embryo being used, but is rather aimed at generally useful and beneficial scientific discoveries. Some laboratory research using embryos is ultimately aimed at discoveries quite unrelated to prenatal life—the understanding, treatment, and prevention of cancer, for example. Other research is aimed at discovering genetic defects in the embryo. This is controversial, since, in the foreseeable future, the probable result of discovering genetic defects in embryos will be to replace diseased embryos with healthy ones in order to prevent the birth of handicapped children. Section III considers how disagreements over the disposition of extracorporeal embryos should be settled.

I. IN VITRO FERTILIZATION AND EMBRYO TRANSFER

The Biological Status of the Extracorporeal Embryo

IVF technology became possible only after the invention of laparoscopy. The laparoscope is an optical surgical instrument that is used to inspect the internal abdominal and pelvic organs. It enables doctors to take ripe eggs from ovarian follicles. Laparoscopy usually requires a general anesthetic. Another technique for egg recovery uses ultrasound to identify the position of a ripe follicle containing an egg. The egg is then retrieved using a needle that is passed through the woman's abdominal wall. This technique can be used under local anesthetic. Eggs are then placed in a culture dish with the father's sperm in the hope that fertilization will occur.

Fertilization, which is marked by the emergence of pronuclei in the inseminated egg and subsequent cleavage, is not instantaneous but occurs gradually over several hours following insemination. Most IVF programs transfer the fertilized egg, or *zygote*, forty-eight to seventy-two hours after insemination, when it has divided into into two, four, six, or eight cells. At this point, the *multicell zygote* is an undifferentiated aggregate of cells called *blastomeres*. In normal conception, the multicell zygote continues to grow and take form as it moves through the fallopian tube into the uterus. In standard IVF/ET, the zygote is transferred directly to the uterus, skipping the fallopian tube. In gamete intrafallopian transfer (GIFT), a recent variation on IVF, eggs taken from the woman are mixed with sperm from the man, and this egg-sperm mixture is immediately transferred into the fallopian tubes, where it is hoped that fertilization will occur. The main difference between GIFT and IVF/ET is that in GIFT fertilization occurs *in vivo* (inside the body), rather than *in vitro,* as in IVF. A possible medical advantage of GIFT is that the fertilized egg spends several days in the fallopian tube before lodging in the uterus, just as in normal conception. On the other hand, GIFT does not allow clinicians to choose which embryos to transfer to the uterus, and to weed out those embryos that are developing abnormally. Obviously, GIFT cannot be performed on women with damaged or absent fallopian tubes.

By the third day after conception, the zygote has reached sixteen cells, which hang together in a loosely packed configuration, similar in appearance to a blackberry, called a *morula.* A fluid-filled space begins to form within the morula, leading to the *blastocyst* stage. During this stage, the zygote is also commonly called a *conceptus.* The blastocyst consists of an inner cell mass, which develops into the embryo proper, and outer cells, which develop into a trophoblastic or feeding layer that becomes the placenta. The developing cellular mass begins to embed itself into the uterine wall. This process, known as *implantation,* marks the beginning of pregnancy as a maternal state. When the blastocyst is well established in the uterine wall (late in the second postfertilization week), a second fluid-filled space, the amniotic cavity, appears within the inner cell mass. This is the embryonic disc; within it the first recognizable features of the embryo proper will appear.

It is not particularly difficult to fertilize the human egg *in vitro.* It is much more difficult to get the fertilized egg to implant in a uterus. As we saw in Chapter 2, even ordinary *in vivo* conception has a relatively high rate of embryo loss, around 31 percent. This rate is comparable to the rate in some *in vitro* fertilization clinics. Because of these difficulties, it is common practice to transfer more than one embryo to the potential mother, and for this reason several eggs need to be recovered. The standard IVF regimen involves giving the woman hormones to induce multiple ovulation, which commonly yields seven or more eggs. Of these, five or more may be fertilized and begin to divide, or cleave. Usually three or four embryos are transferred.

Discarding Surplus Embryos

To avoid adverse publicity and controversy with right-to-life groups, most American IVF programs do not fertilize more eggs than they plan to place in the uterus.[8] This avoids the problem of what to do with surplus embryos, but at a price. Avoiding discard may mean reducing an already fairly slim chance of achieving a viable pregnancy. To avoid having surplus embryos, doctors extract only three or four eggs with each cycle of hormone therapy and laparoscopy. If more than three or four embryos are transplanted, there is an increased risk of multiple births, which is risky both for mother and offspring. However, there is no guarantee that the three or four embryos transferred will implant. If implantation fails to occur, another treatment cycle to extract eggs is necessary—at added expense, discomfort, and risk to the patient. If IVF doctors did not have to worry about discarding surplus embryos, they could extract more eggs—perhaps as many as twenty or thirty—and fertilize all of them. This would enable them to select the embryos with the best chance of implanting, improving the chances of achieving a viable pregnancy. Moreover, any other healthy embryos could be frozen for future use by the couple, in case none of the first batch implanted. Any embryos that appeared not to be developing normally could be discarded or used in research. If the couple did not need the surplus frozen embryos because pregnancy was achieved the first time, or because they decided not to pursue having a child via IVF/ET, the extra embryos could be donated, discarded, or used in research.

If embryos are human persons, with the same right to life as any other person, then discarding them or using them for research purposes because they are unwanted or defective is seriously wrong. Of course, the interest view denies that embryos are persons or that they have moral standing. However, even some who find the sentience criterion of the interest view overly restrictive, and who regard fetuses as having moral standing, are unwilling to regard preimplantation embryos in the same way. They argue that the enormous biological and developmental differences between fetuses and preimplantation embryos justify different moral status. Three features of the preimplantation embryo are regarded as salient. First, the preimplantation embryo lacks even the precursor of a nervous system. Sentience is not merely highly unlikely, but physically impossible. Second, it is not yet a unique individual, since, prior to the development of the primitive streak, twinning might still occur. The third difference, unique to the extracorporeal embryo, has to do with potentiality.

In Chapter 2, I considered the argument that the developing embryo has human moral status because of its potential to develop into a human being. The claim is that embryos, unlike gametes, are potential people because they will develop into people, all by themselves, without further intervention. I noted that, whatever appeal this argument has in the context of normal fertilization and pregnancy, it does not seem to apply in the case of extracorporeal fertilization. The fertilized egg *in vitro* cannot develop into a fetus "all by itself." Unless someone intervenes and transfers the embryo into a uterus, it cannot develop into a person. Therefore, using the criterion advanced by most potentiality theorists to distinguish embryos and gametes—namely, the ability to develop into a person "all by itself"—the extracorporeal embryo is not a potential person, any more than an ovum or a sperm is. This lack of potentiality is held by some to distinguish the extracorporeal preimplantation embryo from an implanted embryo or fetus. Others reject this argument, holding that a distinction must be made between what capability the entity has within itself, and what it receives from the environment.[9] Admittedly, the extracorporeal embryo must be put in the right environment (a uterus) to develop into a person. Nevertheless, it has within itself the capacity to develop into a person in that environment. By contrast, no matter what environment a gamete is put in, it cannot develop into a person all by itself. However, it is not clear that the distinction between internal capacity and environment works to show that fertilized eggs are potential persons but that gametes are not. It could be argued that a sperm *does* have the capacity within itself to develop into a person, so long as it is put in the right environment: a petri dish containing a ripe ovum. At least in the IVF context, embryos are not clearly potential persons any more than gametes are.

The interest view does not regard the biological differences between fertilized ova and nonsentient fetuses as being directly relevant to moral status. Neither embryos nor nonsentient fetuses have interests or a welfare of their own, and so neither has moral status. However, even nonsentient fetuses are visually and developmentally much closer to the kinds of entities that do have a claim to our moral attention—namely, late-gestation fetuses and babies. They evoke a protective response that is not likely to be invoked by blastocysts. As I argued in Chapter 5, there are good psychological reasons against adopting policies that might weaken these sorts of responses.

The Risks of Abnormality

When IVF was in its infancy, a number of critics objected to the procedure on the grounds that it was immoral to run the risk of producing a congenitally abnormal baby, a risk that was at that time unknown. In response, defenders of IVF pointed first to animal studies that indicated that the risk of abnormality was no greater with IVF than with normal conception. Second, they argued that the risk of a deformity's developing is by far the greatest after implantation. A significantly damaged zygote would be unlikely to implant in the first place. Even if chromosomal abnormalities should result from the new technologies, they would be unlikely to result in the birth of abnormal children. The natural process by which most abnormal early embryos are lost during the early weeks of pregnancy would presumably be operative following *in vitro* fertilization as well.[10]

The critics replied that animal studies provided insufficient information. Knowledge about risk requires long-range human studies, decades in which to follow up children conceived through the new technologies through a normal life span. Nor were they convinced that the spontaneous elimination of most abnormalities before birth would occur, even assuming that such loss is reassuring and of little moral relevance. Theologian Hans O. Tiefel characterized LeRoy Walters's conclusion that the procedures do not pose unreasonable risk as "both sanguine and premature."[11]

In the more than a decade since the birth of the first IVF baby, the fears that offspring will be physically handicapped or damaged have not proved to be well-founded. IVF has shown no higher rate of congenital deformity than coital reproduction.[12] A study published in August 1989 in *The Journal of Pediatrics* revealed that babies conceived in a laboratory were as healthy and mentally alert as those conceived normally.[13] Researchers compared the development of eighty-three children born as the result of IVF with ninty-three children born after normal conception. The children in both groups were subjected to a battery of tests that could detect internal abnormalities, and tests measuring mental development. Dr. James L. Mills, one of the researchers, said that the study should reassure parents that babies conceived *in vitro* have no increased risk of abnormal development.[14]

It is of course possible that long-range studies will reveal risks so far unknown. To be more certain, it would be necessary to study larger numbers of children and to study long-term psychological as well as physical development. However, the mere possibility that increased risk will be discovered is not a sufficient reason for abandoning a technology, especially when the evidence so far indicates that there is no increased risk. Couples who opt for IVF now cannot be accused of exposing their offspring to unreasonable risks. A more interesting question is whether it was morally justifiable for people to use IVF while the risks to the resulting offspring were still unknown. Some ethicists condemned the selfishness of parents so bent on having children that they were willing to risk the birth of handicapped children.[15] Tiefel argues that "every parent owes every child-to-be reasonable care not to take chances with its health . . . And the uncertain risks inherent in *in vitro* fertilization are definitely avoidable by abstinence from this particular technology."[16]

John Robertson agrees that parents are obligated not to take avoidable risks with the health of their children, but he argues that the risks in IVF are not avoidable. If the parents abstain from this particular technology, the child will not be born at all.

> From the child's perspective, the only alternative to the action that allegedly violates his right not to be harmed is even less desirable, for it means no existence at all. One does not respect a person's rights by refraining from an activity that prevents his existence altogether.[17]

According to Robertson, the resulting offspring is wronged only if the damage caused by IVF is so severe, so fraught with pain and suffering, that the child might find death preferable. Such severe damage is highly unlikely with noncoital conception, but, Robertson says, "If it did occur, the remedy and obligation would be to limit further damage by immediately ceasing all sustaining efforts."[18]

I have already argued against such a restrictive conception of "wrongful life" (see Chapters 2 and 3). I maintain that children are wronged when they are knowingly brought into existence when there is a substantial chance of their having lives that fall below a decent minimum. It is *unfair* to have a child under such conditions. This unfairness is not mitigated even if the child, once born, wants to go on living. For people often do want to go on living, even under the most miserable conditions. This does not make it right knowingly to bring people into existence under such conditions.

Tiefel agrees. He sees an enormous difference between deciding to bring into existence a child who cannot be reasonably ensured a fair chance at health, and terminating the life of an already existing child. Once the child exists, the moral choice should generally be for life. However, no such preference for life is mandatory before the child exists. Potential parents are not morally required to bring children into existence, and indeed are morally required not to bring children into existence if they are likely to suffer significant setbacks to their health and well-being. "No one has the moral right to endanger a child while there is still the option of whether the child shall come into existence."[19]

Although we now know that children conceived through IVF have as good a chance of being physically and psychologically healthy as children conceived coitally, the question of physical risk with certain IVF variations, such as freezing and thawing of sperm, eggs, and embryos, embryo biopsy, and other manipulations, remains to be resolved. What degree of risk is it permissible to take with the health of future offspring? It should be pointed out that we do not require fertile couples to refrain from procreation, even if they are at serious risk of passing on genetic diseases. Nor do we forbid women to use fertility drugs, even though some of these increase the risk of multiple births, which increase the risk of prematurity and respiratory distress in the offspring. It does not seem fair to require of infertile couples that they refrain from exposing their potential children to any risks at all, if this is not required of couples able to reproduce coitally. Moreover, it is not as if we have no idea of the safety of the new variations. We can refer to animal models, as well as to the experience of researchers in other parts of the world. In addition, couples who conceive noncoitally have the same opportunity as couples who conceive normally of undergoing genetic testing, and aborting fetuses with serious abnormalities. Indeed, they have the additional option of discarding abnormal embryos prior to transfer, thus eliminating the need for abortion.

Politics and IVF Research

Opposition from right-to-life groups has made the funding of IVF research in the United States politically unfeasible. A de facto moratorium on such research has existed for over ten years, despite a recommendation from the Ethics Advisory Board (EAB) in 1979 that such research was ethically acceptable and should not be prohibited. Soon afterward, the EAB was allowed to dissolve. Despite repeated requests from NIH scientists, Public Health Service officials, and the scientific community, five successive Health and Human Services secretaries have refused to appoint members to the EAB. As a result, research that involves fertilization of human sperm and eggs has been excluded from federal support, because these same HHS secretaries have claimed that such research cannot be approved in the absence of an EAB! Without government funding, relatively little research on reproductive technology has been done in the United States. The effect has been costly, ineffective treatment for infertile couples. According to a congressional committee on infertility:

> It is an embarrassment to the U.S. Department of Health and Human Services, and especially to the Public Health Service, that the last five Secretaries of HHS, including the current Secretary, Dr. Louis Sullivan, have ignored HHS regulations to appoint an Ethics Advisory Board. It is a tragedy for the millions of American couples who are infertile, some of whom spend their life savings for treatment that is ineffective.[20]

II. EMBRYOS IN LABORATORY RESEARCH

Extracorporeal embryos provide an opportunity for studying disease or developmental processes unrelated to clinical IVF. There are many possible goals of embryo research, including developing more adequate contraceptives, determining causes of infertility, investigating the development and potential transformation of moles into malignant tumors, evaluating the effect of teratogens on the early embryo, and understanding normal and abnormal cell growth and differentiation.[21] Embryo research may be particularly valuable for understanding, preventing, and treating cancers, and for studying and treating genetic disease.

Although little embryo research is taking place in the United States, it is being done in other countries, including Australia, Canada, France, Italy, and Sweden. In England, the Warnock Report's approval of embryo research initially generated strong opposition, leading the House of Lords in 1985 to pass a bill banning all embryo research. However, in a complete turnaround in 1990, the House of Lords decided by a vote of 234 to 80 to allow research on human embryos to continue. In November 1990, the Human Fertilisation and Embryology Act was enacted. The Act provides a statutory framework for the control and supervision of research involving human embryos. It created the Human Fertilisation and Embryology Authority (HUFEA), which has the authority to issue research licenses. A research license permits the creation of embryos *in vitro,* and their use for specified projects of research. The research must be directed toward certain defined aims (the treatment of infertility, knowledge about the causes of congenital disease and miscarriage, more effective techniques of contraception, and detecting abnormalities prior to embryo implantation), and only where HUFEA is satisfied that the research is necessary or desirable.[22] Following the recommendation of the Warnock Committee, it permits research on human embryos until the appearance of the primitive streak, at about 14 days.[23]

Detecting Genetic Disease in Embryos

One kind of research is aimed at discovering the causes of chromosomal abnormalities in human embryos. Perhaps one-quarter to one-third of all embryos, whether conceived *in vitro* or *in vivo,* have chromosomal imbalances, and there is only limited knowledge of the causes. For example, in the case of Down syndrome, it is known that the defect mostly arises in the oocyte, before fertilization occurs, but it is not known how this happens. The defect could arise as the oocytes are formed in the ovary, when the mother is herself a fetus, or during the final stages of the growth of the oocyte in the adult mother. "Studies on the chromosomes of embryos should help to decide between these possible causes, and might help to promote methods or treatments which can help to limit or prevent such disordered growth.''[24]

Some researchers are working to find out if embryos can be typed for specific forms of inherited disease. Further advances in this field await the development of DNA probes specific for particular gene defects. If such probes are discovered, couples at risk for having a baby with an inherited disorder might choose not to attempt pregnancy in the ordinary way, but might instead choose IVF, so that afflicted embryos could be discarded and a healthy embryo implanted.

Some people disapprove of research aimed at, or likely to be used for, selecting healthy embryos and discarding defective or diseased ones. Obviously, pro-lifers (or at least those who regard human life as beginning at conception) oppose this sort of research. They do not regard the discarding of diseased embryos as a means of preventing genetic disease any more than they would so regard the killing of a born child with a genetic disease.

Even some people who are generally pro-choice are opposed to the idea of prenatal testing and abortion for genetic indications.[25] One such person is Barbara Katz Rothman, author of *The Tentative Pregnancy*.[26] Most of Rothman's objections stem from the fact that currently prenatal testing is done around 16 weeks of gestation, after the pregnancy is already well established. This places the pregnant woman in a peculiar and stressful psychological situation. She's committed to this pregnancy and this fetus, and yet she isn't, because she is prepared to abort if the fetus is affected. This concern may be alleviated by earlier prenatal testing, such as chorionic villus sampling (CVS), which can be done in the first trimester. Embryo replacement would not raise any concern about "tentative pregnancies," since the embryos are created *in vitro* and any diseased ones are discarded around five days after fertilization, prior to being implanted in the woman's uterus, and the establishment of a clinical pregnancy. Thus, the detecting of abnormalities in the embryo would have the advantage of sparing some couples the emotional trauma of an abortion in the fifth month of pregnancy.[27] However, Rothman has another objection to "eugenic" abortion, one that is not alleviated by very early prenatal testing or embryo replacement following IVF. She worries that the "option" of prenatal testing will become a requirement, even for mild diseases and less-than-totally-disabling impairments. She is concerned that there will be increased social pressure not to bring a child with a disability into the world:

> Blame begins to insinuate itself. The birth of a severely disabled child, when the disability could have been prenatally diagnosed and the pregnancy terminated, begins to be seen as an act of irresponsibility. The stan-

dards of production rise, and we are to be held accountable by those standards.[28]

Disabled children themselves may come to be seen as unfortunate mistakes. This fear has led some advocates for the disabled who are generally pro-choice to oppose abortion of impaired fetuses.[29] Adrienne Asch says:

> I believe that genetic screening and prenatal diagnosis followed by abortion differ morally and psychologically from . . . all other abortions save those for sex selection. . . . At the point one ends such a pregnancy, one is indicating that one cannot accept and welcome the opportunity to nurture a life that will have . . . impairments perceived as deficits and problems. What differentiates abortion after prenatal diagnosis (and abortion for sex selection) from all other abortions is that the abortion is a response to characteristics of the fetus and would-be child and not to the situation of the woman.[30]

Asch sees disability as a social, rather than a medical, problem. "Social services, financial support, education, employment, and recreational opportunities will not improve for disabled children or adults until we genuinely believe that it is acceptable to be a person with a disability, and to claim a share of familial and societal resources at least as great as that claimed by those without disabilities."[31] Asch views the acceptance of abortion to prevent disability as evidence of—indeed, reinforcement of—an attitude that disabled people are not fully human, not full-fledged members of society.

While wholeheartedly sympathizing with Asch's goal of a society of equal opportunity for the abled and disabled alike, I think that her position is flawed on two counts. First, it is simply not true that when abortion or embryo discard is chosen to prevent the birth of a child with a genetic defect, the abortion is not chosen because of the woman's own situation. The woman must ask herself whether she (and her family) are prepared to undertake the care of a child with a serious disability. This as much concerns her own situation as having an abortion because she already has five children, or because she is unmarried, or because she is forty-five. All of these situations may prompt a woman to say, "I can't. This asks too much of me." Asch generously acknowledges that the desire to avoid raising a disabled child is not necessarily callous or selfish:

> It is an honest, understandable, if perhaps misinformed, response to the fears that a disabled child will not fulfill what most women seek in mothering—to give ourselves to a new being who starts out with the best we can give, and who will enrich us, gladden others, contribute to the world, and make us proud.[32]

Asch is quite right to point out that the mere fact that a child has a disability does not make parenthood necessarily disappointing or unfulfilling. Parenting a child with a disability may turn out to be an enriching experience, but it can also be the source of extra burdens, disappointment, and grief.[33] Parenting is hard enough with healthy children. Why are parents morally required to accept additional burdens from the outset?

It may be said that parents cannot avoid the risk of such burdens. A fetus free of genetic disease may be injured during birth and develop cerebral palsy; a child who is healthy at birth may contract an infection that destroys the brain. At any time, our children are subject to accident and disease, to disability and dependence. Being willing to care for and love our children even when (especially when) they have problems is part of being a good parent. Therefore, it may be asked, how good a mother is a woman likely to be if she is unwilling to bear a child with a disability?

However, from the fact that parenthood is not risk-free, it does not follow that individuals cannot attempt to avoid or minimize risks *before they become parents*. The obligations of *parents* to undertake burdens, to risk disappointment and grief, for the sake of their children, are not the obligations of potential or prospective parents. If one thinks of the fetus as already being a child, then of course its parents are morally required to care for it, to make large sacrifices to ensure its health and well-being. But this view of the fetus is not open to someone who, like Asch, is generally pro-choice. In essence, Asch equates the decision *to become* a mother, which is implicit in intentionally or willingly becoming pregnant, with already *being* a mother. By contrast, I maintain that even after becoming pregnant, the woman still has a choice to continue or terminate the pregnancy, because the fetus is not yet a child. If, as Asch agrees, it is morally permissible for women to abort to avoid such burdens as unmarried motherhood, the termination of an education, or the disruption of a career, it is equally justified to abort to avoid the burdens that may come from having a seriously disabled child.

The key word here is "seriously." We may well doubt the parenting ability of someone who would abort a fetus because of a minor disability, such as a cleft palate or clubfoot. An individual who would be unwilling to have a child with even a minor defect may be rightly criticized as wanting a "perfect child." But many genetic disorders are not minor. Furthermore, some disorders revealed by prenatal testing have a wide range of possible disability. Prenatal testing can reveal that a fetus has spina bifida, for example, but it cannot reveal the severity of the impairment. It cannot predict whether the child will be of normal intelligence or severely retarded, ambulatory or completely paralyzed. These factors will affect the likelihood of the child's having a worthwhile life, a life that will be a good to her. Prospective parents should be aware that people with serious disabilities can have happy and productive lives, but it is dishonest to pretend that this is always the case, or that the only obstacles such children face are social ones. When we consider both the extra burdens imposed by having a severely disabled child on its parents (in particular, its mother), and the risk that the child may be so severely impaired that its life will be a burden rather than a blessing to it, the decision to abort for genetic indications is at least as justifiable as other reasons for aborting. Advocacy for the disabled should not lead us to "guilt-trip" women who choose abortion in this situation.

Respect for Embryos as a Form of Human Life

Some people object to any research using human embryos, because they consider embryos to be human subjects incapable of giving consent. Others see nothing special about embryo research and would allow it within the confines of the current research review system. That is, since embryo research involves human tissue and would require the consent of the gamete providers, research proposals would have to be reviewed by an institutional review board or ethics committee to ensure that standards for risk-benefit ratios and informed consent are met. A third position is that embryo research is acceptable in principle, but should be subjected to special limitations to protect offspring and to demonstrate "profound respect" for embryos as a form of human life. This third position has been the view of several important official bodies. The Ethics Advisory Board in the United States (1979) found that "the human embryo is entitled to profound respect; but this respect does not necessarily encompass the full legal and moral rights attributed to persons."[34] The Warnock Committee in Great Britain (1984) maintained that "the embryo of the human species ought to have a special status" and "should be afforded some protection in law." A majority of the Committee agreed that research on human embryos should continue, but that embryos should not be "frivolously or unnecessarily used in research."[35]

John Robertson is a leading proponent of the third position on the status of the embryo. He maintains that the human embryo can be accorded respect, not for what it is in its own right, but for the symbolic meaning it has for us:

> Although neither a person nor an entity possessing interests, it may be
> the subject of duties created to demonstrate a commitment to human life

and persons generally. Justice may not require that we grant the embryo rights, but we may choose to treat the embryo differently than other human tissue as a sign of respect for human life generally.[36]

This interpretation of the third position is compatible with the interest view. However, the interest view diverges from the characterization of the third position given by the Warnock Committee in that the interest view does not confer a "special status" on the human embryo. On the interest view, moral status is limited to beings who can have interests of their own. Special moral status might be ascribed to interested beings whose lives are reasonably regarded as having less moral significance than the lives of persons (e.g., animals). But embryos, even human ones, do not have interests of their own. Therefore, they do not have moral status, and it is more accurate to acknowledge their importance for us by ascribing to them moral value (see Chapter 5). However, as I argued in the last chapter, symbolic value should not take precedence over the interests of real people. John Harris makes this point when he says:

> When we bear in mind that . . . most of the secrets of the development of life are contained in early embryos, and that we are extremely likely to be able to use what we learn from such embryos to save many lives and ameliorate many conditions which make life miserable, we would not only be crazy but wicked to cut ourselves off from these benefits unless there are the most compelling moral reasons to do so.[37]

Other questions regarding the interpretation of respect for human embryos remain. For example, does respect for the embryo preclude creating embryos for research? This issue split the members of the Warnock Committee.

Creating Embryos for Research

A distinction can be drawn between "spare embryos" and "research embryos." Spare embryos are those created for the purpose of placement in a woman's uterus but not used for this purpose, either because of a defect in the embryo, or because the patient no longer requires the embryos, and so can be donated for research. Research embryos are conceived purely for research by asking a patient to donate an egg, which is fertilized by a spermatozoon from any man. The resulting embryo is then used in an experimental protocol.

The moral acceptability of creating research embryos was discussed at great length by the Warnock Committee. Once again, three positions emerged. Some members were opposed to all experimentation on human embryos, based on the potential of the embryo to become a person.[38] This group was even more adamantly opposed to the deliberate creation of embryos for the purpose of experimentation. A second group did not distinguish between spare and research embryos. For them, the important question was not the origin of the embryos, but the permissibility of embryo research and the appropriate restrictions to be placed on it. A third group saw a clear moral distinction between using spare embryos and creating embryos for the purposes of research alone. They argued that "it cannot be consonant with the special status that the Inquiry as a whole has agreed should be afforded to the human embryo, to cause it to exist, yet to allow it no possibility of implantation."[39]

The members of the Warnock Committee who differentiated between research and spare embryos based their opposition to creating research embryos on two arguments. The first is a slippery-slope argument. It notes that frivolous and unnecessary embryo research is supposed to be prohibited. However, if it is thought permissible to create embryos with the sole intention that they be used for research, this will open the way for ever-increasing use of human embryos for routine and less valid research. "Once a foot is set on the 'slippery slope' of deliberate creation of embryos, no end can be set to the dangers."[40] But this simply assumes that the deliberate creation of embryos will lead to less valid research. No reason is given why this is likely to occur. Even putting aside general problems with slippery-slope arguments (see Chapter I), this argument begs the question.

The second argument appeals to the doctrine of the double effect, which holds that:

> . . . an act which would be wrong if chosen for its own sake may be justified if it occurs as a by-product of some other, well-intentioned act. According to this view, therefore, there would be no general acceptance of research on embryos, but acceptance only in the limited circumstance of the existence of spare embryos.[41]

On this view, it is not morally acceptable to create embryos simply for the purpose of research. However, if embryos are created for a legitimate purpose (establishing a pregnancy), and then cannot be used for that purpose, it is morally permissible to use them in research, rather than discard them.

The plausibility of the double-effect argument depends on acceptance of the premise that there is something wrong with creating embryos solely for the purpose of research. For if this is not wrong, then there is no need to explain why it is permissible to experiment on spare embryos. Unfortunately, the wrongness of creating embryos for research was not explained, but only asserted as inconsistent with the special status of the human embryo. But why should this be so? Perhaps the idea is that embryos, while not quite persons, are sufficiently like persons to make it wrong to experiment on them without their consent. But surely this argument would also rule out experimenting on spare embryos. Another argument is that it is "surely repugnant to create human life solely for the purpose of destroying it in embryo experiments."[42] However, research embryos are not created solely for the purpose of destroying them. Rather, the purpose is to gain knowledge that will enable us to save lives and prevent misery. Why isn't this purpose as legitimate as establishing a pregnancy? I think the idea must be that creating an embryo to be used in research, even beneficial research, is to treat it as a mere thing, which is wrong. By contrast, creating an embryo that will be implanted and develop into a baby is to benefit it, to act in its interest. This argument depends on the assumption that embryos *have* interests, an assumption rejected by the interest view. If embryos do not have interests of their own, they cannot be harmed *or* benefited. The idea that an embryo is benefited by being allowed to develop into a person is a mistake. So, IVF/ET does not benefit embryos, but neither does laboratory research harm them. If this is right, then it is as permissible to create embryos with the intention of using them in valuable scientific research as it is to create them with the intention of transferring them for implantation.

III. DISPOSITIONAL PROBLEMS

Some of the thorniest problems posed by the new reproductive technologies concern who has jurisdiction over extracorporeal embryos in the event of the parents' death or divorce. The technological advance that has created the problem is the ability to freeze embryos for later implantation. This is a great advantage, since it means that patients can have a second or third chance at pregnancy without having to undergo another laparoscopy. However, this leaves the problem of what should be done with surplus frozen embryos. Should they be donated to a woman who cannot produce her own eggs? Discarded? Or used in research?

Most jurisdictions have not faced this issue. Laboratories simply keep embryos frozen in liquid nitrogen; there are probably thousands of frozen embryos in Europe, Australia, Great Britain, and the United States. Their disposition becomes an issue only when property rights or custody must be resolved.

The Rios Case

Property rights were involved in the case of Mario and Elsa Rios, a couple from Los Angeles who went to Melbourne, Australia, for IVF treatment in 1981. An embryo was transferred to Mrs. Rios, but the pregnancy ended in an early miscarriage. Two other embryos were frozen. The couple returned to America and decided to adopt a baby in Mrs. Rios's native Argentina. All three were killed in a plane crash in Chile in 1983.

The Rioses left an estate of about one million dollars. The sole heir was Michael Rios, the son of Mario Rios by a previous marriage. The couple had died without leaving wills and Michael Rios was not aware of the frozen embryos. Nor was the Queen Victoria Medical Center aware of the deaths of the Rioses until June 1984. Michael Rios's lawyer said that the embryos were not heirs, but John Noonan, at the time a law professor at Boalt and an active member of California's right-to-life organization, claimed that embryos had rights under California law. Meanwhile, in Melbourne, a right-to-life organization pressed the Victorian attorney general to appoint an independent legal guardian for the embryos. A Roman Catholic theologian said that a surrogate should be found to bear the children; several women were reported to have volunteered. The medical center then announced that the embryos were not Mario Rios's biological offspring after all. Donor sperm had been used. Moreover, the embryos were doubtfully viable. No pregnancies had occurred from embryos frozen at that time, and no pregnancies have occurred from embryos frozen over two years.

The Victorian government committee on ethical issues in IVF recommended that the embryos be destroyed, since the couple had not specified what they wanted done. But in November 1984 the Victorian Parliament passed laws regulating IVF; among its provisions was one stipulating that "orphaned" embryos should be anonymously donated to a woman who cannot produce her own eggs. Presumably this would be done only if the embryos in question were viable, which was extremely unlikely of the Rios embryos.

Writing in 1984, Peter Singer and Deane Wells acknowledged that cryopreservation of embryos creates legal problems that need to be clarified. These problems are especially difficult if the couple divorces and there has been no agreement about what should be done with the frozen embryos. However, Singer and Wells were not particularly troubled by this prospect:

> We shall not attempt to predict the evolution of the law in this new area. New solutions will have to be found to unusual problems. For most couples, however, the problems will not arise. If a couple has been well

counseled and has signed statements covering the most likely eventualities, few of these disputes should need to go to court to be resolved.[43]

This is a little like saying that few disputes over inheritance should need to go to court, since people can make wills. The fact is that people often do not make wills, and so inheritance matters often end up in court. Still, it should be easier to require people to consult lawyers about the disposition of embryos than to require them to make wills. In fact, this is standard operating procedure for most IVF centers, and could be made a legal requirement, as it is in the 1990 British Human Fertilisation and Embryology Act.[44] This might not completely obviate the need for courts to adjudicate in such cases. Just as wills and prenuptial agreements can be challenged, so can advance agreements on the disposition of frozen embryos. When such cases come before the courts, judges will have to decide how to consider extracorporeal embryos. Is the embryo the property of the couple concerned? Or should the embryos be considered to be ''preborn children'' and a custody model employed? This was the issue in the case of *Davis* v. *Davis*.[45]

Davis *v.* Davis

Mary Sue Davis and Junior Lewis Davis married in 1980. They very much wanted to have a family, but after Mrs. Davis suffered five tubal pregnancies, she had her fallopian tubes severed to prevent further risk to her. She and her husband thereafter decided to resort to *in vitro* fertilization. After six unsuccessful attempts at IVF, the Davises tried to adopt a child. This too was unsuccessful, and the Davises returned to the IVF program.

In the fall of 1988, Mrs. Davis learned about a new technique, cryopreservation. On December 8, 1988, nine eggs were aspirated from Mrs. Davis by laparoscopy, fertilized with Mr. Davis's sperm, and allowed to mature *in vitro* to the eight-cell cleavage stage. Two of the embryos were implanted in Mrs. Davis on December 10, 1988, neither of which resulted in a pregnancy. The remaining seven were placed in cryogenic storage for future implantation purposes.

The Davises discussed the fact that the storage life of the embryos probably would not exceed two years. They also considered the possibility of donating the remaining seven embryos, should Mrs. Davis become pregnant as a result of her implant on December 10, but the couple made no decision about that matter. Nor did they sign a consent form stipulating how the embryos should be disposed of in the event of future contingencies, such as their deaths or divorce. Apparently, the clinic had such forms, but the staff did not think it necessary that the Davises sign one, as they were "old customers" and were regarded as a very stable couple.

The couple filed for divorce in February 1989. Mr. Davis's filing papers requested an order enjoining the fertility clinic from releasing the embryos to Mrs. Davis or others for the purposes of thawing and implantation. With divorce impending, Mr. Davis did not want to become a parent. Mrs. Davis contended that she was the mother of the embryos, and that she had the right to try to establish a pregnancy with them. Moreover, she contended that the embryos were "preborn children" with rights of their own.

A circuit court judge, W. Dale Young, ruled in favor of Mrs. Davis. The judge framed the issue not as who should get the embryos, but rather whether the embryos were people or products. Judge Young concluded that the embryos *in vitro* were people, and therefore that a "best-interest" analysis was the appropriate one. He held that it was in the manifest best interest of these "children" that they be available for implantation and that their mother be permitted to bring them to term.

The judge's decision that the embryos are people was based exclusively on the testimony of one witness, French right-to-life physician Jerome Lejeune. The testimony of the other witnesses was rejected primarily because they all termed the embryos "pre-embryos." The judge held that he could not find the term in any encyclopedia or dictionary, and hence concluded that there is no such term, and that the seven cryopreserved entities were human embryos. Since, in his view, human life begins at conception, the embryos were human beings, with all the rights of other human beings.

A number of commentators have objected to the term "pre-embryo" as a recent verbal invention, created for self-serving reasons. John Marshall, a professor of clinical neurology and member of the Warnock Committee, writes:

> The term "pre-embryo" was not heard of prior to all this debate [on embryo experimentation]. From the time of fertilization up to about the eighth week the entity was called "embryo." Suddenly this term "pre-embryo" is now in every paper and every symposium. Some scientists are saying that they had been thinking along these lines already in 1975. It is surprising that if they had been thinking about it as far back as 1975, they never actually used the term until now. It seems like a public relations manoeuvre to make people think that the experts are against *embryo* experimentation, but that it is alright to experiment on the "pre-embryo," as if the latter was somehow different.[46]

Certainly, moral status should not depend on what the entity is called. However, it can be argued that the term "pre-embryo" is more accurate than "embryo" in characterizing the initial phase of mammalian and human development. The earliest stages of development after fertilization do not establish the embryo proper, but a feeding layer or trophoblast, which begins to function before the embryonic disc forms. For this reason, the zygote, morula, and early blastocyst stages can be regarded as pre-embryonic stages, with the term "embryo" reserved for the entity that appears at the end of the second week after fertilization, when the primitive streak, the precursor of the nervous system, appears.[47] Moreover, many commentators would argue that the term "pre-embryo" is not only scientifically more accurate, but that certain features of the pre-embryo—its lack of a nervous system, its ability to turn into more than one individual, and its inability to develop into a person without further intervention (transfer to a uterus)— justify ascribing to the pre-embryo a different moral status from that of the implanted embryo. The interest view does not regard these features as morally decisive, but nevertheless it is unfair and inaccurate to view the term "pre-embryo" as a mere verbal maneuver, and worse to claim, as did Judge Young, that the term does not exist.

Like so many other right-to-life advocates, Judge Young assumed that the issue was the genetic humanity of the embryos. But no one has ever disputed that the embryos are genetically human. The issue, totally missed by Judge Young, is whether these human embryos have the moral or legal status of born human beings. John Robertson expresses the point this way: "While the preimplantation embryo is clearly human and living, it does not follow that it is also a 'human life' or 'human being' in the crucial sense of a person with rights or interests."[48] Robertson calls the judge's conclusion that four-celled preimplantation human embryos are children "unprecedented and unwarranted."[49]

To show how ludicrous it is to equate blastocysts with children, George Annas gives the following example. If a fire broke out in a laboratory where the seven embryos were stored, and a two-month-old child was also in the laboratory, and only the embryos or the child could be saved, would anyone hesitate before saving the child? Of course not. This shows that no one really does equate embryos and children.[50]

Annas notes that if the judge really believed that he had to decide this case based on the "best interests of the children," he would have had at least to determine if Mrs. Davis was a fit mother to gestate them. "Given her past history of inability to carry a fetus to term, there is little probability of her successfully gestating any of the seven embryos. Requiring her to hire a surrogate mother to gestate them would almost certainly enhance their chances to be born."[51] Annas also points out that despite the fact that Judge Young spent all his time deciding that the embryos are people, not property, he ended up treating them like property. "Instead of deciding custody, visitation, and support issues (which he would have to do if the embryos *were* children), he awards them to Mrs. Davis in exactly the way he would award a dresser or a painting."[52]

Judge Young's decision was bad law and bad bioethics. This was recognized by the Tennessee Court of Appeals, an intermediate-level appeals court that overturned Judge Young's decision. The ruling was widely reported as giving both Junior Davis and his ex-wife, who has since remarried and is now Mary Sue Stowe, "joint custody" of the embryos. In fact, Mrs. Stowe and Mr. Davis were given joint *control* of the fertilized ova and equal voice over their disposition. The distinction is important. Joint custody suggests that the embryos were children; joint control does not. At this writing, the case is before the Tennessee Supreme Court, which heard oral arguments in May 1991.

If the embryos are not "preborn children," are they property? Some maintain that these are the only two possibilities currently in the law.[53] The property model is extremely repugnant to many people, not just right-to-lifers, for it suggests that embryos can be bought and sold, as sperm can be sold, or perhaps marketed for use in cosmetics.[54] However, there is an alternative to viewing extracorporeal embryos either as children or as property. George Annas expresses it this way:

> . . . embryos could just as easily be considered *neither* products nor people, but put in some other category altogether. There are many things, such as dogs, dolphins, and redwoods that are neither products nor people. We nonetheless legally protect these entities by limiting what their owners or custodians can do with them. Every national commission worldwide that has examined the status of the human embryo to date has placed it in this third category: neither people nor products, but nonetheless entities of unique symbolic value that deserve society's respect and protection.[55]

What are the implications of this view for deciding *Davis* v. *Davis?* The interests to be considered are not those of the preimplantation embryos, for preconscious, presentient entities do not yet have interests of their own. Rather, the relevant interests belong to the couple. The question is whose interests are most important and should prevail: Mrs. Stowe's interest in becoming a mother or Mr. Davis's interest in avoiding becoming a father?

While acknowledging that both parties have significant interests, John Robertson argues that, in the absence of advance instructions, the party wishing to avoid reproduction—in this case, Mr. Davis—should prevail. He writes:

A way out of the dilemma exists if we consider the irreversibility of the respective losses at issue and the essential fungibility of the embryos. The party who wishes to avoid offspring is irreversibly harmed if embryo transfer and birth occur, for the burdens of unwanted parenthood cannot then be avoided. On the other hand, frustrating the ability of the willing partner to reproduce with these embryos will—in most instances—not prevent that partner from reproducing at a later time with other embryos. As long as the party wishing to reproduce could without undue burden create other embryos, the desire to avoid biologic offspring should take priority over the desire to reproduce with the embryos in question.[56]

The burdens of unwanted parenthood include risks of financial liability. This risk could be removed by statute, relieving the party wishing to avoid reproduction of rearing rights and responsibilities, as has been done with donor insemination. As things stand now, however, a man providing sperm for insemination is the legal father, with rearing rights and duties, including support requirements. Mrs. Stowe has said that she has no interest in securing child support from her husband, but that would not prevent the children themselves or the state from seeking child support at a future date.

Mr. Davis's primary objection to becoming a father was not fear of financial liability. Rather, he objected to being "raped of his reproductive rights" and also to having a child produced to live in a single-parent home. His own life was shattered when, at the age of six, his parents were divorced and he and his three brothers were sent to a boys' home. Robertson refers to such considerations as the "psychosocial impact of unwanted biologic offspring," and argues that these should be given appropriate weight in deciding individual disputes. He maintains that Mr. Davis would be irreversibly harmed if embryo transfer and birth occur, as he would be forced to accept the psychosocial and financial burdens of parenthood. By contrast, Mrs. Stowe would not be irreversibly harmed by being denied embryo transfer, as she could reproduce at a later time with other embryos. Admittedly, she has undergone many painful, physically tiring, and emotionally taxing procedures. This is not determinative, according to Robertson, "since the burdens of any one additional retrieval cycle are moderate and acceptable, at least relative to the irreversible burdens of imposing fatherhood on the husband."[57]

The question of whose interests should prevail is extremely difficult to resolve. The procreative liberty of both parties is at stake. If these frozen embryos in fact represent Mrs. Stowe's last chance to give birth, her desire to become a mother should be given at least as much weight as Mr. Davis's desire to avoid fatherhood. The case would have to be settled by attempting to determine which party would be more badly harmed by frustration of his or her reproductive interests. Robertson suggests that the desire to avoid reproduction should take priority, so long as the party wishing to reproduce could, without undue burden, create other embryos. It seems to me that it would impose an "undue burden" to require Mrs. Stowe to undergo another round of treatment. She has already undergone serious physical burdens and risks, including being subjected to drugs and hormones to induce superovulation, the long-term effects of which have not been determined; laparoscopy, which carries a significant risk of mortality or morbidity; and the possibility of infection, physical damage, or an ectopic pregnancy through the placement of the zygotes in her uterus. In addition to the physical burdens, Mrs. Stowe has undergone severe emotional trauma from her seven failed attempts at IVF. To ask her to undergo yet another treatment cycle in order to have a chance at pregnancy would be unduly burdensome and unfair.

However, the situation changed when Mrs. Stowe decided not to try to have the pre-embryos implanted in her uterus, but to retain custody of the pre-embryos because they are "potential life" and she wants that potential realized. An appellee brief filed by her lawyer in May 1990 said that she now wants to donate the eggs to another infertile couple. This move prompted one of the judges on the state appeals court panel to question Mrs. Stowe's motives for still wanting the embryos. "Is this a case of a party wanting to win at any cost?" Judge Franks asked.[58]

From a right-to-life perspective, Mrs. Stowe's motives are noble. Her concern is solely for the welfare of her "preborn children." She is willing to renounce her claim to the frozen embryos, and her chance to become a mother, in order to enhance their chance of live birth. On the interest principle, however, the welfare of the embryos is not the issue, because fertilized eggs do not have a welfare or interests of their own. Nor does the case any longer involve a conflict of interests in reproductive liberty, since Mrs. Stowe no longer has any intention of becoming pregnant with the embryos. Mrs. Stowe's desire to have her genetic offspring brought to birth by someone else, who will then become the rearing parent, should have no weight at all. The only reproductive interest is Mr. Davis's interest in avoiding paternity. His interest should prevail. As Judge Franks wrote for the court:

> It would be repugnant and offensive to constitutional principles to order Mary Sue to implant these fertilized ova against her will. It would be equally repugnant to order Junior to bear the psychological, if not the legal, consequences of paternity against his will.[59]

Obviously, it would be better for everyone concerned if such matters never, or rarely ever, reached the courts. The British solution has been to allow storage of embryos only with the effective consent (i.e., written consent that has not been withdrawn) of both parties providing gametes. As Derek Morgan and Robert G. Lee interpret the Act, "Withdrawal of the consent of either donor to the embryo's creation appears to mean that it must be allowed to perish, although this does not appear explicitly stated."[60] Some American commentators have made similar recommendations.[61] The trouble with this solution is that it is unduly biased in favor of the party wishing to avoid reproduction. What if Mrs. Stowe wanted to attempt another pregnancy but was unable to produce more eggs, so that the frozen embryos represented her last chance at gestating a child? Should her ex-husband be able to thwart her procreative interest for no good reason, perhaps out of spite? A fairer solution is Robertson's proposed principle, which determines whose interests should prevail in terms of the relative burdens that will be imposed. The crucial point is that the relevant interests are not those of the embryos but those of the disputing parties. These cases will rarely be easy to resolve, but without conceptual clarity about the nature and status of extracorporeal embryos, they will be hopeless.

Notes

INTRODUCTION

1. Joel Feinberg, *Harm to Others* (New York, Oxford: Oxford University Press, 1984), p. 18.

CHAPTER 1

1. See Kurt Baier, *The Moral Point of View* (New York: Random House, 1965), especially Chapter Five.

2. Joel Feinberg, "The Rights of Animals and Unborn Generations," in William T. Blackstone, *Philosophy & Environmental Crisis* (University of Georgia Press, 1974), pp. 43–68. Reprinted in Thomas A. Mappes and Jane S. Zembaty, eds., *Social Ethics,* 3rd edition (New York: McGraw-Hill, 1987), pp. 484–493.

3. See, for example, Peter Singer, *Animal Liberation* (New York: Avon Books, 1975).

4. Immanuel Kant, "Duties to Animals," in Tom Regan/Peter Singer, eds., *Animal Rights and Human Obligations* (Englewoods Cliffs, N.J.: Prentice-Hall, 1976), pp. 122–123.

5. Louis B. Schwartz, "Moral Offenses and the Model Penal Code," *Columbia Law Review* 63 (1963), p. 669. Reprinted in Joel Feinberg and Hyman Gross, eds., *Philosophy of Law,* 3rd edition (Belmont, Calif.: Wadsworth, 1986), pp. 236–237.

6. Albert Schweitzer, "The Ethics of Reverence for Life,"

in Regan/Singer, *Animal Rights and Human Obligations* (see note 4), pp. 133–138.

7. Ibid., p. 134.

8. Ibid., p. 137.

9. Joel Feinberg, *Harm to Others* (New York: Oxford University Press, 1984), p. 34.

10. Ibid.

11. See H.L.A. Hart, "Are There Any Natural Rights?" *The Philosophical Review* 64 (1955). Reprinted in A.I. Melden, ed., *Human Rights* (Belmont, Calif.: Wadsworth Publishing Company, Inc., 1970.) Hart argues that if X promises Y that he will look after Y's aged mother, then it is Y, and not Y's mother, to whom performance is owed. Y's mother is a person *concerning whom* X has an obligation and a person who will benefit by its performance, but the person *to whom* X has an obligation is Y. "It is important for the whole logic of rights that, while the person who stands to benefit by the performance of a duty is discovered by considering what will happen if the duty is not performed, the person who has a right (to whom performance is *owed* or *due*) is discovered by examining the transaction or antecedent situation or relations of the parties out of which the 'duty' arises." (*Human Rights,* p. 66.)

12. Tom Regan, "Feinberg on What Sorts of Beings Can Have Rights," *The Southern Journal of Philosophy* 14 (1976), pp. 485–498.

13. Ibid., p. 490.

14. Ibid., pp. 492–493.

15. Feinberg, *Harm to Others* (see note 9), p. 491.

16. Ibid., p. 490.

17. R.G. Frey, *Interests and Rights: The Case Against Animals* (Oxford: Clarendon Press, 1980).

18. Stephen Stich, "Do Animals Have Beliefs?" *Australasian Journal of Philosophy* 57 (March 1979), p. 18.

19. Donald Davidson, "Rational Animals," 36 *Dialectica* (1982), pp. 320–321. Reprinted in Ernest LePore and Brian P. McLaughlin, eds., *Action and Events: Perspectives on the Philosophy of Donald Davidson* (Oxford: Basil Blackwell, 1985), p. 475.

20. Stich (see note 18), p. 27.

21. Ibid., p. 26.

22. In fact, as Stich points out, Davidson's view seems to restrict beliefs not only to language-users, but to language-users who share a significant number of our background beliefs. For, according to Davidson, we can say what someone believes only if there is a shared fund of background beliefs. This means that people from radically different cultures, or very distant eras, could not be said to have beliefs. Stich comments, "But surely all this is perverse and amounts to no more than a reduction of the principle that beliefs must have specifiable content." "Do Animals Have Beliefs?" (see note 18), p. 25.

23. Thomas Nagel, *The Possibility of Altruism* (Oxford: Clarendon Press, 1970).

24. A number of philosophers emphasize the importance of sentience to moral status. See especially L. W. Sumner, *Abortion and Moral Theory* (Princeton, N.J.: Princeton University Press, 1981). See also Mary Anne Warren, "Do Potential People Have Moral Rights?" in R.I. Sikora and Brian Barry, eds., *Obligations to Future Generations* (Philadelphia, Penn.: Temple University Press, 1978), pp. 22–24, and Samuel Gorovitz, *Doctors' Dilemmas: Moral Conflict and Medical Care* (New York: Oxford University Press, 1982). Peter Singer argues that not only must the interests of all sentient beings be considered, but the comparable interests of all sentient beings must count equally. *Animal Liberation* (see note 3), pp. 8–9 and 23–24.

25. Feinberg, *Harm to Others* (see note 9), p. 83.

26. Ibid., p. 90 (borrowing these categories from George Pitcher, "The Misfortunes of the Dead," *American Philosophical Quarterly* 21 (1984), p. 184.

27. W.D. Ross, *Foundations of Ethics* (Oxford: Clarendon Press, 1939), p. 300. Cited in Feinberg, *Harm to Others* (see note 9), p. 84.

28. Feinberg, *Harm to Others* (see note 9), p. 91.

29. Several critics have found this paradoxical. See, for example, Joan Callahan, "On Harming the Dead," *Ethics* 97 (1987), Nancy K. Rhoden, "Litigating Life and Death," *Harvard Law Review* 102 (December 1988), and Judith Thomson, "Feinberg on Harm, Offense, and the Criminal Law: A Review Essay," *Philosophy & Public Affairs* 15 (Fall 1986), pp. 381–395.

30. I owe this way of explaining postmortem harm to Professor Robert Meyers.

31. It goes without saying that not all interests are—or should be—protected by law. For example, under Anglo-American law, one cannot libel the dead; that is, the estate of a dead person cannot recover damages for libel. The rationale for this is a societal interest in free speech that might be hampered if authors and publishers had to be concerned about lawsuits. The dead no longer can suffer from a loss of reputation; they don't have to worry about losing their jobs or their friends. Therefore, their interest in maintaining a good reputation, real as it is, can be outweighed by the interest society has in the unrestricted flow of ideas. Nevertheless, someone who maliciously and knowingly sets out to defame a dead person not only acts wrongly; he wrongs and harms the once-living person who is now dead.

32. Ronald E. Cranford, "The Persistent Vegetative State: The Medical Reality (Getting the Facts Straight)" (hereafter "The Persistent Vegetative State"), *Hastings Center Report* 18 (February/March 1988), p. 31.

33. Ibid., p. 27.

34. Ibid., p. 31. The longest recorded PVS was that of Elaine Esposito: thirty-seven years, 111 days. Norris McWhirter, ed., *The Guinness Book of World Records* (New York: Bantam Books, 1981), p. 42.

35. *Brophy* v. *New England Sinai Hospital, Inc.* 398 Mass. 417, 497 N.E.2d 626 (1986).

36. *Brophy,* Amicus Curiae Brief, American Academy of Neurology, Minneapolis, MN (1986). Cited in Cranford (see note 32), p. 31.

37. A.B. Fletcher, "Pain in the Neonate," *New England Journal of Medicine* 217 (1987), pp. 1347–1348.

38. Cranford (see note 32), p. 29.

39. I have written about a dramatic illustration of medical fallibility regarding PVS in "Recovery from Persistent Vegetative State? The Case of Carrie Coons," *Hastings Center Report* 19 (July/August 1989), pp. 14–15.

40. President's Commission for the Study of Ethical Problems in Medicine and Biomedical and Behavioral Research, *Deciding to Forego Life-Sustaining Treatment* (New York: Concern for Dying, 1983), p. 179.

41. Telephone conversation with Dr. Ronald Cranford, May 31, 1988. Dr. Cranford is a neurologist in Minneapolis, a past president of the American Society of Law and Medicine, and a consultant to the White House on right-to-die issues.

42. The distinction between biological life (being alive) and biographical life (having a life) is drawn by James Rachels in *The End of Life: Euthanasia and Morality* (Oxford University Press, 1986), p. 25.

43. This view was taken by the President's Commission in *Deciding to Forego Life-Sustaining Treatment* (see note 40), pp. 181–182.

44. The case of Helga Wanglie, widely reported in the newspapers, may be a case in point. After a heart attack in May 1990, Mrs. Wanglie was diagnosed as being in a persistent vegetative state, with no hope of regaining consciousness. In 1991, when the hospital sought to remove her life-support system, her husband and two children strenuously objected, saying that she was a devout Lutheran who told them that she favored every effort to maintain life. A judge agreed with Mr. Wanglie that he was in the best position to know his wife's beliefs, and gave him the power to make medical decisions for her. Although Mrs. Wanglie remained on life support, she died anyway within a few days.

45. Fred Rosner et al., "The Anencephalic Fetus and Newborn as Organ Donors," *New York State Journal of Medicine* (July 1988), pp. 360–365, at 360.

46. Ibid.

47. Sue A. Meinke, "Anencephalic Infants as Potential Organ Sources: Ethical and Legal Issues," Scope Note 12, National Reference Center for Bioethics Literature, Kennedy Institute of Ethics, citing Michael Harrison, "Organ Procurement for Children: the Anencephalic Fetus as Donor," *Lancet* 2:8520, December 1986, pp. 1383–1386, and Robert C. Cefalo and H. Tristram Engelhardt, "The Use of Anencephalic Tissue for Transplantation," *Journal of Medicine and Philosophy* 14:1 (February 1989), pp. 25–43.

48. Joyce L. Peabody, Janet R. Emery, and Stephen Ashwall, "Experience with Anencephalic Infants as Prospective Organ Donors," *The New England Journal of Medicine* 321:6 (August 10, 1989), pp. 344–350, at 344.

49. Alexander M. Capron, "Anencephalic Donors: Separate the Dead from the Dying," *Hastings Center Report* 17:1 (February 1987), p. 6.

50. Ronald E. Cranford and John C. Roberts, "Use of Anencephalic Infants as Organ Donors: Crossing a Threshold," in Howard H. Kaufman, ed., *Pediatric Brain Death and Organ Tissue Retrieval: Medical, Ethical and Legal Aspects* (New

York and London: Plenum Medical Book Company, 1989), Chapter 20, pp. 191–197.

51. See John Arras and Shlomo Shinnar, "Anencephalic Newborns as Organ Donors: A Critique," *Journal of the American Medical Association* 259:15 (April 15, 1988), pp. 2284–2285; Alexander Capron, "Anencephalic Donors" (see note 49); and D. Alan Shewmon, Alexander Capron, Warwick J. Peacock, and Barbara L. Shulman, "The Use of Anencephalic Infants as Organ Sources: A Critique," *Journal of the American Medical Association* 261:12 (March 24/31, 1989), pp. 1773–1781.

52. Shewmon et al., "The Use of Anencephalic Infants as Organ Sources" (see note 51), p. 1775.

53. Samuel Gorovitz, *Doctors' Dilemmas* (MacMillan Publishing Co., Inc., 1982), pp. 167–168.

54. Cranford and Roberts, "Use of Anencephalic Infants as Organ Donors" (see note 50), p. 193.

55. Arthur L. Caplan, "Should Fetuses or Infants Be Utilized as Organ Donors?" *Bioethics* 1:2 (1987), p. 122.

56. Cranford and Roberts, "Use of Anencephalic Infants as Organ Donors" (see note 50), p. 193.

57. Shewmon et al., "Anencephalic Infants as Organ Sources" (see note 52), p. 1776.

58. Ibid.

59. Cranford and Roberts, "Anencephalic Infants as Organ Donors" (see note 50), p. 193.

60. D. A. Shewmon, "Anencephaly: Selected Medical Aspects," *Hastings Center Report* 18:5 (October/November 1988), pp. 11–19.

61. Ibid., p. 13.

62. Ibid., p. 17.

63. Capron, "Anencephalic Donors" (see note 49), p. 8.

64. See Allen E. Buchanan, "The Limits of Proxy Decisionmaking for Incompetents," *UCLA Law Review* 29:2, December 1981.

65. Caplan, "Should Fetuses or Infants Be Utilized as Organ Donors?" (see note 55), p. 138.

66. See Richard T. De George, "Do We Owe the Future Anything?" in *Law and the Ecological Challenge* (1978). Reprinted in James P. Sterba, ed., *Morality in Practice*, 2nd edition (Belmont, California: Wadsworth, 1988), pp. 108–115.

67. Derek Parfit, *Reasons and Persons* (Oxford: Clarendon Press, 1984), p. 356.

68. Ibid., p. 357.

69. Ibid., p. 361.

70. Douglas MacLean, "A Moral Requirement for Energy Policies," in Douglas MacLean and Peter G. Brown, eds., *Energy and the Future* (Totowa, N.J.: Rowman & Littlefield, 1983), pp. 180–197.

71. Feinberg agrees. He argues that a pact on the part of all human beings

never to have children would not violate the rights of those who would otherwise have been born. "My inclination then is to conclude that the suicide of our species would be deplorable, lamentable, and a deeply moving tragedy: but that it would violate no one's rights." *Harm to Others* (see note 9), p. 493.

CHAPTER 2

1. *Roe* v. *Wade,* 410 U.S. 113 (1973).

2. Technically, the term "fetus" refers to the unborn after eight weeks of gestation. Many writers on abortion use the term "fetus" to refer generally to the unborn throughout pregnancy. I will follow this convention except where necessary to distinguish the different phases of gestation.

3. Kristin Luker, *Abortion and the Politics of Motherhood* (Berkeley, Calif.: University of California Press, 1984), especially Chapter 7.

4. Ruth Macklin, "Personhood and the Abortion Debate," in Jay Garfield and Patricia Hennessey, eds., *Abortion: Moral and Legal Perspectives* (Amherst, Mass.: The University of Massachusetts Press, 1984), p. 97.

5. A good example is Don Marquis, "Why Abortion is Immoral," *The Journal of Philosophy* 76:4 (April 1989), pp. 183–202.

6. See, for example, Sandra Harding, "Beneath the Surface of the Abortion Dispute," in Sidney Callahan and Daniel Callahan, eds., *Abortion: Understanding Differences* (New York and London: Plenum Press, 1984).

7. Ibid., p. 214.

8. Judith Jarvis Thomson, "A Defense of Abortion," *Philosophy & Public Affairs* 1:1 (1971). Reprinted in Joel Feinberg, ed., *The Problem of Abortion,* 2nd edition (Belmont, Calif.: Wadsworth Publishing Company, 1984), pp. 173–187.

9. John T. Noonan, Jr., "An Almost Absolute Value in History," in John T. Noonan, Jr., ed., *The Morality of Abortion: Legal and Historical Perspectives* (Cambridge, Mass.: Harvard University Press, 1970). Reprinted in John D. Arras/ Nancy K. Rhoden, eds., *Ethical Issues in Modern Medicine,* 3rd edition (Mountain View, Calif.: Mayfield Publishing Company, 1989), pp. 261–265.

10. *Roe* v. *Wade* (see note 1), p. 160.

11. Noonan, "An Almost Absolute Value in History" (see note 9), p. 10.

12. Richard Warner, "Abortion: The Ontological and Moral Status of the Unborn," *Social Theory and Practice* 3:4 (1974). Revised and reprinted in Richard A. Wasserstrom, ed., *Today's Moral Problems,* 2nd edition (New York: Mac-Millan Publishing Company, Inc., 1979), p. 55.

13. Obstetricians date the beginning of a pregnancy from the woman's last menstrual period, which can be more reliably fixed than conception. This adds approximately two weeks to the fetus's age. Thus, a fetus that is 14 weeks g.a. is actually about 12 weeks old.

14. Baruch Brody, *Abortion and the Sanctity of Life* (Cambridge, Mass.: The MIT Press, 1975), p. 111.

15. Ibid., p. 83.

16. K.J.S. Anand and P.R. Hickey, "Pain and Its Effects in the Human Neo-

nate and Fetus," *The New England Journal of Medicine* 317:21, Nov. 19, 1987, p. 1322.

17. Mary Warnock, *A Question of Life: The Warnock Report on Human Fertilization and Embryology* (Oxford: Basil Blackwell, 1985), pp. 59–60.

18. Cited in Michael Lockwood, "Warnock versus Powell (and Harradine): When Does Potentiality Count?" *Bioethics* 2:3 (July 1988), p. 190.

19. I borrow this term from Rosalind Hursthouse, *Beginning Lives* (Oxford: Basil Blackwell in association with the Open University), 1987.

20. Mary Anne Warren, "On the Moral and Legal Status of Abortion," *The Monist* 57 (1973). Reprinted in Joel Feinberg, ed., *The Problem of Abortion* (see note 8), pp. 102–119.

21. Ibid., p. 109.

22. It may be that in calling abortion morally neutral, Warren intended only to claim that abortion is a private decision, and not one with which the State ought to be concerned. With this claim, I of course agree. I suspect that her comparison of abortion with having one's hair cut was largely hyperbole, a reaction against right-to-lifers who maintain that abortion is murder.

23. Jean Bethke Elshtain, "Commentary to Chapter 5," in Sidney Callahan and Daniel Callahan, eds., *Abortion: Understanding Differences* (see note 6), p. 139.

24. Joel Feinberg makes this point in "Abortion," in Tom Regan, ed., *Matters of Life and Death: New Introductory Essays in Moral Philosophy,* 2nd edition (New York: Random House, 1986), p. 259.

25. H. Tristram Engelhardt, "Viability and the Use of the Fetus," in W.B. Bondeson, H. Tristram Engelhardt, Jr., S.F. Spicker, and D.H. Winship, eds., *Abortion and the Status of the Fetus* (Dordrecht, Holland: D. Reidel Publishing Company, 1983), p. 185.

26. Ruth Macklin, "Personhood and the Abortion Debate" (see note 4), p. 97.

27. Michael Tooley, *Abortion and Infanticide* (Oxford: Clarendon Press, 1983), p. 100.

28. Tooley, "A Defense of Abortion and Infanticide," in Joel Feinberg, ed., *The Problem of Abortion* (see note 8), p. 73.

29. Ibid., p. 120.

30. Dr. Benjamin Spock, *Baby and Child Care* (New York: Pocket Books, 1976), p. 9.

31. A similar argument is made by Carson Strong, "Delivering Hydrocephalic Fetuses," *Bioethics* 5:1 (January 1991), pp. 7–11.

32. Stephen Buckle, "Arguing from Potential," *Bioethics* 2:3 (July 1988), p. 227.

33. Ibid.

34. Stanley Benn, "Abortion, Infanticide, and Respect for Persons," in Feinberg, ed., *The Problem of Abortion* (see note 8), p. 143.

35. Don Marquis, "Why Abortion is Immoral" (see note 5), pp. 183–202.

36. See Paul Bassen, "Present Sakes and Future Prospects: The Status of Early

Abortion,'' *Philosophy & Public Affairs* 11:4 (1982), pp. 314–337. Bassen argues on grounds similar to mine that embryos are not the sorts of things that can be victims.

37. Clifford Grobstein, *Science and the Unborn* (New York: Basic Books, Inc., 1988), p. 76.

38. John Harris, *The Value of Life: An Introduction to Medical Ethics* (London: Routledge & Kegan Paul, 1985), pp. 11–12.

39. R. M. Hare may be the only potentiality theorist who does not hinge his argument on a morally significant difference between embryos and gametes. On Hare's version of the argument from potential, abortion is *prima facie* morally wrong, but so are contraception and abstention from procreation. See "Abortion and the Golden Rule," *Philosophy & Public Affairs* 4:3 (Spring 1975).

40. "Study Finds 31% Rate of Miscarriage," *The New York Times,* Wednesday, July 27, 1988, p. A14.

41. Hursthouse, *Beginning Lives* (see note 19), p. 80.

42. Warner, "Abortion: The Ontological and Moral Status of the Unborn" (see note 12), p. 57.

43. Peter Singer and Karen Dawson, "IVF Technology and the Argument from Potential," *Philosophy & Public Affairs* 17:2 (Spring 1988), p. 96.

44. Stephen Buckle, "Arguing from Potential" (see note 32), p. 241.

45. Ibid., p. 230.

46. Ibid., p. 237.

47. Ibid., p. 238.

48. Joel Feinberg, "Abortion" (see note 24), p. 267.

49. Tooley, *Abortion and Infanticide* (see note 27), p. 193.

50. Angela Neustatter, with Gina Newson, *Mixed Feelings: the Experience of Abortion* (London: Pluto Press, 1986), p. 10.

51. Hursthouse, *Beginning Lives* (see note 19).

52. However, a recent study showed that more than a third of women denied abortions confessed to strongly negative feelings toward their children, and that children born to women whose requests for abortion were refused are much likelier to be troubled and depressed, to drop out of school, to commit crimes, to suffer from serious illnesses, and to express dissatisfaction with life than are the offspring of willing parents. See Natalie Angier, "Study Says Anger Troubles Women Denied Abortions," *The New York Times,* May 29, 1991, C10.

53. Hare, "Abortion and the Golden Rule" (see note 39), pp. 220–221.

54. Feinberg, *Harm to Others* (Oxford: Oxford University Press, 1984), pp. 81–82.

55. This view is also taken by John Bigelow and Robert Pargetter, in "Morality, Potential Persons and Abortion," *American Philosophical Quarterly* 25:2 (April 1988), pp. 173–181.

56. Don Locke, "The Parfit Population Problem," *Philosophy* 62 (April 1987), pp. 131–157, p. 137.

57. Ibid., p. 138.

58. R. B. Brandt, "The Morality of Abortion," in Robert L. Perkins, ed., *Abortion: Pro and Con* (Cambridge, Mass.: Schenkman Publishing Company, 1974), p. 163.

59. Mary Anne Warren, "Do Potential People Have Moral Rights?" in R. I. Sikora and Brian Barry, eds., *Obligations to Future Generations* (Philadelphia, Pa.: Temple University Press, 1978), p. 25.

60. In *Reasons and Persons,* Parfit argues that the usual principles offered to justify our moral convictions are inadequate. They are too narrow, or they conflict with one another, or they yield extremely counterintuitive judgments. We need, according to Parfit, a new theory of beneficence, or *Theory X.* Theory X would have acceptable implications when applied to both Same People and Different People Choices. It would solve both the Non-Identity Problem and what he calls "the Repugnant Conclusion" (that it is better to have many more marginally happy people than fewer much happier people). Parfit has not yet found Theory X, but remains optimistic that either he or someone else will.

61. John D. Arras, "AIDS and Reproductive Decisions: Having Children in Fear and Trembling," *The Milbank Quarterly* 68:3 (1990), pp. 353–382, at 355. A more recent article places the risk at 13 to 30 percent (Mireya Navarro, "Women With AIDS Virus: Hard Choices on Motherhood," the *The New York Times,* July 23, 1991, A1.

62. Ibid., p. 365.

63. Thomson, "A Defense of Abortion" (see note 8).

64. Ibid., p. 174.

65. The claim that individuals do not have a legal obligation to donate body parts to others, even when they are needed for life itself, has been upheld in several cases. The first recorded case, to my knowledge, is *Shimp* v. *McFall,* 10 Pa. D. & D.3d 90 (1978), which I discuss in Chapter 4.

66. Thomson, "A Defense of Abortion" (see note 8), p. 182.

67. The burdens of even normal pregnancies are well detailed by Donald Regan, "Rewriting *Roe* v. *Wade,*" *Michigan Law Review* 77 (1979).

68. Thomson, "A Defense of Abortion" (see note 8), p. 184.

69. Warren, "On the Moral and Legal Status of Abortion" (see note 20), p. 108.

70. *Roe* v. *Wade* (see note 1), p. 161.

71. Ibid., p. 154.

72. Ibid., p. 163–164.

73. *Webster* v. *Reproductive Health Services,* 492 U.S. 490 (July 3, 1989).

74. Roberto Suro, "Nation's Strictest Abortion Law Enacted in Louisiana Over Veto," *The New York Times,* June 19, 1991, A1.

75. "U.S. Judge Strikes Down Louisiana Abortion Law," *The New York Times,* Thursday, August 8, 1991, A16.

76. The Supreme Court did not reconsider its decision in *Roe* in deciding *Webster,* because it did not consider the Missouri statute to be in conflict with *Roe.* In her concurring opinion, Sandra Day O'Connor wrote, "When the constitutional

invalidity of a State's abortion statute actually turns on the constitutional validity of *Roe* v. *Wade,* there will be time enough to reexamine *Roe.* And to do so carefully.''

The first abortion law reviewed by the Supreme Court was Pennsylvania's, on April 22, 1992. A decision is expected by July. Under the state law, a woman seeking an abortion must wait 24 hours after applying for one; doctors must tell women seeking abortions about fetal development and alternatives to abortion; minors in most cases must obtain approval from at least one parent, and married women in most cases must notify their husbands of their plans for an abortion. In October 1991, a federal appeals court upheld most of the law's abortion restrictions, but found the spousal notice provision unconstitutional. Significantly, the court held that the abortion right was no longer fundamental and abortion restrictions were to be reviewed under an "undue burden" test rather than strict scrutiny.

77. For such a discussion, see Ronald Dworkin, "The Great Abortion Case," *The New York Review of Books* 36:11, June 29, 1989, pp. 49–52.

78. See, for example, George J. Annas (Counsel of Record), Leonard H. Glantz, and Wendy K. Mariner, Brief for Bioethicists for Privacy as Amicus Curiae Supporting Appellees, *Webster* v. *Reproductive Health Services,* No. 88–605, March 30, 1989.

79. *Eisenstadt* v. *Baird,* 405 U.S. 438, 453 (1972).

80. Regan, "Rewriting *Roe* v. *Wade*" (see note 67).

81. *Roe* v. *Wade* (see note 1), p. 153.

82. Ibid., p. 163.

83. John Hart Ely, "The Wages of Crying Wolf: A Comment on *Roe* v. *Wade,*" *Yale Law Journal* 82:920, at 924 (1973).

84. Norman Fost, David Chudwin, and Daniel Wikler, "The Limited Moral Significance of 'Fetal Viability,' " *Hastings Center Report* (December 1980), pp. 12–13.

85. Patricia A. King, "The Juridical Status of the Fetus: A Proposal for Legal Protection of the Unborn," *Michigan Law Review* 77 (1979).

86. *Akron* v. *Akron Center for Reproductive Health,* 462 U.S. 416, 458 (1983).

87. Gina Kolata, "Survival of the Fetus: A Barrier is Reached," *The New York Times,* Tuesday, April 18, 1989, C1–C5.

88. Nancy K. Rhoden, "Trimesters and Technology: Revamping *Roe* v. *Wade,*" *Yale Law Journal* 95:4 (March 1986), pp. 639–697, at 661.

89. Ibid., p. 658.

90. Ibid., p. 671.

91. Ibid., p. 684.

92. Ibid., pp. 658–662.

93. For an argument that fetuses begin to acquire sentient capacity as early as 6 weeks, and certainly by 9 to 10 weeks of gestation, see Peter McCullagh, *The Fetus as Transplant Donor: Scientific, Social and Ethical Perspectives* (Chichester: John Wiley & Sons, 1987), Chapter 9.

94. Gary B. Gertler, "Brain Birth: A Proposal for Defining When a Fetus is

Entitled to Human Life Status,'' *Southern California Law Review* 59 (1986), pp. 1061–1078. Other scholars have also suggested a ''brain-birth'' standard. At an international symposium held at the University of Iowa, November 4–7, 1990, Hans-Martin Sass, a professor of philosophy and senior research fellow at the Kennedy Institute of Ethics at Georgetown University, proposed a model piece of legislation that would extend legal protection to fetuses at a point when integrated brain functioning begins to emerge—at 10 weeks after conception. This point was chosen as ''a morally conservative'' point in development, when the connections between nerve cells first appear in the area that will become the embryo's cerebral cortex. Peter Steinfels, ''Scholar Proposes 'Brain Birth' Law,'' *The New York Times,* November 8, 1990, A28.

95. Gertler, ''Brain Birth'' (see note 94), p. 1069. Gertler apparently does not notice that, taken literally, his proposal commits him to ascribing full and equal protection against homicide to chimpanzees and gorillas. All primates, not just humans, have neocortical activity.

96. Tooley, *Abortion and Infanticide* (see note 27), p. 407.

97. Nan D. Hunter, ''Time Limits on Abortion,'' in Sherrill Cohen and Nadine Taub, eds., *Reproductive Laws for the 1990s* (Clifton, New Jersey: Humana Press, 1989), p. 130. Citing Henshaw, Binkin, Blaine and Smith, ''A Portrait of American Women Who Obtain Abortions,'' *Family Planning Perspectives* 17 (1985), p. 91.

98. Ibid., pp. 132–133.

99. Ibid., p. 147.

100. Robert D. Goldstein, *Mother-love and Abortion: A Legal Interpretation* (Berkeley and Los Angeles, California: University of California Press), p. 47.

101. In ''Trimesters and Technology'' (see note 88, p. 690), Nancy Rhoden persuasively argues that abortions for fetal indications present different problems, and that the time period for such abortions should be longer than for elective abortions.

CHAPTER 3

1. *Roe* v. *Wade,* 410 U.S. 113, 161.

2. *State* v. *Beale,* 64PA88–Cumberland, Feb. 9, 1989.

3. George Gombossy, ''Viable Fetus Isn't Human, Judge Rules in Shooting Case,'' *The National Law Journal,* Monday, June 30, 1986, p. 8.

4. *O'Grady* v. *Brown,* 64734, Supreme Court of Missouri, Aug. 16, 1983.

5. Minn. Stat., Sect. 609.2661(1), 609.2662(1). In *State* v. *Merrill* (C7–89–766), the Supreme Court of Minnesota ruled that the state's fetal homicide statutes do not violate the equal-protection or due-process clauses of the U.S. Constitution.

6. *Craig* v. *IMT Insurance Co.,* 118/86–535.

7. Dawn Johnsen, ''The Creation of Fetal Rights: Conflicts with Women's Constitutional Rights to Liberty, Privacy, and Equal Protection,'' *Yale Law Journal* 95 (1986) (hereafter ''Women's Rights/Fetal Rights''), p. 603.

8. *Bonbrest* v. *Kotz,* 65 F. Supp. 138 (1946).

9. The same result was reached earlier in Canada in *Montreal Tramways* v. *Leveille* (4 D.L.R. 337, 345 (S.C.C. 1933). In England the same result has been reached by statute through the Congenital Disabilities Act (1976). The act totally supersedes the common law.

10. Three jurisdictions (Nebraska, Arizona, and Virginia) do not allow recovery for prenatal injuries. Ten states (South Dakota, North Dakota, Alaska, Hawaii, Idaho, Colorado, Arkansas, Montana, Maine, and Wyoming) have not been confronted with the issue of whether live-born children can recover for prenatal injuries. It can be safely assumed that when these states are confronted, the majority will allow recovery at least from viability if not conception because no court has explicitly rejected the theory in modern times. See Ron Beal, " 'Can I Sue Mommy?' An Analysis of a Woman's Tort Liability for Prenatal Injuries to her Child Born Alive" (hereafter "Prenatal Injuries"), *San Diego Law Review* 21 (1984).

11. *Dietrich* v. *Northampton,* 138 Mass. 14 (1884).

12. *Allaire* v. *St. Luke's Hospital,* 184 Ill. 359, 56 N.E. 638 (1900).

13. Ibid., p. 642.

14. Ibid., p. 641.

15. Ibid., p. 642.

16. See, for example, *Amann* v. *Faidy,* 415 Ill. 422, 430–31, 114 N.E.2d 412.

17. *Kelly* v. *Gregory,* 282 A.D. 542, 125 N.Y.S.2d 696 (1953).

18. *Smith* v. *Brennan,* 31 N.J. 353, 367, 157 A.2d 497, 504 (1960).

19. Harper and James, *Law of Torts,* Vol. 2 (1956), p. 1030, emphasis added.

20. 483 F.2d 237 (10th Cir. 1973). Cited in David L. Runner, "The Prenatal Plaintiff and the *Feres* Doctrine: Throwing Baby Out with the Bath Water?" *Willamette Law Review* 20 (1984), p. 502.

21. *Renslow* v. *Mennonite Hospital,* 67 Ill.2d 348, 367 N.E.2d 1250 (1977) [alleged that negligent blood transfusion to plaintiff's mother eight years prior to her conception caused injuries to plaintiff's brain, nervous system, and other organs]; *Bergstresser* v. *Mitchell,* 577 F.2d 22 (8th Cir. 1978) [infant plaintiff alleged that due to a negligent cesarean performed two years before his conception, he was born with brain damage and other severe injuries].

22. *Albala* v. *City of New York,* 54 N.Y.2d 269, 429 N.E.2d 786, 445 N.Y.S.2d 108 (1981).

23. *Enright* v. *Lilly & Co.,* 155 A.D.2d 64 (1990).

24. Ibid., p. 70.

25. In *Hymowitz* v. *Lilly & Co.,* 155 A.D.2d 64 (1990), the New York Court of Appeals held that liability could be imposed upon DES manufacturers in accordance with their share of the national DES market, notwithstanding the plaintiff's inability to identify the manufacturer particularly at fault for her injuries.

26. *Enright* v. *Lilly & Co.* (see note 23), p. 69.

27. Ibid., p. 71.

28. *Enright by Enright* v. *Lilly & Company,* 568 N.Y.S.2d 550 (Ct.App. 1991).

29. Ibid., p. 555.

30. *The National Law Journal,* Monday, October 21, 1991, p. 6.

31. See, for example, John A. Robertson, "Procreative Liberty and the Control of Conception, Pregnancy and Childbirth," *Virginia Law Review* 69 (1983), p. 438.

32. *Hewellette* v. *George*, 68 Miss. 703, 9 So. 885 (1891).

33. *Stallman by Stallman* v. *Youngquist*, 152 Ill.App.3d 683, 504 N.E.2d 920, 924 (1987).

34. *Goller* v. *White*, 20 Wis.2d 402, 122 N.W.2d 193 (1963).

35. Beal, "Prenatal Injuries" (see note 10), p. 336.

36. Ibid., p. 357.

37. The phrase is Janet Gallagher's. See "Prenatal Invasions & Interventions: What's Wrong with Fetal Rights," *Harvard Women's Law Journal* 10 (1987), p. 13.

38. *Grodin* v. *Grodin*, Mich.App., 301 N.W.2d 869 (1981).

39. Robertson, "Procreative Liberty" (see note 31), p. 441, footnote 114.

40. Johnsen, "Women's Rights/Fetal Rights" (see note 7), p. 607.

41. Beal, "Prenatal Injuries" (see note 10), p. 340.

42. *Stallman* v. *Youngquist*, 125 Ill.2d 267, 531 N.E.2d 355 (1988).

43. *Stallman* v. *Youngquist*, 504 N.E.2d 920, 925 (1987), citing *Sorensen* v. *Sorensen*, 369 Mass. 350, 359, 339 N.E.2d 907, 912 (1975).

44. For a more extensive treatment of wrongful-death actions, see my "Prenatal Wrongful Death," *Bioethics* 1:4 (October 1987), pp. 301–320.

45. Stuart M. Speiser and Stuart S. Malawer, "An American Tragedy: Damages for Mental Anguish of Bereaved Relatives in Wrongful Death Actions," *Tulane Law Review* 51 (1976).

46. See, for example, *Kwaterski* v. *State Farm Mutual Automobile Insurance Company*, 34 Wis.2d 14, 201, 148 N.W.2d 107, 110 (1967), holding that barring prenatal wrongful death ". . . would produce the absurd result that an unborn child who was badly injured by the tortious acts of another, but who was born alive could recover while an unborn child, who was more severely injured and died as a result of the tortious acts of another, could recover nothing."

47. *Moen* v. *Hanson*, 85 Wn. 597, 537 P.2d 266 (1975).

48. *Torigian* v. *Watertown News Co.*, 352 Mass. 446, 225 N.E.2d 926 (1967).

49. *Wallace* v. *Wallace*, 120 N.H. 675, 679, 421 A.2d 134, 137 (1980).

50. *Toth* v. *Goree*, 65 Mich. App. 296, 304, 237 N.W.2d 297, 301 (1975).

51. "Recovery for the Tortious Death of the Unborn," *South Carolina Law Review* 33 (1982), p. 802.

52. David Westfall, "Beyond Abortion: The Potential Reach of a Human Life Amendment," *American Journal of Law & Medicine* 8:2 (Summer 1982), p. 112.

53. See, for example, Margery Shaw, "Conditional Prospective Rights of the Fetus," *Journal of Legal Medicine* 5 (1984); John E. B. Myers, "Abuse and Neglect of the Unborn: Can the State Intervene?" *Duquesne Law Review* 23 (1984); and "Comment: Criminal Liability of a Prospective Mother for Prenatal Neglect of a Viable Fetus," *Whittier Law Review* 9 (1987) (hereafter "Prenatal Neglect").

54. "Prenatal Neglect" (see note 53), p. 387.

55. See J. C. Smith and Brian Hogan, *Criminal Law,* 4th ed. (London: Butterworths, 1978), pp. 4–8, 20–21.

56. *Commonwealth* v. *Cass,* 392 Mass. 799, 467 N.E.2d 1324, 1328 (Mass. 1984).

57. See John T. Shannon, "A Fetus is Not a 'Person' as the Term is Used in the Manslaughter Statute" (hereinafter "Born Alive Rule"), *University of Arkansas Law Review* 10 (1987–88) and Clarke D. Forsythe, "Homicide of the Unborn Child: The Born Alive Rule and other Legal Anachronisms," *Valparaiso University Law Review* 21 (1987).

58. Forsythe, "Homicide of the Unborn Child" (see note 57), p. 564.

59. Edward Coke, *The Third Part of the Institutes of the Laws of England* 50 (1628) (Garland Pub. reprint 1979). Cited in Forsythe, "Homicide of the Unborn Child" (see note 57), p. 583.

60. W. Blackstone, *Commentaries on the Laws of England* 198 (1765 ed.) (University of Chicago Press Facsimile 1979). Cited in Forsythe, "Homicide of the Unborn Child" (see note 57), p. 585.

61. Forsythe, "Homicide of the Unborn Child" (see note 57), p. 586.

62. Shannon, "Born Alive Rule" (see note 57), p. 407.

63. *Hollis* v. *Commonwealth,* 652 S.W.2d 61 (Kentucky 1983).

64. *People* v. *Greer,* 79 Ill.2d 103, 402 N.E.2d 203 (1980).

65. *Keeler* v. *Superior Court of Amador County,* 2 Cal.3d 619, 470 P.2d 617, 87 Cal. Rptr. 481 (1970).

66. Ibid., p. 631, 87 Cal. Rptr. at 488 (1970).

67. Ibid., p. 633–34, 87 Cal. Rptr. at 489–90.

68. *State* v. *Horne,* 282 S.C. 444, 319 S.E.2d 703 (1984).

69. See Ga. Code Ann. Sect. 26–1105 (1983); Ill. Rev. Stat. ch. 38, 9–1.2, 12–3.1 (1986 Supp.); Iowa Code Ann. Sect. 707.7 (West 1979); Mich. Comp. Laws Ann. Sect. 750.322 (West 1968); Minn. Stat. Ann. Sect 609.266 (1987 Supp.).

70. California Penal Code, sect. 187(a) (West Supp. 1987).

71. *People* v. *Carlson,* 37 Cal. App.3d 349, 358, 112 Cal. Rptr. 321, 327 (1974) ("[T]here is no crime constituting manslaughter of a fetus.").

72. For example, see *People* v. *Smith,* 59 Cal. App.3d 751, 129 Cal.Rptr. 498 (1976).

73. *People* v. *Apodaca,* 76 Cal. App. at 486, 142 Cal. Rptr. at 836. Cited in "Prenatal Neglect" (see note 53), p. 379.

74. Technically, assault is an act by which a person, intentionally or recklessly, causes another to apprehend immediate and unlawful personal violence. The actual infliction of such violence is a battery. In ordinary usage, the term "assault" is used to cover both assault and battery.

75. For example, Arkansas has amended its battery statute to include pregnant women in the class against whom intentionally or recklessly causing physical injury is battery in the first degree. (Act of March 31, 1987, No. 482, 1987 Ark. Acts 1365 (Adv. Leg. Serv.), amending Ark. Stat. Ann. Sect. 41–1601 (1977).)

76. *Commonwealth* v. *Cass*, 392 Mass. 799, 467 N.E.2d 1324, 1329 (Mass. 1984). Emphasis added.

77. William E. Schmidt, "Murder Trial Now Focus of Abortion Debate," *The New York Times*, Friday, June 15, 1990, B5.

78. Shannon, "Born Alive Rule" (see note 57), p. 409. See, e.g., *State* v. *Beale*, 376 S.E.2d 1, 4 (N.C. 1989); *State* v. *Trudell*, 755 P.2d 511, 516 (Kan. 1988); *People* v. *Vercelletto*, 514 N.Y.S.2d 177, 179–180 (Co. Ct. 1987); *Meadows* v. *State*, 722 S.W.2d 584, 586 (Ark. 1987); *State* v. *Evans*, 745 S.W.2d 880, 884 (Tenn. Cr. App. 1987).

79. *Cass* (see note 76), 467 N.E.2d at 1325.

80. *Mone* v. *Greyhound Lines*, 368 Mass. 354, 331 N.E.2d 916 (1975).

81. *Cass* (see note 76), 467 N.E.2d at 1326.

82. Ibid., p. 1329.

83. Ibid.

84. See, for example, Bruce Palmer, "State Protection of Future 'Persons': *Commonwealth* v. *Cass*," *Connecticut Law Review* 18 (Winter 1986); Henn, "Vehicular Homicide of a Viable Fetus—Judicial Statutory Amendment," *Massachusetts Law Review* (Winter 1986).

85. *State ex rel. Atkinson* v. *Wilson*, 332 S.E.2d 807, 813 (W. Va. 1984).

86. *Commonwealth* v. *Elizabeth A. Levey*, Commonwealth of Massachusetts, Middlesex, SS., Superior Court Department, Ind. No. 89–2725.

87. *Commonwealth* v. *Elizabeth Levey*, Superior Court Department, Nos. 89–2725 -2729, *Memorandum in Support of Motion to Dismiss*, p. 9.

88. Ibid., p. 3.

89. Ibid., p. 9.

90. Ibid., p. 19.

91. Much of the material in this section comes from my article, "The Logical Case for 'Wrongful Life'," *Hastings Center Report* 16:2 (April 1986), pp. 15–20, and from a report prepared under contract for the Office of Technology Assessment, U.S. Congress, Washington, D.C., "Ethical Implications of Population Screening for Cystic Fibrosis: The Concept of Harm and Claims of Wrongful Life."

92. See, for example, *Berman* v. *Allan*, 80 N.J. 421, 404 A.2d 8 (1979); *Speck* v. *Finegold*, 497 Pa. 77, 439 A.2d 110 (1981); *Karlsons* v. *Guerinot*, 57 App.Div.2d 73, 394 N.Y.S.2d 933 (1977); *Becker* v. *Schwartz*, 46 N.Y.2d 401, 413 N.Y.S.2d 895, 386 N.E.2d 807 (1978); *Harbeson* v. *Parke-Davis, Inc.*, 98 Wash.2d 460, 656 P.2d 483 (1983).

93. *Zepeda* v. *Zepeda*, 41 Ill. App.2d 240, 190 N.E.2d 849 (1963).

94. *Curlender* v. *Bio-Science Laboratories*, 106 Cal.App.3d 811, 165 Cal.Rptr. 477 (1980).

95. *Gleitman* v. *Cosgrove*, 49 N.J. 22, 227 A.2d 689 (1967).

96. Dawn Currier, "The Judicial System's Wrongful Conception of Wrongful Life," *Western New England Law Review* 6 (1983).

97. *Berman* v. *Allan,* 80 N.J. 421, 404 A.2d 8 (1979).

98. *Procanik* v. *Cillo,* 97 N.J. 339; 478 A.2d 755 (1984), p. 5.

99. Alexander M. Capron, "Tort Liability in Genetic Counseling," *Columbia Law Review* 79 (1979); K. J. Jankowski, "Wrongful Birth and Wrongful Life Actions Arising from Negligent Genetic Counseling: The Need for Legislation Supporting Reproductive Choice," *Fordham Urban Law Journal* 27 (1989).

100. Joel Feinberg, *Harm to Others* (New York, Oxford: Oxford University Press, 1984), p. 101.

101. Joel Feinberg, "Wrongful Life and the Counterfactual Element in Harming" (hereafter, "Wrongful Life"), *Social Philosophy & Policy* 4:1 (1987).

102. I say "ordinarily" because it is possible that someone irrationally prefers death when he has, as we say, "everything to live for." Such a person would not be "better off dead," though he might irrationally believe this to be the case. Similarly, someone might be "better off dead," but irrationally prefer not to die. This would be the case when the person must choose between a relatively painless death now and a far more terrible death in the very near future, and, out of fear, opts for the later and worse death. See Philippa Foot, "Euthanasia," *Philosophy and Public Affairs* 6 (Winter 1977), pp. 85–112.

103. See Allen E. Buchanan, "The Limits of Proxy Decisionmaking for Incompetents," *UCLA Law Review* 29 (December 1981).

104. Moreover, when handicapped individuals have lives that are not worth living, their substandard lives are often not inevitable, but rather due to the failings of the larger society in regulating them to poorly funded institutions without opportunities for education or training. See John Robertson, "Involuntary Euthanasia of Defective Newborns: A Legal Analysis," *Stanford Law Review* 27 (1974–75), p. 253.

105. Feinberg, "Wrongful Life" (see note 101), p. 164.

106. The parents' judgment was challenged by a right-to-life lawyer, but ultimately the parents prevailed. See Bonnie Steinbock, "Baby Jane Doe in the Courts," *Hastings Center Report* 14:1 (1984), pp. 13–19.

107. The example of Baby Jane Doe herself is a case in point. The prognosis given her parents turns out to have been unduly pessimistic. According to a story in *Newsday* in late 1987, Keri-Lynn (her real name) "talks and laughs; she smiles and hugs and screams and plants kisses firmly on a stranger's cheek." She goes to a school for the physically and neurologically handicapped, where she takes classes in speech, and physical and occupational therapy. Although Keri-Lynn is handicapped, her life is undoubtedly worth living. The problem of "prognostic uncertainty" complicates the determination of which lives will be lives not worth living.

108. Robertson, "Involuntary Euthanasia" (see note 104), p. 254.

109. John D. Arras, "Ethical Principles for the Care of Imperiled Newborns: Toward an Ethic of Ambiguity" (hereafter, "Ethic of Ambiguity") in Thomas Murray and Arthur Caplan, eds., *Which Babies Shall Live?* (Clifton, NJ: Humana Press, 1985).

110. Several writers have suggested criteria similar to the "minimally decent existence" standard. For example, on Richard McCormick's "relational potential" standard, life is to be preserved only insofar as it contains some potential for human relationships. "To Save or Let Die: the Dilemma of Modern Medicine," *Journal of the American Medical Association* 229:2 (1974), pp. 172–176.

111. Feinberg, "Wrongful Life" (see note 101), p. 174.

112. John Harris makes this point in "The Wrong of Wrongful Life," *Journal of Law and Society* 17:1 (Spring 1990), pp. 1–16.

CHAPTER 4

1. Arlene Eisenberg, Heidi Eisenberg Murkoff, and Sandee Eisenberg Hathaway, *What to Expect When You're Expecting* (New York: Workman Publishing, 1984), pp. 331–333.

2. Rorie Sherman, "Keeping Baby Safe From Mom," *The National Law Journal,* Monday, October 3, 1988, p. 25.

3. Sherman Elias and George J. Annas, *Reproductive Genetics and the Law,* (Chicago: Yearbook Medical Publishers, Inc., 1987), p. 196.

4. Ibid., p. 208.

5. Ibid.

6. A. P. Streissguth, H.M. Barr, H.M. Sampson et al., "IQ at Age 4 in Relation to Maternal Alcohol Use and Smoking During Pregnancy," *Developmental Psychology* 25:1 (1989), p. 9.

7. Robert Weir, *Selective Nontreatment of Handicapped Newborns* (New York: Oxford University Press, 1984), p. 40.

8. A. Revkin, "Crack in the Cradle," *Discover,* September 1989, pp. 63–69.

9. Michel Marriott, "After 3 Years, Crack Plague in New York Only Gets Worse," *The New York Times,* February 20, 1989, A1.

10. Jane E. Brody, "Cocaine: Litany of Fetal Risks Grows," *The New York Times,* Tuesday, September 6, 1988, C1.

11. A study done by the National Center for Perinatal Addiction Research and Education assessed the prevalence of drug use in pregnancy by collecting urine samples from all pregnant women who visited public health clinics or private obstetricians' offices in Pinellas County, Florida, for one month in 1989. In Florida, all drug use during pregnancy must be reported to health departments. The researchers found that about 15 percent of both the white and the black women used drugs, but black women were 10 times as likely as whites to be reported to the authorities, and poor women were more likely to be reported than middle-class women. "Racial Bias Seen on Pregnant Addicts," *The New York Times,* Friday, July 20, 1990, A13.

12. Celia W. Dugger, "Infant Mortality in New York City Declines for First Time in 4 Years," *The New York Times,* April 20, 1991, p. 1.

13. Brody, "Cocaine" (see note 10), C8.

14. See, for example, Tatiana M. Doberczak, M.D., Stefan Shanzer, M.D.,

Ruby T. Senie, Ph.D., and Stephen R. Kandall, M.D., "Neonatal Neurologic and Electroencephalographic Effects of Intrauterine Cocaine Exposure," *Journal of Pediatrics* 113:2 (1988), pp. 354–358.

15. Elias and Annas, *Reproductive Genetics and the Law* (see note 3), p. 209.

16. Streissguth et al., "IQ at Age 4" (see note 6), pp. 7–8.

17. Daniel Goleman, "Lasting Costs for Child Are Found From a Few Early Drinks," *The New York Times,* Thursday, February 16, 1989, B16.

18. Some feminists and civil libertarians think that even warning labels go too far. In April 1991, the New York State chapter of the National Organization for Women joined liquor sellers in lobbying against a bill that would require restaurants, taverns, and package-stores to post signs warning pregnant women of the dangers of alcohol consumption. New York NOW views the warning-sign legislation as an attack on a woman's right to choose. They argue that it sends a message that the rights of the fetus exceed those of the woman carrying it. Kevin Sack, "Unlikely Union in Albany: Feminists and Liquor Sellers," *The New York Times,* April 5, 1991, B1.

19. Sherman, "Keeping Baby Safe From Mom" (see note 2), p. 24.

20. Tamar Lewin, "When Courts Take Charge of the Unborn," *The New York Times,* Monday, January 9, 1989, A11.

21. Ibid.

22. *In the Matter of Sharon Fletcher, Lisa Flynn Respondent,* N-3968/88.

23. Felicia R. Lee, "Breaking Up Families, Crack Besieges a Court," *The New York Times,* Thursday, February 9, 1989, A1.

24. Jan Bays, "Substance Abuse and Child Abuse: Impact of Addiction on the Child," *Pediatric Clinics of North America* 37:4 (August 1990), pp. 881–904.

25. The 1989 Child Fatality Review Panel of New York City recommended that proof of parental substance abuse alone should create a presumption of abuse or neglect. D.J. Besharov, P.L. Dempsey, R.G. Dudley, et al., "1988 Report of the Child Fatality Review Panel" (New York: The City of New York Human Resources Administration, 1989).

26. Sherman, "Keeping Baby Safe From Mom" (see note 2), p. 24.

27. "Woman Convicted of Abuse of Fetus," *The New York Times,* May 5, 1989, A25. (Despite the misleading headline, the woman was not "convicted" of anything, as no criminal charges were brought. Rather, a petition in the name of the minor child alleging abuse and neglect was brought by state officials. The petition was granted, and an order of protection was granted.)

28. Telephone conversation with Paul Logli, May 5, 1989.

29. "Mother Charged In Baby's Death From Cocaine," *The New York Times,* Wednesday, May 10, 1989, A18.

30. Telephone conversation (see note 28).

31. Angela Bonavoglia, "The Ordeal of Pamela Rae Stewart," *Ms.,* Vol. XVI, Nos. 1 & 2, July/August 1987, p. 196.

32. For example, in *Reyes* v. *Superior Court,* 75 Cal.App.3d 214 (1977), the court declined to punish prenatal conduct under the felony child-endangering stat-

ute, Section 273 (a). The defendant was addicted to heroin and pregnant. Despite warnings from a public health nurse that if she continued to use heroin and failed to seek prenatal medical care, the health and life of any child born would be endangered, the defendant continued using heroin and failed to seek prenatal medical care. She gave birth to twin boys, who were both addicted to heroin and suffering withdrawal at birth. The court concluded that Section 273(a) contemplates a born child, and so did not apply to defendant's conduct while pregnant.

33. Defendant's Memorandum of Points and Authorities, *People* v. *Pamela Rae Stewart,* Case No. M508197, February 23, 1987, p. 18.

34. See, for example, John E. B. Myers, "Abuse and Neglect of the Unborn: Can the State Intervene?" *Duquesne Law Review* 23 (1984), p. 76, and Note, "Maternal Substance Abuse: The Need to Provide Legal Protection for the Fetus," *Southern California Law Review* 60, (1987), p. 1235.

35. See, for example, N.J. section 30, 4C-11, 1981. Cited in Larry Gostin, "Waging a War on Drug Users: An Alternative Public Health Vision," *Law, Medicine & Health Care* 18:4 (Winter 1990), pp. 385–394.

36. Note, "Maternal Rights and Fetal Wrongs: The Case Against the Criminalization of 'Fetal Abuse,' " *Harvard Law Review* 101 (1988).

37. Women's Rights Project, American Civil Liberties Union, Memorandum: Legislative Update on Drug Use During Pregnancy, September 16, 1991.

38. Rorie Sherman, "Split Rulings for Fetal Abuse Cases," *The National Law Journal,* Monday, February 24, 1992, p. 3.

39. Tamar Lewin, "Drug Use in Pregnancy: New Issue for the Courts," *The New York Times,* February 5, 1990, A14.

40. *State* v. *Johnson,* 89–890CFA (Cir. Ct. Seminole Co.).

41. Tamar Lewin, "Appeals Court in Florida Backs Guilt for Drug Delivery by Umbilical Cord," *The New York Times,* April 20, 1991, p. 6.

42. Wendy Chavkin, "Drug Addiction and Pregnancy: Policy Crossroads," *American Journal of Public Health* 80:4 (April 1990), p. 485.

43. Sherman, "Keeping Baby Safe From Mom" (see note 2), p. 25.

44. Jan Hoffman, "Pregnant, Addicted—and Guilty?" *The New York Times Magazine,* August 19, 1990, p. 53

45. Isabel Wilkerson, "Court Backs Woman in Pregnancy Drug Case," *The New York Times,* April 3, 1991, A15.

46. Sherman, "Keeping Baby Safe From Mom" (see note 2), p. 25.

47. Letter, *The National Law Journal,* Monday, December 5, 1988, p. 12.

48. Sherman, "Keeping Baby Safe From Mom" (see note 2), p. 25.

49. *Harris* v. *McCarthy* (85–6002) (C.D. California) (1985).

50. Barry, "Quality of Prenatal Care for Incarcerated Women Challeged," *Youth Law News* 6 (November–December 1985), pp. 1–4. Cited in Defendant's Memorandum (see note 33), p. 25.

51. Women's Rights Project, American Civil Liberties Union, Memorandum: "Update of State Legislation Regarding Drug Use During Pregnancy," May 22, 1990, p. 11.

52. Fifteen to twenty million jobs is the estimate of the Bureau of National Affairs, *Pregnancy and Employment* 57 (1987), limited to injury caused by chemicals. The number would be far greater if it included jobs where there is exposure to X rays or emissions from video display terminals.

53. Joan E. Bertin, "Reproductive Hazards in the Workplace," in Sherrill Cohen and Nadine Taub, eds., *Reproductive Laws for the 1990s* (Clifton, New Jersey: Humana Press, 1989), p. 280.

54. Elias and Annas, *Reproductive Genetics and the Law* (see note 3), p. 215.

55. Bertin, "Reproductive Hazards" (see note 53), p. 279, citing Minutes of the Environmental Health Committee of the Lead Industries Ass'n, Inc., Sept 9, 1974.

56. Similar conclusions were reached in a 1988 study conducted by the Massachusetts Department of Public Health and the University of Massachusetts Occupational Health Program of 198 large chemical and electronics companies in Massachusetts (Cynthia Daniels, Maureen Paul, and Robert Rosofsky, *Family, Work & Health,* November 1988). The study was the first of its kind to analyze systematically employer practices regarding reproductive hazards. It found that nearly one in five of the companies restrict women's work options on the ground of potential risk to their reproductive health, but most ignore the reproductive hazards faced by men.

57. Bertin (see note 53), pp. 281–282.

58. Elias and Annas, *Reproductive Genetics and the Law* (see note 3), p. 219.

59. *UAW* v. *Johnson Controls, Inc.,* 886 F.2d 871 (7th Cir. 1989) (en banc).

60. Ibid., p. 912.

61. Ibid., p. 913.

62. Linda Greenhouse, "Court Backs Right of Women to Jobs With Health Risks," *The New York Times,* March 21, 1991, A1.

63. Elias and Annas (see note 3), p. 220.

64. *Family, Work & Health* (see note 56), p. 41.

65. Bertin, "Reproductive Hazards" (see note 53), p. 295.

66. See Gina Kolata, *The Baby Doctors: Probing the Limits of Fetal Medicine* (New York: Delacorte Press, 1990).

67. Gina Kolata, "Lifesaving Surgery On a Fetus Works For the First Time," *The New York Times,* Thursday, May 31, 1990, A1.

68. "Saving Lives Not Yet Begun," *People,* June 18, 1990, p. 40.

69. Kolata, "Lifesaving Surgery On a Fetus" (see note 67), B8.

70. Nancy K. Rhoden, "The Judge in the Delivery Room: The Emergence of Court-Ordered Cesareans," *California Law Review* 74 (December 1986), p. 1959.

71. Nancy K. Rhoden, "Cesareans and Samaritans," *Law, Medicine & Health Care,* 15:3 (Fall 1987), p. 118.

72. See, for example, Patricia A. King, "The Juridical Status of the Fetus: A Proposal for Legal Protection of the Unborn," *Michigan Law Review* (August 1979), pp. 1647–1687; John Robertson, "The Right to Procreate and In Utero Fetal Therapy," *Journal of Legal Medicine* 3 (1982); and Margery Shaw, "Conditional Prospective Rights of the Fetus," *Journal of Legal Medicine* 5 (1984).

73. See, for example, George Annas, "Forced Cesareans: The Most Unkindest

Cut of All," *Hastings Center Report,* June 1982; Janet Gallagher, "Prenatal Invasions & Interventions: What's Wrong with Fetal Rights," *Harvard Women's Law Journal* 10 (1987); Dawn Johnsen, "The Creation of Fetal Rights: Conflicts with Women's Constitutional Rights to Liberty, Privacy, and Equal Protection," *Yale Law Journal* 95 (January 1986); Lawrence J. Nelson and Nancy Milliken, "Compelled Medical Treatment of Pregnant Women," *Journal of the American Medical Association* 259 (Feb. 19, 1988), pp. 1060–1066; and Nancy Rhoden (see notes 70 and 71).

74. Veronika E. D. Kolder, Janet Gallaher, and Michael T. Parsons, "Court-Ordered Obstetrical Interventions," *New England Journal of Medicine* 316 (May 7, 1987), pp. 1192–1196.

75. Jurow and Paul, "Cesarean Delivery for Fetal Distress Without Maternal Consent," *Obstetrics & Gynecology* 63 (1984).

76. George J. Annas, "Protecting the Liberty of Pregnant Patients," *New England Journal of Medicine* 316 (May 7, 1987).

77. Gregory L. Goyert, Sidney F. Bottoms, Majorie C. Treadwell, and Paul C. Nehra, "The Physician Factor in Cesarean Birth Rates," *The New England Journal of Medicine* 320 (March 16, 1989), p. 706.

78. Gina Kolata, "New York Seeks to Reduce Rate of Caesarean Births," *The New York Times,* Friday, January 27, 1989, B2.

79. *Jefferson* v. *Griffin Spalding County Hospital Authority,* 247 Fa. 86, 274 S.E.2d 457 (1981).

80. George J. Annas, "Forced Cesareans" (see note 73), p. 16.

81. Elias and Annas, *Reproductive Genetics and the Law* (see note 3), p. 255; Rhoden, "The Judge in the Delivery Room" (see note 70), p. 1960.

82. Ronni Sandroff, "Invasion of the Body Snatchers: Fetal Rights vs. Mothers' Rights," *Vogue* (October 1988), p. 331. The case was originally reported by Janet Gallagher in "The Fetus and the Law—Whose Life Is It Anyway?" *Ms.* (1984), pp. 134–135.

83. J. Pritchard, P. MacDonald, and N. Gant, *Williams Obstetrics* 3 (17th ed. 1985), pp. 868–869.

84. National Institutes of Health, U.S. Department of Health and Human Services, Pub. No. 82–2067, *Cesarean Childbirth: Report of a Consensus Development Conference* 51 (1981), p. 268.

85. *Jefferson* (see note 79) 247 Ga. at 87, 89, 274 S.E.2d at 458, 460.

86. John E. B. Myers, "Abuse and Neglect of the Unborn" (see note 34), p. 18.

87. Ibid., p. 75.

88. Rhoden, "The Judge in the Delivery Room" (see note 70), pp. 2013–2015, footnotes omitted.

89. For example, Lawrence J. Nelson, Brian P. Buggy, and Carol J. Weil, "Forced Medical Treatment of Pregnant Women: 'Compelling Each to Live as Seems Good to the Rest,' " *Hastings Law Journal* 37 (May 1986), and Nancy K. Rhoden, "The Judge in the Delivery Room" (see note 70).

90. *Colautti* v. *Franklin,* 439 U.S. 379 (1979).

91. Ibid. at 400, cited in Rhoden, "The Judge in the Delivery Room" (see note 70), p. 1990.

92. *Thornburgh* v. *American College of Obstetricians & Gynecologists,* 737 F.2d 283 (3rd Cir. 1984), *aff'd* 106 S. Ct. 2101 (1986).

93. Ibid., p. 300. Cited in Nelson et al (see note 89), p. 744.

94. Nelson et al., "Forced Medical Treatment" (see note 89), p. 745.

95. *Shimp* v. *McFall,* 10 Pa. D. & C.3d 90 (1978).

96. Ibid., p. 92 (emphasis in original).

97. Angela Holder, *Legal Issues in Pediatrics and Adolescent Medicine,* 2nd edition (New Haven: Yale University Press, 1985), p. 171.

98. See e.g., *Hart* v. *Brown,* 29 Conn. Supp. 368, 289 A.2d 386 (1972); *Strunk* v. *Strunk,* 445 S.W.2d 145 (Ky. 1969).

99. See In re *Richardson,* 284 So.2d 185 (La. Ct. App. 1973); In re *Pescinski,* 67 Wis. 2d 4, 226 N.W.2d 180 (1975).

100. Lance Morrow, "Ethics: Sparing Parts," *Time,* June 17, 1991, pp. 54–58.

101. Rhoden, "The Judge in the Delivery Room" (see note 70), footnote 273, p. 2004, citing a statement by Dr. Norman Fost, Presentation on Fetal Therapy at the Hastings Center, Conference on Abortion and Scientific Change, Hastings-on-Hudson, New York (May 24, 1985).

102. W. A. Bowes and B. Selgestad, "Fetal versus Maternal Right: Medical and Legal Perspectives," 58 *American Journal of Obstetrics & Gynecology* (1981), p. 209. The case is In re *Unborn Baby Kenner,* No. 79 JN 83 (Col. Juv. Ct. March 6, 1979).

103. Annas, "Forced Cesareans" (see note 73), p. 45.

104. In re *Angela Carder,* Transcript of Testimony and Proceedings, no. 87–609, Tuesday, June 16, 1987, p. 33.

105. Ibid., p. 15.

106. Ibid., p. 65.

107. Ibid., p. 70.

108. Ibid., p. 92.

109. Ibid., p. 60.

110. Ibid., p. 97.

111. Annas, "Protecting the Liberty of Pregnant Patients" (see note 76).

112. In re *Angela Carder,* no. 87–609, District of Columbia Court of Appeals, Tuesday, June 16, 1987, p. 6.

113. *In the Matter of A.C.,* No. 87–609, Amended Brief on the Merits, p. 22. The Death Certificate of Angela Carder lists as a contributing cause of death the "status post-Cesarean section."

114. In re *A.C.,* 533 A.2d 611, 617 (D.C.App. 1987).

115. George J. Annas, "She's Going to Die: The Case of Angela C," *Hastings Center Report* 18:1 (February/March 1988), p. 25.

116. In re: *A.C., Appellant,* No. 87–609, District of Columbia Court of Appeals (en banc) (Decided April 26, 1990), p. 1130.

117. Ibid., p. 1123.

118. Ibid., p. 1142.

119. "And whatsoever man there be of the house of Israel, or of the strangers that sojourn among you, that eateth any manner of blood: I will even set my face against that soul that eateth blood, and will cut him off from among his people. . ." (Lev. 17:10–14), cited by Ruth Macklin, "Consent, Coercion, and Conflicts of Rights," *Perspectives in Biology and Medicine* 20:3 (Spring 1977), pp. 360–371. Reprinted in Thomas A. Mappes and Jane S. Zembaty, eds., *Biomedical Ethics,* 2nd edition (McGraw-Hill, 1986), pp. 348–354.

120. *Application of President and Directors of Georgetown College,* 331 F.2d 1000, 1010 (D.C. Cir. *cert. denied* 377 U.S. 978 (1964).

121. *Prince* v. *Massachusetts,* 321 U.S. 158 (1944), p. 170.

122. See, e.g., In re *Green,* 448 Pa. 338, 292 A.2d 387 (1972); *Wallace* v. *Labranz,* 411 Ill. 618, 104 N.E.2d 769 (1952); *State* v. *Perricone,* 37 N.J. 483, 181 A.2d 751 (1962).

123. There have been several cases in recent years of Christian Scientists being convicted of manslaughter or neglect in cases where their children have died. For example, in July 1990, in Boston, Massachusetts, two Christian Scientists, David and Ginger Twitchell, were convicted of manslaughter in the death of their two-year-old son. The Twitchells relied on prayer instead of seeking conventional medical care to treat their son, Robyn, who died in 1986 of a bowel obstruction. *The New York Times,* Sunday, July 8, 1990, E9.

124. Alan R. Fleischman and Ruth Macklin, "Fetal Therapy: Ethical Considerations, Potential Conflicts," in William B. Weil, Jr., and Martin Benjamin, eds., *Ethical Issues at the Outset of Life* (Boston: Blackwell Scientific Publications, 1987), p. 144.

125. See, for example, *Application of President and Directors of Georgetown College* (note 121).

126. This is suggested in Bruce L. Miller, "Autonomy and the Refusal of Lifesaving Treatment," *Hastings Center Report* (August 1981). Reprinted in John D. Arras and Nancy K. Rhoden, eds., *Ethical Issues in Modern Medicine,* 3rd ed. (Mountain View, California: Mayfield Publishing Company, 1989), pp. 167–176.

127. Sandroff, "Invasion of the Body Snatchers: Fetal Rights vs. Mothers' Rights" (see note 82), p. 330.

128. Ibid.

129. E.g., see my "Preterm Labor and Prenatal Harm," *Hastings Center Report* 19:2 (March/April 1989), pp. 32–33.

130. American College of Obstetricians and Gynecologists Committee Opinion Number 55, "Patient Choice: Maternal-Fetal Conflict" (October 1987).

131. John A. Robertson and Joseph D. Schulman, "Pregnancy and Prenatal Harm to Offspring: The Case of Mothers with PKU," *Hastings Center Report* 17:4 (August/September 1986), pp. 23–33.

132. Ibid., p. 32.

CHAPTER 5

1. Cf. Joel Feinberg, "The Mistreatment of Dead Bodies," *Hastings Center Report* 15:1 (February 1985), p. 32.

2. Alexander M. Capron, "Bioethics on the Congressional Agenda," *Hastings Center Report* 19:2 (March/April 1989), p. 22.

3. Ibid., p. 23.

4. The National Commission for the Protection of Human Subjects of Biomedical and Behavioral Research, *Research on the Fetus: Report and Recommendations* (hereafter *Research on the Fetus*), DHEW Publication No. (OS) 76–127, 1975, pp. 73–76.

5. Michele Simon, "The Politics of Fetal Research" (unpublished manuscript), p. 5.

6. Legislative History, Public Law 99–158, Health Research Extension Act of 1985, p. 719. Cited in John C. Fletcher and Kenneth J. Ryan, "Federal Regulations for Fetal Research: A Case for Reform," *Law, Medicine & Health Care* 15:3 (1987), pp. 126–138, p. 133.

7. Capron, "Bioethics on the Congressional Agenda" (see note 2), p. 22.

8. Philip Boffey, "White House Backs Away From Ban on Fetal Tissue Research," *The New York Times,* September 6, 1988, p. 6.

9. *Report of the Human Fetal Tissue Transplantation Panel* (hereafter *Report*), Vol. II, December 1988, p. 1.

10. Ibid., Appendix A, Summary and Conclusion, p. A25.

11. Philip J. Hilts, "Abortion Debate Clouds Research on Fetal Tissue," *The New York Times,* Monday, October 16, 1989, A19.

12. Philip J. Hilts, "Citing Abortion, U.S. Extends Ban on Grants for Fetal Tissue Work," *The New York Times,* Thursday, November 2, 1989, p. A1.

13. Gwen Ifill, "House Approves Fetal Tissue Use in Federally Financed Research," *The New York Times,* July 26, 1991, A11.

14. Presentation of Robert Auerbach, Ph.D., Director of the Center for Developmental Biology, University of Wisconsin, Madison, in *Report* (see note 9), Vol. II, pp. D27–D31.

15. "Hope of Parkinson's Drug," *Manchester Guardian Weekly,* August 13, 1989, p. 5.

16. Presentation of Lars Olsen in *Report* (see note 9), Vol. II, pp. D220 and D223.

17. Sandra Blakeslee "Fetal Cell Transplants Show Early Promise In Parkinson Patients," *The New York Times,* November 12, 1991, C3.

18. Larry Rohter, "Implanted Fetal Tissue Aids Parkinson's Patients," *The New York Times,* January 7, 1988, B13.

19. Presentation of Dr. Olson in *Report* (see note 9), Vol. II, p. D224. Emphasis added.

20. Summary of the Panel meeting prepared by science writer Jeffrey Fox in *Report* (see note 9), Vol. II, pp. A9–10.

21. Statement of Carol Lurie to the Panel in *Report* (see note 9), Vol. II, p. D157.

22. Peter McCullagh, *The Fetus as Transplant Donor: Scientific, Social and Ethical Perspectives* (Chichester, New York, Brisbane, Toronto, Singapore: John Wiley & Sons, 1987).

23. Ibid., p. 49.

24. Ibid., p. 45.

25. Ibid., p. 78.

26. "Embryos and Parkinson's Disease," *The Lancet,* May 14, 1988, p. 1087.

27. George J. Annas and Sherman Elias, "Sounding Board: The Politics of Transplantation of Human Fetal Tissue," *New England Journal of Medicine* 320:16 (April 20, 1989), p. 1081.

28. Testimony of Bernard M. Dickens, Ph.D., LL.D., in *Report* (see note 9), Vol. II, p. D92.

29. *Report* (see note 9), Vol. I, p. 7.

30. James Bopp and James Burtchaell, Statement of Dissent, *Report* (see note 9), Vol. I, p. 47.

31. See John A. Robertson, "Fetal Tissue Transplants," *Washington University Law Quarterly* 66 (1988), pp. 464–465.

32. Testimony of Alan Meisel in *Report* (see note 9), Vol. II, p. D183.

33. Robertson, "Fetal Tissue Transplants" (see note 31), p. 465.

34. Kathleen Nolan, "Genug ist Genug: A Fetus is Not a Kidney," *Hastings Center Report* 18:6 (1988), pp. 13–19.

35. Philip J. Hilts, "Fetal Tissue Use: Personal Agony in Medical First," *The New York Times,* April 16, 1991, A1.

36. Bopp and Burtchaell, Statement of Dissent (see note 30), p. 52.

37. Testimony of Mrs. Kay C. James in *Report* (see note 9), Vol. II, p. D258.

38. Statement by J. Fred Voss, Vice-President for Research and Development for Hana Biologics, in *Report* (see note 9), Vol. II, p. D258.

39. The Stanford University Medical Center Committee on Ethics, "Special Report: The Ethical Use of Human Fetal Tissue in Medicine," *The New England Journal of Medicine* 320:16 (April 20, 1989), pp. 1093–1096, at 1094.

40. Annas and Elias, "The Politics of Transplantation" (see note 27), p. 1082.

41. Bopp and Burtchaell, Statement of Dissent in *Report* (see note 9), Vol. I, p. 53.

42. Ibid., pp. 53–54. Others disagree. Jane Friedman, citing precisely the same data as Bopp and Burtchaell, concludes that "the number of women who initially seek an abortion and subsequently change their minds is infinitesmal." "The Federal Fetal Experimentation Regulations: An Establishment Clause Analysis," *Minnesota Law Review* 61 (1977), p. 1000.

43. Ibid., p. 56.

44. *Report* (see note 9), Vol. I, p. 2.

45. John A. Robertson, "Rights, Symbolism, and Public Policy in Fetal Tissue Transplants," *Hastings Center Report* 18:6 (December 1988), p. 6.

46. Statement of James T. Burtchaell. Report of the Advisory Committee to the Director, National Institutes of Health, Human Fetal Tissue Transplantation Research, December 14, 1988, p. C24.

47. Annas and Elias, "The Politics of Transplantation of Human Fetal Tissue" (see note 27), p. 1080.

48. Kristine Moe, "Should the Nazi Research Data Be Cited?" *Hastings Center Report* 14:6 (December 1984), p. 5.

49. Ibid., p. 7.

50. Willard Gaylin, "Commentary. Nazi Data: Dissociation from Evil," *Hastings Center Report* 19:4 (July/August 1989), p. 18.

51. Hilts, "Fetal Tissue Use" (see note 35), p. C2.

52. Testimony of Carol Lurie in *Report* (see note 9), Vol. II, p. D155.

53. Quoted in Tamar Lewin, "Medical Use of Fetal Tissues Spurs New Abortion Debate," *The Sunday New York Times,* August 16, 1987, p. 1.

54. Alan Fine, "The Ethics of Fetal Tissue Transplants," *Hastings Center Report* 18:3 (June/July 1988), p. 6.

55. Ibid., p. 6.

56. Robertson, "Fetal Tissue Transplants" (see note 31), p. 456.

57. Ibid., p. 458.

58. Ibid.

59. Ibid., p. 460.

60. Jane M. Friedman, "The Federal Fetal Experimentation Regulations: An Establishment Clause Analysis" (see note 42) pp. 963–964.

61. Maurice J. Mahoney, "The Nature and Extent of Research Involving Living Human Fetuses" (hereafter "Research Involving Living Fetuses") in *Research on the Fetus,* Appendix (see note 4), p. 1–3.

62. Sherman Elias and George J. Annas, *Reproductive Genetics and the Law* (Chicago, London, Boca Raton: Yearbook Medical Publishers, Inc., 1987), p. 69.

63. Mahoney, "Research Involving Living Human Fetuses" (see note 61), p. 1–7. Emphasis added.

64. Elias and Annas, *Reproductive Genetics and the Law* (see note 62), p. 140.

65. Ibid., p. 195.

66. John P. Wilson, "A Report on Legal Issues Involved in Research on the Fetus," *Research on the Fetus,* Appendix (see note 4), p. 14–14.

67. Paul Ramsey, "The Enforcement of Morals: Nontherapeutic Research on Children," *Hastings Center Report* 6:4 (August 1976), pp. 21–30.

68. Richard A. McCormick, "Proxy Consent in the Experimentation Situation," *Perspectives in Biology and Medicine* 18 (1974), pp. 2–20.

69. Richard A. McCormick, "Experimentation on the Fetus: Policy Proposals," in *Research on the Fetus,* Appendix (see note 4), p. 5–4–5. McCormick adds that he believes that most induced abortions are wrong, and that he personally views experimenting on fetuses from such abortions as complicitous with the wrong of abortion. Therefore, he thinks that fetal experimentation is clearly justified only where the abortion is spontaneous or has been justifiably induced (e.g., to save the

mother's life). However, recognizing that society in general does not share his view of abortion, McCormick maintains that opposition to abortion cannot serve as the basis for public policy regarding fetal experimentation.

70. Joseph Fletcher, "Fetal Research: An Ethical Appraisal," in *Research on the Fetus*, Appendix (see note 4), p. 3–3.

71. Ibid.

72. Jane English makes this point in "Abortion and the Concept of a Person," *Canadian Journal of Philosophy* 5:2 (October 1975).

73. *Research on the Fetus: Report and Recommendations* (see note 4), p. 66.

74. Ibid., p. 67.

75. Mahoney, "Research Involving Living Human Fetuses" (see note 61), p. 1–21.

76. Strictly speaking, the nonviable fetus *ex utero* is not a fetus at all, since fetal life ends with expulsion from the uterus. However, to call the organism a "baby" is misleading, since a nonviable fetus cannot survive for long outside the womb. A fetus that shows some signs of life after abortion, but lacks the capacity for independent life, is thus often termed a "nonviable" or "previable fetus *ex utero*." The term "premature baby" is reserved for those beings capable of surviving outside the womb. It is important to recognize that a fetus may be alive but nonviable.

77. Mahoney, "Research Involving Living Human Fetuses" (see note 61), p. 1–4. Citing Humphrey, T., "The Development of Human Fetal Activity and Its Relation to Postnatal Behavior," *Advances in Childhood Developmental Behavior* 5:1 (1970).

78. Ibid., citing Adam, P.A.J.; Raiha, N.; Rahiala, E.L., et al., "Cerebral Oxidation of Glucose and D-BOH-Butyrate by the Isolated Perfused Fetal Head," *Pediatric Research* 7 (1973).

79. John C. Fletcher and Kenneth J. Ryan, "Federal Regulations for Fetal Research: A Case for Reform," *Law, Medicine & Health Care* 15:3 (Fall 1987), pp. 126–138, at 126–127.

80. Ibid., p. 134.

81. A. M. Capron, "The Law Relating to Experimentation with the Fetus," *Research on the Fetus*, Appendix (see note 4), p. 13–1.

82. Ibid., pp. 13-12–13-13.

83. *Research on the Fetus* (see note 4), p. 57.

CHAPTER 6

1. The story of the first IVF baby is recounted in Peter Singer and Deane Wells, *Making Babies: The New Science and Ethics of Conception* (New York: Charles Scribner's Sons, 1985), Chapter 1.

2. Philip J. Hilts, "U.S. Urged to End Ban on In Vitro Birth Research," *The New York Times*, Sunday, December 3, 1989, p. 37. The figure of 12,000 IVF births comes from Mary Carrington Coutts, "Ethical Issues in In Vitro Fertilization," *Scope Note 10*, Kennedy Institute of Ethics, December 1988.

3. Congregation for the Doctrine of the Faith. *Instruction on Respect for Human Life in its Origin and on the Dignity of Procreation: Replies to Certain Questions of the Day*. Vatican City: The Congregation, February 22, 1987. Reprinted in Ronald Munson, ed., *Intervention and Reflection: Basic Issues in Medical Ethics*, 3rd ed. (Belmont, California: Wadsworth Publishing Company, 1988), pp. 459–460.

4. See, for example, Gena Corea, *The Mother Machine: Reproductive Technologies from Artificial Insemination to Artificial Wombs* (New York: Harper and Row, 1985).

5. This objection is discussed by John A. Robertson, "Embryos, Families, and Procreative Liberty: The Legal Structure of the New Reproduction" (hereafter, "The New Reproduction"), *Southern California Law Review* 59 (1986), p. 1027, and Mary Anne Warren, "IVF and Women's Interests: An Analysis of Feminist Concerns," *Bioethics* 2:1 (January 1988), pp. 37–57.

6. There is wide variation in the success rates of IVF clinics. In 1988, the average success rate for all institutions reporting nationwide was 13 percent. Nearly half of IVF clinics in the United States have yet to achieve a live birth. See Warren E. Leary, "In Vitro Fertilization Clinics Vary Widely in Success Rates, " *The New York Times,* Friday, March 10, 1989, A16.

7. Clinics may mislead prospective patients by giving success statistics for achieving a *pregnancy,* rather than a live birth, or they may give nationwide success statistics, rather than their own success in producing a live birth. See United States Congress, Office of Technology Assessment, *Infertility: Medical and Social Choices. Summary*. Washington, DC: U.S. Government Printing Office, May 1988, p. 10.

8. Robertson, "The New Reproduction" (see note 5), p. 948.

9. See, for example, John Marshall, "The Case Against Experimentation," in Anthony Dyson and John Harris, eds., *Experiments on Embryos* (London and New York: Routledge, 1990), pp. 55–64, especially p. 61.

10. Ethics Advisory Board, Department of Health, Education and Welfare, *Report and Conclusions: HEW Support of Research Involving Human In Vitro Fertilization and Embryo Transfer* (hereafter, *EAB Report*). Washington, D.C.: U.S. Government Printing Office, May 4, 1979.

11. Hans O. Tiefel, "Human In Vitro Fertilization: A Conservative View," *Journal of the American Medical Association* 247 (1982), pp. 3235–3242. Reprinted in Richard T. Hull, ed., *Ethical Issues in the New Reproductive Technologies* (Belmont, California: Wadsworth Publishing Company, 1990), p. 124.

12. Robertson, "The New Reproduction" (see note 5), p. 991.

13. N.C. Morin, F.H. Wirth, D.H. Johnson, et al., "Congenital Malformations and Psychosocial Development in Children Conceived by In Vitro Fertilization," *Journal of Pediatrics* 115 (1989), pp. 222–227.

14. "Reassuring Study on In Vitro Babies," *The New York Times,* August 11, 1989, p. A17.

15. See Paul Ramsey, "Manufacturing Our Offspring: Weighing the Risks," *Hastings Center Report* 8:5 (October 1978), p. 7; Leon Kass, " 'Making Babies' Revisited," *Public Interest* 54 (1979), pp. 34–48; Hans Tiefel (see note 11).

16. Tiefel (see note 11), p. 126.

17. John A. Robertson, "In Vitro Conception and Harm to the Unborn," *Hastings Center Report* 8:5 (October 1978), p. 14.

18. Robertson, "The New Reproduction" (see note 5), p. 989.

19. Tiefel (see note 11), p. 126.

20. United States Congress, Committee on Government Operations, "Infertility in America: Why is the Federal Government Ignoring a Major Health Problem?" Washington, DC: U.S. Government Printing Office, 1989, p. 7.

21. *EAB Report* (see note 10), p. 22.

22. Derek Morgan and Robert G. Lee, *Blackstone's Guide to the Human Fertilisation & Embryology Act* (London: Blackstone Press Limited, 1991), pp. 26–27.

23. Ibid., p. 82.

24. Robert Edwards, "Ethics and Embryology: The Case for Experimentation," in Anthony Dyson and John Harris, eds., *Experiments on Embryos* (see note 9), pp. 42–54, at p. 47.

25. Not all prenatal testing is performed with the idea of aborting affected fetuses. For example, approximately 20 percent of women who discover that their fetus has spina bifida continue their pregnancies. Nevertheless, the overwhelming majority seek prenatal testing in order to terminate the pregnancy if the fetus has a serious disorder.

26. Barbara Katz Rothman, *The Tentative Pregnancy* (New York: Viking, 1986).

27. This position is taken by Robert Edwards (see note 24), p. 48.

28. Rothman (see note 26), p. 227.

29. Steven A. Holmes, "Abortion Issue Divides Advocates for Disabled," *The New York Times,* July 4, 1991, A11.

30. Adrienne Asch, "Reproductive Technology and Disability," in Sherrill Cohen and Nadine Taub, eds., *Reproductive Laws for the 1990s* (Clifton, New Jersey: Humana Press, 1989), p. 82.

31. Ibid., p. 77.

32. Ibid., p. 86.

33. See Helga Kuhse and Peter Singer, *Should the Baby Live?* (Oxford: Oxford University Press, 1985).

34. *EAB report* (see note 10), pp. 35–36.

35. Mary Warnock, *A Question of Life: The Warnock Report on Human Fertilisation and Embryology* (hereafter *The Warnock Report*) (New York: Basil Blackwell, 1985) pp. 63–64.

36. Robertson, "The New Reproduction" (see note 5), p. 974.

37. John Harris, "Embryos and Hedgehogs: On the Moral Status of the Embryo," in Dyson and Harris (see note 9), pp. 65–81, at p. 80.

38. This position was taken by Madeline Carriline, John Marshall, and Jean Walker in their dissent from paragraph 18 of Chapter Eleven in *The Warnock Report* (see note 35), pp. 90–93.

39. *The Warnock Report* (see note 35), p. 67.

40. Ibid.

41. Ibid., p. 68.

42. This argument was put forward by Lord Jackobovits in support of an unsuccessful amendment to the Human Fertilisation and Embryology Act 1990. Reported in Morgan and Lee, *Blackstone's Guide to the Human Fertilisation and Embryology Act 1990* (see note 22), p. 26.

43. Singer and Wells, *Making Babies* (see note 1), p. 89.

44. Morgan and Lee, *Blackstone's Guide to the Human Fertilisation & Embryology Act 1990* (see note 22), p. 137.

45. Junior L. Davis vs. Mary Sue Davis vs. Ray King, M.D., d/b/a Fertility Center of East Tennessee, *In the Circuit Court for Blount County, Tennessee, at Maryville, Equity Division (Division I),* No. E-14496, September 21, 1989.

46. John Marshall, "The Case Against Experimentation" (see note 9), p. 63.

47. John A. Robertson, "The New Reproduction" (see note 5), pp. 969–970.

48. John A. Robertson, "Resolving Disputes Over Frozen Embryos," *Hastings Center Report* 19:6 (November/December 1989), p. 11.

49. Ibid.

50. George J. Annas, "A French Homunculus in a Tennessee Court," *Hastings Center Report* 19:6 (November/December 1989), p. 22.

51. Ibid.

52. Ibid., p. 21.

53. See, for example, Douglas Cusine, "Experimentation: Some Legal Aspects," in Dyson and Harris (see note 9), p. 123.

54. "Embryos to Lipsticks?" *New Scientist* (October 10, 1985), p. 21. Cited in Alan Fine, "The Ethics of Fetal Tissue Transplants," *Hastings Center Report* 18:3 (June/July 1988), p. 7.

55. Annas, "A French Homunculus" (see note 50), p. 20.

56. Robertson, "Resolving Disputes over Frozen Embryos" (see note 48), p. 8.

57. Ibid., p. 9.

58. "Chill in Custody Fight," *The National Law Journal,* June 18, 1990, p. 6.

59. Duncan Mansfield, "Joint Custody Granted in Embryo Appeal," Associated Press, *The Times Union,* Friday, September 14, 1990, A7.

60. Morgan and Lee, *Blackstone's Guide to the Human Fertilisation and Embryology Act 1990* (see note 22), p. 137.

61. See Developments in the Law, "Medical Technology and the Law," *Harvard Law Review* 103 (1990), p. 1545.

Index

Abortion
conservative position, 46–48: genetic-
humanity criterion, 46, 48, 51; and
argument from potential, 55
emotional significance of, 52, 67
equal-protection basis for, 81–82
for genetic indications, 205–8
gradualist approach to, 62
and infanticide, 52–53
late-gestation, 87–88
person view, 51–58
Akron v. *Akron Center for Reproductive
Health,* 83
Albala v. *City of New York,* 93–95
Allaire v. *St. Luke's Hospital,* 91
Anand, K. J. S., 49
Anencephalic infants, 13, 30–36, 69
A. C., in re, 155–60
Animals
cruelty to, 11
experiments on, 167, 189
and interests, 21–24
moral status of, 21–24, 52, 68
Annas, George, 131, 154, 158, 159, 175,
179, 188, 215, 216
Arras, John, 75–76, 122

Asch, Adrienne, 206–7
Autonomous goodness, 19–20
in embryos, 40
in plants, 19, 21
Autonomy, 161–62, 165

Baby Jane Doe, 121, 236 *n.* 107
Baby Jeffries, in re, 149
Bassen, Paul, 227 *n.* 36
Beal, Ron, 95
Becker v. *Schwartz,* 117
Beliefs
in animals, 21–23
as explanations of behavior, 22
as propositional attitudes, 22–23
and truth, 23
Bentham, Jeremy, 23
Benn, Stanley, 59
Bertin, Joan, 143, 145
Bigelow, John, 228 *n.*55
Blackstone, William, 106
Bonbrest v. *Kotz,* 91, 112
Bopp, James, 176, 178, 180
Bork, Robert, 81
Bosze, Jean-Pierre, 153
"Brain birth," 85–87

251

Brain death, 31. *See also* Uniform
    Determination of Death Act
    and "brain absence," 31
Brandt, Richard, 74
Brody, Baruch, 48–50
Brophy, Paul *(Brophy* v. *New England
    Sinai Hospital, Inc.),* 27
Brown, Louise, 195
Buckle, Stephen, 59, 64–66
Buggy, Brian P. *See* Nelson, Lawrence J.
Burtchaell, James, 176, 178, 180, 181

Caplan, Arthur, 33
Capron, Alexander, 31, 32, 34, 117–18
Cesarean sections, compulsory, 147–62
    attitudes of physicians toward, 147
    communitarian approach toward, 154
    and court orders, 148–49
    for fetal distress, 151
Chavkin, Wendy, 138
Child abuse, applied to fetuses, 133–36.
    See also Fetus
Coke, Edward, 106
Colautti v. *Franklin,* 151, 156, 158
Commonwealth v. *Cass,* 109, 110–11,
    112
Commonwealth v. *Elizabeth A. Levey,*
    111–13
Conscious awareness, 14, 18. *See also*
    Consciousness; Sentience
    absence of in plants, 20
    in anencephalics, 33
    and fetuses, 13, 40
    and interests, 13
    as necessary for a worthwhile life, 122
Consciousness, 13–14, 24
Cook, Robin, 35, 179
Cranford, Ronald E., 31, 34
Curlender v. *Bio-Science Laboratories,*
    115

Davidson, Donald, 22–23, 222 *n.* 22
Davis v. *Davis,* 213–18
Dawson, Karen, 64
Dead people, 13
    as antemortem people, 25–26
    dead bodies, 24, 25
    interests of, 24–26

possibility of harming, 26
DES (diethylstilbestrol), 93–94. *See also*
    Preconception torts
Dietrich v. *Northhampton,* 91
"Different People Choices," 13, 72. *See
    also* "Same People Choices"
Double effect, doctrine of, 210
Down syndrome, 116, 124, 204–5
Drug use during pregnancy
    as criminal offense, 138–39
    as dangerous to fetal health, 130–31
    incarceration to protect fetus from,
        140–42
    treatment for, 138–39
Dworkin, Ronald, 230 *n.* 77

Eisenstadt v. *Baird,* 81
Elias, Sherman, 131, 175, 179, 188
Elshtain, Jean, 53
Ely, John Hart, 82
Embryo
    dispositional problems with, 211–19
    extracorporeal, 194, 196, 200, 213,
        219
    implantation of blastocyst, 198
    impossibility of sentience in, 196, 199
    moral status of, 196, 199, 200, 209
    preimplantation, 196, 199, 215, 216;
        potentiality of, 199–200, 210
    research on, 203–205: creating for
        purposes of, 209–11
    surplus, 198–199: frozen, 211
    as symbol of human life, 197, 208,
        216
Engelhardt, H. Tristram, Jr., 54
English, Jane, 246 *n.* 72
Enright v. *Lilly & Co.,* 94–95
Environmental ethic, 21
Ethics Advisory Board (EAB), 168, 208

Feinberg, Joel, 8, 10, 14, 16, 20, 21, 25,
    26, 55, 66, 71, 118–19, 121, 123,
    225 *n.* 71, 227 *n.* 24
Fetal-abuse statutes, 138, 140
Fetal alcohol syndrome (FAS). *See* Fetal
    health, dangers to
Fetal health, dangers to
    fetal alcohol syndrome (FAS), 129–30:

from moderate alcohol consumption, 131
from cocaine, 130–31
from lead, 143
from tobacco, 130
Fetal-protection policies, 142–46
Fetal research. *See also* Fetal-tissue transplantation
on living fetuses *ex utero,* 192–94
moral objections to, 188–90, 193: equality principle, 190–91
moratorium on, 167–68
recommendations of National Commission, 168
scientific and medical benefits of, 186–88
Fetal rights, 129. *See also* Fetus
Fetal surgery, 146–47
Fetal-tissue transplantation, 167, 169
feminist objection to, 183–84
Human Tissue Fetal Transplant Research Panel (U.S.A.), recommendations of, 169
and morality of abortion, 167, 170, 171, 180–83, 184
moratorium on, 169–71, 178
and Nazi experiments, 182–83
scientific justification for, 171–75
as treatment for diabetes, 172, 173
as treatment for Parkinson's disease, 169, 172–73, 174, 189
Fetus
appearance of brain waves in, 48: and capacity for conscious experience, 49–50
as child abuse victim, 133–36, 138, 238 *n.* 25
as homicide victim, 89–90, 105–10
and moral status, 44, 69–70: of to-be-aborted fetuses, 191
neocortical activity in, 85: *See also* "Brain birth"
recognizable human appearance of, 47–48
as research tool, 166, 186–94
sentience in, 48–50, 188–89, 193–94
as symbol of humanity, 167, 190
Fleischman, Alan, 160–61

Fletcher, Joseph, 190
Foot, Philippa, 236 *n.* 102
Forsythe, Clarke, 105–6
Frey, R. G., 21, 23
Future people, 13, 37–40

Gamete intrafallopian transfer (GIFT), 197–98
Gaylin, Willard, 182
Gertler, Gary, 85, 231 *n.* 95
Gleitman v. *Cosgrove,* 115
Goldstein, Robert, 88
Goller v. *White,* 95
Good Samaritans, 81, 82, 153, 154, 184
minimally decent, 79
Gorovitz, Samuel, 32, 223 *n.* 24
Grobstein, Clifford, 62
Grodin v. *Grodin,* 96–97

Harding, Sandra, 44, 226 *n.* 6
Hare, R. M., 71, 228 *n.* 39
Harm. *See also* Wrongful life
and abortion, 41
in coming to exist, 117
counterfactual condition in harming, 119–20
of death, 71
to future people, 41
as making worse off, 39, 119
posthumous, 25–26
Harris, John, 62, 209, 236 *n.* 112
Hart, H. L. A., 222 *n.* 11
Hewellette v. *George,* 95
Hickey, P. R. *See* Anand, K. J. S.
HIV-infected women. *See* Wrongful life
Holder, Angela, 153
Hollis v. *Commonwealth,* 107, 109
Holmes, Oliver Wendell, 91, 106
Homicide, criminal
and "born alive rule" (BAR), 105–7, 111: contrasted with aggravated-assault approach, 110
applied to fetuses, 108–10
vehicular, 110–14
Human Fertilisation and Embryology Act (Great Britain), 204, 213
Hunter, Nan, 87–88
Hursthouse, Rosalind, 63, 67

Interest principle, 10, 55
Interests
    and beliefs, 12, 21
    and consciousness, 12, 14–15, 16
    and a good of one's own, 16–18
    and linguistic ability, 13, 21
    and moral status, 9, 10, 21, 24
    and rights, 10, 21
    as stakes in things, 14
In vitro fertilization (IVF), 195–203
    Catholic objections to, 196
    feminist objections to, 196
    risk in abnormality in, 200–203

Jefferson v. *Griffin Spalding County Hospital Authority,* 149, 150
Jehovah's Witnesses, 160–61
Johnsen, Dawn, 97
Johnson, Jennifer, 138–39
Jorgensen v. *Meade Johnson Laboratories,* 93

Keeler v. *Superior Court of Amador County,* 108, 109
Kelly v. *Gregory,* 92
Kilpatrick, James, 103
King, Patricia, 82

Lee, Robert G. *See* Morgan, Derek
Lejeune, Jerome, 214
Locke, Don, 72–73
Logli, Paul, 136
Lord Campbell's Act. *See* Wrongful-death actions
Luker, Kristin, 44

Macklin, Ruth, 44, 54, 161
Marquis, Don, 60, 226 *n.* 5
Marshall, John, 214
MacLean, Douglas, 225 *n.* 70
McCormick, Richard, 189–90, 236 *n.* 110, 246 *n.* 69
McCullagh, Peter, 173–74, 230 *n.* 93
McFall v. *Shimp,* 152–53, 159–60
Meisel, Alan, 176
Meyers, Robert, 223 *n.* 30
Miller, Bruce L., 243 *n.* 126
Mills, James L., 201
Moe, Kristine, 182

Moral status, 9–10, 11, 13
    definition, 10
    of human beings, 10, 69
    and interests, 10
    and moral value, 166
    and rationality, 24
    relevance of species to, 24
    scale, 24, 38, 41, 68, 70
    and sentience, 24
Morgan, Derek, 219
Myers, John, 150–51

Nagel, Thomas, 23
Natural-function view, 18–21
Nelson, Lawrence J., 152
Nolan, Kathleen, 177
Noonan, John, 46, 63, 212

O'Connor, Sandra Day, 83, 229 *n.* 76

Parfit, Derek, 38–40, 72, 74–75, 229 *n.* 60
Pargetter, Robert. *See* Bigelow, John
Park v. *Chessin,* 117
People v. *Apodaca,* 108, 109
People v. Greer, 107, 109
Persistent vegetative state (PVS), 13, 27–30
    differentiated from death, 27
    interests of people in, 24, 29
    and pain, 28
    recovery from, 28
Person-affecting Restriction, 72–73. *See also* Possible Persons Principle
Person view. *See* Abortion
Personhood
    descriptive sense of, 51, 53–54
    as normative concept, 36, 54, 68, 86
    and quickening, 106
    and sentience, 52
    and special moral status, 51–52, 54
    and viability: for insurance purposes, 90; in law of homicide, 90, 108, 110; in vehicular homicide, 110–11, 113
    and wrongful-death actions, 89, 103–4, 111
Phenylketonuria (PKU), 162
Placenta previa, 137, 148, 149, 151

Plants, 19–21. *See also* Autonomous
  goodness
Possible people, 40, 71–76
  Possible Persons Principle, 73: *see also*
  Person-affecting Restriction
Potentiality
  argument from potential, 59–68: and
  contraception, 62–68; and interest
  view, 66
  consequentialist conception of, 64–65
  deontological conception of, 65–66
  moral relevance of, 68, 167
Preconception torts, 90, 92–95
Prenatal torts, 90, 91–96
  parental immunity from, 95–96: and
  automobile insurance coverage, 98–
  100
Privacy
  constitutional right of, 46, 81, 165: in
  Roe v. *Wade*, 80, 150; and civil
  liability for behavior during
  pregnancy, 96–97; threatened by
  fetal rights, 129
  and moral right to bodily self-
  determination, 45, 70, 76–79, 165
Procanik v. *Cillo*, 117
Procreative liberty. *See* Reproductive
  liberty

Rachels, James, 224 *n.* 42
Radical discontinuity thesis, 48, 50, 56–
  57
Ramsey, Paul, 189
Raymond, Janice, 183–84
Regan, Donald, 81, 229 *n.* 67
Regan, Tom, 16–18
Reproductive liberty, 103, 217–18. *See
  also* Rights, reproductive
Rhoden, Nancy, 83–84, 147, 151, 152,
  231 *n.* 101
Right to life, 43, 45, 55
  and ability to enjoy life, 57
  as desire for one's own continued
  existence, 56
  of newborns, 58, 68, 69
  and right to use another person's body,
  77–79
Rights
  as based on interests, 10, 21

noncontingent, 41
  reproductive, 217. *See also*
  Reproductive liberty
Rios, Mario and Elsa, 212
Roberts, John C. *See* Cranford, Ronald
Robertson, John, 97, 122, 162–63, 180–
  81, 185–86, 201–2, 208, 215, 216–
  19
Roe v. *Wade*, 43, 46, 79–82, 103
  implications for court-ordered
  cesareans, 150–52, 156
Rolling Stones, 25
Ross, W. D., 25
Rothman, Barbara Katz, 205
RU 486, 51, 185

"Same People Choices," 13, 38–40, 72.
  See also "Different People Choices"
Sass, Hans-Martin, 230 *n.* 94
Schulman, Joseph. *See* Robertson, John
Schweitzer, Albert, 11–13
Sentience
  as restriction on abortion, 84–87
  in anencephalic infants, 35
  in fetuses, 40, 58, 69–70, 84–85,
  188–89, 193–94
  and interests, 23
  and moral status, 20, 23–24, 70,
  223 *n.* 24
  and right to life, 58
Shaw, George Bernard, 25
Shewmon, D. Alan, 32, 33, 34
Silent Scream, 58
Singer, Peter, 23, 64, 212, 223 *n.* 24
Slippery-slope arguments, 32, 210
Smith v. *Brennan,* 92
Speciesism, 10. *See also* Animals.
Stallman v. *Youngquist,* 98–100
Steinberg, Joel, 177
Stewart, Pamela Rae, 136–37
Stich, Stephen, 22–23, 222 *n.* 22
Strong, Carson, 227 *n.* 31
Sumner, L. W., 223 *n.* 24

Thomson, Judith, 46, 76–79
Thornburgh v. *American College of
  Obstetricians & Gynecologists,* 152,
  156, 158

Tiefel, Hans O., 201, 202
Tooley, Michael, 53, 55–58, 66, 86

UAW v. *Johnson Controls, Inc.,* 144
Unborn Baby Kenner, in re, 154
Uniform Anatomical Gift Act (UAGA), 168, 176, 179
Uniform Determination of Death Act (UDDA), 31, 36

Value, symbolic, 7, 41, 167, 190, 197, 208, 216. *See also* Embryo; Fetus
Vehicular homicide. *See* Homicide
Viability
  as basis for legal protection, 82–83
  definition, 47
  determination of, 85, 193
  and late gestation, 84
  moral significance of, 47, 82, 84
  and prenatal torts, 91–92
  and research on living fetus, 193
  in *Roe* v. *Wade,* 80, 82–84
  and technological advances, 83

Walters, LeRoy, 201
Wanglie, Helga, 224 *n.* 44
Warner, Richard, 63
Warnock, Mary, 50

Warnock Committee (Great Britain), 204, 208, 209, 214
Warren, Mary Anne, 51–55, 74, 79, 223 *n.* 24, 227 *n.* 22
Webster v. *Reproductive Health Services,* 80, 103
Weil, Carol J. *See* Nelson, Lawrence J.
Wells, Deane, 212
Wilson, John P., 188
Wrongful-death actions, 100–101
  prenatal, 90, 100: and abortion, 102–4; as redressing a wrong to the parents, 101–2; and reproductive liberty, 103; significance of viability in, 101–2
Wrongful-birth suits, 114. *See also* Wrongful life
Wrongful life, 114–25, 202
  and being "better off unborn," 120–24
  lawsuits, 114–25: difficulty of determining damages in, 115–16; logical problems with, 117–18; and value of life, 116–17
  and principle of parental responsibility, 73–75: application to HIV-infected women, 75–76
  and right not to be born, 118–19

Zepeda v. *Zepeda,* 115